Coronary Artery Disease: Advances in Cardiovascular Medicine

Coronary Artery Disease: Advances in Cardiovascular Medicine

Edited by Owen Cooper

hayle
medical

New York

Hayle Medical,
750 Third Avenue, 9th Floor,
New York, NY 10017, USA

Visit us on the World Wide Web at:
www.haylemedical.com

ISBN: 978-1-63241-559-2

Cataloging-in-Publication Data

Coronary artery disease : advances in cardiovascular medicine / edited by Owen Cooper.
   p. cm.
Includes bibliographical references and index.
ISBN 978-1-63241-559-2
1. Coronary heart disease. 2. Cardiovascular system--Diseases.
3. Coronary artery bypass. 4. Cardiology. I. Cooper, Owen.
RC685.C6 C67 2019
616.123--dc23

Table of Contents

Preface

Coronary artery disease (CAD) is a common cardiovascular disease. It is of various types, such as stable and unstable angina, myocardial infarction and cardiac death. It may lead to complications such as abnormal heartbeat and heart failure. The risk factors that contribute to the incidence of coronary artery diseases include smoking, diabetes, high blood pressure, obesity, lack of exercise, blood cholesterol, poor diet, alcohol consumption, etc. Individuals may have a predisposition to coronary artery disease depending on their genetics. MRI, exercise ECG, echocardiology, intravascular ultrasound, etc. are used for determining coronary artery disease. Stress echocardiography is used for diagnosing obstructive coronary artery disease. It can be treated through lifestyle changes, coronary interventions such as coronary stent, angioplasty, coronary artery bypass grafting, using drugs such as beta-blockers, nitroglycerin, cholesterol lowering medications, etc. Research in this domain is focused on stem cell therapies and new angiogenic treatment modalities. This book is compiled in such a manner, that it will provide in-depth knowledge about coronary artery disease. From theories to research to practical applications, case studies related to all contemporary topics of relevance to this field have been included herein. The topics covered herein offer the readers new insights in this field.

This book has been the outcome of endless efforts put in by authors and researchers on various issues and topics within the field. The book is a comprehensive collection of significant researches that are addressed in a variety of chapters. It will surely enhance the knowledge of the field among readers across the globe.

It gives us an immense pleasure to thank our researchers and authors for their efforts to submit their piece of writing before the deadlines. Finally in the end, I would like to thank my family and colleagues who have been a great source of inspiration and support.

Editor

Diabetes and Coronary Artery Disease – Pathophysiologic Insights and Therapeutic Implications

David Fridman, Amgad N. Makaryus, John N. Makaryus, Amit Bhanvadia, Erion Qaja, Alina Masters and Samy I. McFarlane

Abstract

Cardiovascular disease is the leading cause of morbidity and mortality among people with diabetes worldwide, accounting for 60% of all deaths in diabetics. Despite advances in our pathophysiologic understanding of diabetic co-morbidities and measures to help counter these, diabetics still remain at increased risk for cardiovascular disease complicating our overall approach to management. Diabetics, in particularly type 2, are often fraught with additional risk factors contributing to their overall propensity for developing cardiovascular disease. These include, but are not limited to, obesity, dyslipidemia, poor glycemic control, lack of physical activity, and hypertension. In response to this, research driven guidelines focusing on primary prevention have continued to arise with new clinical targets and goals substantially changing our approach with the diabetic population. It is important to note early on, type 1 diabetics carry a higher risk of cardiovascular disease for which the pathophysiology is only recently being elucidated. The underlying relationship between cardiovascular events and risk factors is, however, not well understood. For this reason, management approaches to risk reduction have been extrapolated from experience in type 2 diabetes mellitus. The purpose of this chapter is to present the conclusions of current literature pertaining to blood pressure and blood glucose control, cholesterol management, aspirin therapy, and lifestyle modification. We present a synthesis of the new guidelines, and clinical targets, including preventative measures for subclinical cardiovascular disease for the contemporary management of patients with diabetes mellitus.

Keywords: Diabetes, atherosclerosis, coronary artery disease, glycemic control, antidiabetic medications

1. Introduction

1.1. Diabetes and cardiovascular risk: Scope of the problem

Cardiovascular disease (CVD) is the major cause of morbidity and mortality in the diabetic population which is rapidly expanding around the globe and is increasing due to the rising epidemic of obesity and increasing sedentary lifestyle along with poor dietary habits.[1] The cardiovascular events associated with type 2 diabetes and the high incidence of other macro-vascular complications, such as strokes and amputations, are major causes of illnesses and a large economic burden. Heart disease and strokes account for over 2/3 of mortality in the diabetic population who are 2–4 times more likely to have atherosclerotic heart disease compared to non-diabetic individuals. In fact, diabetes itself is considered a cardiovascular risk equivalent and the diabetic population is less likely to survive when they develop CVD, compared to their non-diabetic counterparts. While the additional risk diabetes confers cannot be completely eliminated, large benefit is seen when multiple risk factors and associated comorbid conditions are addressed globally in this patient population and addressed specifically with respect to treatment targets and goals.

1.2. Risk factors for cardiovascular disease in diabetes

Risk factors for increased CVD among people with diabetes include traditional ones such as insulin resistance, hypertension, dyslipidemia, central obesity, and cigarette smoking. Non-traditional risk factors include microalbuminuria, increased inflammation, oxidative stress, hyperuricemia, hypercoagulable states, endothelial dysfunction, decrease nitric oxide function, increase vascular reactivity and permeability, increased glycated end products, as well as stimulation of the renin angiotensin aldosterone (RAAS) system.

Modifiable Risk Factors	Non-modifiable Risk Factors
Overweight/obesity	Family history of diabetes or premature coronary disease
Sedentary lifestyle	Latino/Hispanic, Non-Hispanic black, Asian American, Native American, or Pacific Islander ethnicity
Hypertension	History of gestational diabetes
Elevated LDL-C and/or triglycerides and/or low HDL-C	History of infant delivery birth weight "/>9 pounds
Psychiatric illness	Polycystic ovarian syndrome
IGT, IFG	Age
HDL-C, high-density lipoprotein cholesterol; LDL-C, low-density lipoprotein cholesterol; IFG, impaired fasting glucose; IGT, impaired glucose tolerance	
Adapted from Diabetes Care Volume 38, Supplement 1, January 2015 [2]	

Table 1. Modifiable and non-modifiable risk factors associated with type 2 diabetes mellitus and cardiovascular disease

1.3. Hypertension

Hypertension is the most common comorbid disease associated with diabetes. It has been found to increase the risk of nephropathy, retinopathy, left ventricular hypertrophy, and cardiovascular events.[3] Prevention of these vascular complications is a worldwide priority as the prevalence of diabetics by 2030 is estimated to be approximately 350 million.[4] As a result, blood pressure (BP) management is arguably one of the more critical aspects of the care of the patient with diabetes. The current 2015 American Diabetes Association (ADA) recommendations are for all diabetics to achieve a systolic blood pressure (SBP) of <140 and a diastolic blood pressure (DBP) of <90. This has been revised to reflect the most recent high-quality evidence that exists to support a goal of DBP, 90 mmHg. Although, it has been traditionally recommended that diabetics achieve a blood pressure of less of 130/80, there is insufficient evidence to justify the benefit of this value.[5] While hypertension therapy is not the main focus of this chapter, it is important to realize that lifestyle therapy for hypertension should be offered to all patients as a reasonable first intervention; this includes weight loss, increased physical activity, and a Dietary Approaches to Stop Hypertension (DASH)–style diet. If despite this the patient is unable to achieve the goal BP pharmacological therapy should comprise a regimen that includes either an angiotensin converting enzyme (ACE) inhibitor or angiotensin receptor inhibitor (ARB)–either of which are effective in preventing the development or progression of microalbuminuria which reduces the incidence of new or worsening nephropathy.[6]

2. Hyperglycemia and cardiovascular risk

Hyperglycemia, even in the non-diabetic range such as impaired fasting glucose and/or impaired glucose tolerance (collectively classified as pre-diabetes) is associated with increased risk of coronary artery disease. This has been shown in several trials and also evidence exists that glycemic control is associated with decreased coronary artery disease. For example, the landmark United Kingdom Diabetes Perspective Study (UKPDS) showed a graded risk reduction in myocardial infarction among the diabetic population with 14% decreased risk for every 1% decrease in A1C. Glucose control is important and associated with decreased microvascular complications such as diabetic nephropathy, retinopathy, as well as neuropathy, with about 30% risk reduction with each 1% decrease in A1C, as evidenced from large trials in type 1 DM such as Diabetes Complication (DCCT) in type 1 diabetes and from UKPDS study in type 2 diabetes in patient with new onset/early onset diabetes.[7]

Long term follow up of these cohorts also provided evidence of decreased macrovascular disease such as in the Epidemiology of Diabetes Interventions and Complications (EDIC), a follow up of the DCCT trial where intensive blood glucose control reduced risk of any CVD event by 42% and the risk of nonfatal myocardial infarction, stroke, or death from cardiovascular causes by 57%.[8] However, tight glycemic control has been shown to be associated with increased mortality among high-risk population. In the large randomized controlled trial, ACCORD (Action to Control Cardiovascular Risk in Diabetes), tight control of blood glucose to a hemoglobin A1C of 6.4%, compared to 7.5% in the control group, was associated with a

22% increased mortality leading to premature termination of the study protocol. Furthermore, there was increased risk of hypoglycemia requiring assistance and an average of 10 kg weight gain in the period of 3.5 years of follow up. This study, as well as others, triggered a Position Statement by the American Diabetes Association (ADA) and the European Association for the Study of Diabetes (EASD) calling for an individualized patient approach with less stringent glycemic control for patients with established vascular complications, as well as those with longer diabetes duration and increased risk of hypoglycemia such as those with CKD and the elderly with long standing diabetes and neuropathy.

2.1. Cardiovascular disease in the high-risk diabetic sub-population

Diabetes disproportionately affects minority populations such as blacks, Hispanics, Native Americans, and South Asians. In these populations, the prevalence of diabetes is much higher compared to Whites and they are disproportionately affected by diabetes complications including chronic kidney disease, strokes, and coronary artery disease.

Premenopausal women with diabetes lose the estrogen protective effects that are partially mediated through nitric oxide and women with diabetes have worse outcomes compared to men when presented with acute coronary syndrome. Despite advances in the diagnosis and treatment of acute coronary syndrome, and through improved medical therapies such as revascularization, improved survival among men and women without diabetes as well as men with diabetes has been observed, but evidence suggests worse prognosis for women with diabetes remains.

2.2. Screening for cardiovascular disease

Screening of asymptomatic patients with high CVD risk is not recommended, as there have been no trials that demonstrate improved outcomes even in the setting of angiographically defined coronary disease. One of the largest trials to address this concern was the Detection of Ischemia in Asymptomatic Diabetics (DIAD) study. DIAD randomized 1,123 subjects into two categories: those who would and would not be screened with stress myocardial perfusion imaging (MPI). Despite abnormal myocardial perfusion imaging in more than one in five patients, cardiac events were lower than expected and equivalent in screened versus unscreened patients.[9] Furthermore, trials including the COURAGE and BARI 2D have shown no difference between revascularization and optimal medical therapy in patients who are effected by stable coronary disease supporting a less invasive approach to management. [10,11] The favorable cardiac outcomes among asymptomatic diabetics can likely be attributed to guideline-driven management of cardiac risk factors. Therefore, the current standard of care for type 2 diabetes should focus on the reduction of cardiovascular risk factors with avoidance of indiscriminate screening.

2.3. Type I diabetes mellitus

Type I diabetes is a challenging clinical entity. It deserves separate mention as its management has lagged in success when compared to type II diabetes.

Type I diabetes is associated with an increased risk of early death with acute diabetes-related complications responsible for the majority of younger deaths and cardiovascular disease the main cause for older patients.[12,13,14] CVD occurs much earlier in type I diabetics than in the general population—often after 2 decades of disease. This can occur as early as 30 years of age disease rates of >3% per year.[15] Poor glycemic control has correlated to cardiovascular risk (Table 2), however, the success rates of achieving optimal A1c levels is far from ideal. In two national registries, only 13% to 15% of patients with type 1 diabetes met a target A1c level of <7%.[16,13] The difficulty partially lies in dietary/insulin regimen adherence and risks of tight blood sugar control (absolute risk of severe hypoglycemia increasing with tighter control).[6]

Mean HbA1c	Death from any cause	Death from cardiovascular disease
≤ 6.9%	2.36 (95%CI: 1.97–2.83)	2.92 (95%CI: 2.07–4.13)
7.0%–7.8%	2.38 (95%CI: 2.02–2.80)	3.39 (95%CI: 2.49–4.61)
7.9%–8.7%	3.11 (95%CI: 2.66–3.62)	4.44 (95%CI: 3.32–5.96)
8.8%–9.6%	3.65 (95%CI: 3.11–4.30)	5.35 (95%CI: 3.94–7.26)
≥ 9.7%	8.51 (95%CI: 7.24–10.01)	10.46 (95%CI: 7.62–14.37)

Adapted from Lind et al [11].

Table 2. Adjusted hazard ratios for death from any cause and death from cardiovascular disease among individuals with type 1 diabetes vs control according to the glycated hemoglobin

Even when target glycemic control is achieved, the risk of death from cardiovascular causes is more than twice the risk in the general population and poor glycemic control portends a risk ten times higher.[17] The issue is complicated by several components highlighted by the Scottish Registry Linkage Study. Unlike type 2 diabetics, type 1 diabetics generally do not suffer from obesity and hypertension/dyslipidemia rates are not in excess of the general population.[18] At this time, there is no clear explanation for the additional risk. It is postulated that earlier onset and severely altered glucose homeostasis produces a variety of oxidative stressors promoting a milieu of underlying vascular disease. This may be especially true in the preadolescent years where subclinical disease manifests, priming the cardiovascular system for accelerated atherosclerosis despite the best efforts at achieving glycemic control later in life.[19] The term coined, *metabolic memory*, has been used to denote this theoretical process. The phenomenon gained support after a significant trend was noted at the conclusion of the DCCT and follow-up EDIC trial in regards to microvascular complications, e.g. nephropathy, retinopathy. In summary, the DCCT trial ended with a transition of participants to an intensive insulin regimen secondary to successful glycemic control and reduction in microvascular complications with this method. Interestingly, as the same patients were followed, those originally on the standard insulin regimen continued to have higher incidences of microvascular disease when compared to their counterpart. This occurred despite achieving near equivalent A1c levels.[20,21,22] The notion of early vascular stress portending a worse prognosis was also echoed in a recent Cochrane review where findings concluded that tight control reduced the risk of developing microvascular diabetes complications (the risk for macrovascular complications was less clear secondary to the younger patient population they examined), but the impact became weaker once complications manifested.[23] Furthermore, during the EDIC study, macrovascular relationship became more apparent. Those participants who initially were under the intensive regimen experienced a 42% reduction in CVD events after 17 years. The ongoing EDIC showed these benefits persisted up to 10 years after the end of the DCCT.[7,24,25,26] These findings are promising as more effort is being placed at identifying subjects and initiating treatment earlier. Early therapy stands to eliminate or reduce a large amount of complications; however, longer-term studies are still needed to realize the full potential. It is also still unclear why cardiovascular complications start so early in the disease history when, presumably, only mild hyperglycemia exists.

3. Multifactorial therapy: A comprehensive evidence based approach

Over the past two decades, diabetes management has evolved substantially as epidemiologic and therapeutic based research has broadened our understanding of this complex disease. As a general principle, diabetes magnifies many of the indolent cardiovascular risk factors for morbidity and mortality amongst non-diabetic patients. As the population of diabetics increases, there is a growing effort to acknowledge the risks and lessen them to the best of our abilities. This begins with addressing modifiable risk factors for late complications in patients which includes hyperglycemia, hypertension, and dyslipidemia—all of which increase the risk of a poor outcomes.

Intensive treatment of multiple cardiovascular risk factors can have a major impact among patients with diabetes. Reduction in glycosylated hemoglobin values, systolic and diastolic blood pressure, fasting serum cholesterol and triglyceride levels, and urinary albumin excretion rate all have their value in reducing cardiovascular morbidity and mortality. Up until the turn of the century, numerous randomized trials investigated the effect of intensified intervention involving a single risk factor in patients with type 2 diabetes demonstrating benefits in terms of both macrovascular and microvascular complications in kidneys, eyes, and nerves.[27,28,29,30,31] This formed the basis of American Diabetes Association recommendations for many years which were finally bolstered by the landmark publication, Steno-2 study, which investigated a multifactorial, goal directed strategy involving lifestyle modification and pharmacologic management addressing all major metrics. An unrivalled 50% reduction in the risk of macro and micro-vascular events was demonstrated in those who received intensive treatment.[32] Since this study, several further trials have replicated these findings and have shown that the benefit of aggressive lifestyle and multi-drug therapy is effective and should be coupled with timely screening to confer a life-long benefit.[33,34,35]

3.1. Dietary management

Diet is one of the most important behavioral aspects of diabetes treatment, slowing and potentially preventing the rate of developing complications. Basic principles of nutritional management have evolved over the past decade from a generalized approach to an individualized one in the form of medical nutrition therapy (MNT). This approach takes scientific evidence, individual goals and abilities into consideration to formulate lifestyle changes that can be maintained. It is monitored and guided by a dietician or nutritionist with regular follow up. Goals of MNT that apply to individuals with diabetes include achieving and maintaining (1) blood glucose levels in the normal range or as close to normal as is safely possible, (2) a lipid and lipoprotein profile that reduces the risk for vascular disease, (3) blood pressure levels in the normal range or as close to normal as is safely possible, (4) to prevent, or at least slow, the rate of development of the chronic complications of diabetes by modifying nutrient intake and lifestyle to address individual nutrition needs, taking into account personal and cultural preferences and willingness to change, and (5) the pleasure of eating by only limiting food choices when indicated by scientific evidence.[36] By the mid-90's diet directed research had bolstered this involved form of dietary intervention with promising results. Randomized controlled trials of MNT have reported decreases in HbA1c (A1C) of 1% in type 1 diabetics and 1–2% in type 2 diabetics, depending on the duration of diabetes. After initiation of MNT, improvements were apparent in 3–6 months.[10,37,38]

3.2. Lipid management

Both types of diabetes associated with a substantially increased risk of atherosclerotic vascular disease, identification of treatments for the prevention of major occlusive vascular events is a public-health priority.[39,40,41] The most recent meta-analyses have underscored the importance of lipid management and have changed the medical communities general approach to risk reduction in the diabetic community. There appears to be an approximately linear relationship between the absolute reductions in LDL cholesterol achieved in these trials and the proportional reductions in the incidence of major vascular events.[42,43] The implications of this is far reaching. What used to be a categorical approach with a goal cholesterol level in mind has broadened considerably. In all patients with diabetes over the age of 40 years moderate intensity statin treatment should be considered, in addition to lifestyle therapy (Table 3). If the patient falls under a 'high-risk' category—those with acute coronary syndromes or previous cardiovascular events, LDL cholesterol > 100mg/dL, high blood pressure, currently smoking and/or overweight should have more aggressive therapy with high doses of statins.[44,45] This strategy should be coupled with medical nutritional therapy.

3.2.1. Aspirin therapy

In general, patients with or without diabetes, who have known occlusive vascular disease, stand to benefit from long-term antiplatelet therapy with aspirin, reducing the yearly risk of serious vascular events. The benefits of antiplatelet therapy substantially exceed the risk of major bleeding events and it is therefore widely accepted as means of secondary prevention. For primary prevention, however, the balance is less clear with no single trial demonstrating a clear benefit.[46,47] In order to reconcile the uncertainty regarding primary prevention the American Diabetes Association performed a meta-analysis that added data from additional trials performed specifically in patients with diabetes to the data from the subgroups of

Age	Risk factors	Recommended statin dose*	Monitoring with lipid panel
< 40 years	None	None	Annually or as needed to monitor for adherence
	CVD risk factor(s)**	Moderate or high	
	Overt CVD***	High	
40-75 years	None	Moderate	As needed to monitor adherence
	CVD risk factors	High	
	Overt CVD	High	
>75 years	None	Moderate	As needed to monitor adherence
	CVD risk factors	Moderate or high	
	Overt CVD	High	

* Moderate-Intensity Statin Therapy: Atorvastatin 10-20 mg, Rosuvastatin 5-10 mg, Simvastatin 20-40 mg, Pravastatin 40-80 mg, Lovastatin 40 mg. High-Intensity Statins Therapy: Atorvastatin 80 mg, Rosuvastatin 20-40 mg.

**CVD risk factors include LDL cholesterol $100 mg/dL (2.6 mmol/L), high blood pressure,

smoking, and overweight and obesity.

***Overt CVD includes those with previous cardiovascular events or acute coronary syndromes.

Adapted from Diabetes Care Volume 38, Supplement 1, January 2015 [2]

Table 3. Recommendations for statin treatment in people with diabetes

patients with diabetes from the six trials included in the ATT (Antiplatelet Trialists' Collaboration Collaborative) meta-analysis. They concluded that aspirin appears to produce a modest-sized reduction in MI and stroke in patients with diabetes, but current evidence remains inconclusive. This was partially rectified by recent 14 trial meta-analysis which found a significant net benefit, but the authors still concluded inconclusiveness in regards to diabetic patients.[48,49,50]

In 2010, a position statement of the ADA, the American Heart Association, and the American College of Cardiology Foundation recommended physicians consider aspirin therapy (75–162 mg/day) as a primary prevention strategy in those with type 1 or type 2 diabetes at increased cardiovascular risk (10-year risk >10%). This includes most men aged >50 years or women aged >60 years who have at least one additional major risk factor (family history of CVD, hypertension, smoking, dyslipidemia, or albuminuria). However, aspirin was no longer recommended for those at low CVD risk (women under age 60 years and men under age 50 years with no major CVD risk factors; 10-year CVD risk under 5%) as the low benefit is likely to be outweighed by the risks of significant bleeding.[27]

3.3. Anti-diabetic medications and cardiovascular disease

Several classes of antidiabetic medications are currently available and effectively decreased hyperglycemia; however, concern regarding increased CVD risk was raised with the publication of the famous metanalysis by Nissen et al (2007) and showed rosiglitazone to be associated with a significant increase in the risk of myocardial infarction and with an increase in the risk of death from cardiovascular causes that had borderline significance. This study eventually, as well as other concerns, led to the withdrawal of the medication from the European Union as well as severe restriction that amounted to effective withdrawal in the United States as well. These findings also prompted the FDA to require cardiovascular safety data prior to approval of new diabetes drugs in the USA. Currently, evidence available regarding cardiovascular safety and even protective effects for metformin either neutral or uncertain effects of others agents due to lack of long-term safety data.

4. Global control of cardiovascular risk in the diabetic population

The estimation and categorization of cardiovascular risk requires close attention to the risks being explored (Table 4). While certain CVD risks are modifiable such as smoking, obesity, hypertension and dyslipidemia, others are non-modifiable such as family history of premature coronary artery disease. Despite evidence for improved CVD outcomes with control of CVD risk factors, data from our group (McFarlane et al., 2002, 2005) conducted at multiple centers in the USA, among various ethnic groups and practice settings, showed largely suboptimal control of glycemia, blood pressure, and cholesterol and also demonstrated gender disparity in the outcomes of diabetic care. For these reasons, a multifactorial targeted and evidence based approach as detailed in this chapter needs to be employed for the appropriate and adequate management of these diabetic patients at risk for cardiovascular disease.

Modifiable Risk Factors	Non-Modifiable Risk Factors
Hypertension	Age
Diabetes	Sex
Dyslipidemia	Race/Ethnicity
Tobacco Use	Family history of premature CAD
Poor dietary habits (high fat, high carbohydrate)	
Sedentary lifestyle	
Obesity (particularly central distribution)	
microalbuminuria	
Increased inflammation	
Stimulation of RAAS	

CAD= Coronary artery disease

RAAS = Renin Angiotensin Aldosterone System

Table 4. Risk Factor Categorization

Author details

David Fridman[1], Amgad N. Makaryus[1,2], John N. Makaryus[1], Amit Bhanvadia[3], Erion Qaja[4], Alina Masters[3] and Samy I. McFarlane[3*]

*Address all correspondence to: smcfarlane@downstate.edu

1 North Shore-LIJ Health System, Hofstra NSLIJ School of Medicine, Manhasset, NY, USA

2 Department of Cardiology, NuHealth, Nassau University Medical Center, East Meadow, NY, USA

3 Division of Endocrinology, Department of Medicine, SUNY Downstate Medical Center, Brooklyn, NY, USA

4 Wyckoff Heights Medical Center, Brooklyn, NY, USA

References

[1] Global Atlas on Cardiovascular Disease Prevention and Control. Mendis S, Puska P, Norrving B editors. World Health Organization (in collaboration with the World Heart Federation and World Stroke Organization), Geneva 2011.

[2] Cardiovascular disease and risk management. Diabetes Care. 2015;38 Suppl:S49–57.

[3] Buse JB, Ginsberg HN, Bakris GL, et al.; American Heart Association; American Diabetes Association. Primary prevention of cardiovascular diseases in people with diabetes mellitus: a scientific statement from the American Heart Association and the American Diabetes Association. Diabetes Care 2007;30:162–172

[4] Wild, G Roglic, A Green, R Sicree, H King. Global prevalence of diabetes; estimates for year 2000 and projections for 2030. Diabetes Care, 21 (2004), pp. 1047–1053

[5] James PA, Oparil S, Carter BL, et al. 2014 evidence-based guideline for the management of high blood pressure in adults: report from the panel members appointed to the Eighth Joint National Committee (JNC 8). JAMA. 2014;311(5):507–20.

[6] Patel A, Macmahon S, Chalmers J, et al. Effects of a fixed combination of perindopril and indapamide on macrovascular and microvascular outcomes in patients with type 2 diabetes mellitus (the ADVANCE trial): a randomised controlled trial. Lancet. 2007;370(9590):829–40.

[7] The effect of intensive treatment of diabetes on the development and progression of long-term complications in insulin-dependent diabetes mellitus. The Diabetes Control and Complications Trial Research Group. N Engl J Med. 1993;329(14):977–86.

[8]   Epidemiology of Diabetes Interventions and Complications (EDIC). Design, implementation, and preliminary results of a long-term follow-up of the Diabetes Control and Complications Trial cohort. Diabetes Care. 1999;22(1):99–111.

[9]   Young LH, Wackers FJ, Chyun DA, et al. Cardiac outcomes after screening for asymptomatic coronary artery disease in patients with type 2 diabetes: the DIAD study: a randomized controlled trial. JAMA. 2009;301(15):1547–55.

[10]   Boden WE, O'Rourke RA, Teo KK, et al.; COURAGE Trial Research Group. Optimal medical therapy with or without PCI for stable coronary disease. N Engl J Med 2007;356:1503–1516 67.

[11]   BARI 2D Study Group; Frye RL, August P, et al. A randomized trial of therapies for type 2 diabetes and coronary artery disease. N Engl JMed 2009;360:2503–2515

[12]   Laing SP, Swerdlow AJ, Slater SD, et al. The British Diabetic Association Cohort Study, I: all-cause mortality in patients with insulin-treated diabetes mellitus. Diabet Med 1999;16:459–65

[13]   Skrivarhaug T, Bangstad HJ, Stene LC, Sandvik L, Hanssen KF, Joner G. Longterm mortality in a nationwide cohort of childhood-onset type 1 diabetic patients in Norway. Diabetologia 2006;49:298–305

[14]   Secrest AM, Becker DJ, Kelsey SF, Laporte RE, Orchard TJ. Cause-specific mortality trends in a large populationbased cohort with long-standing childhood-onset type 1 diabetes. Diabetes 2010;59:3216–22.

[15]   Secrest AM, Becker DJ, Kelsey SF, Laporte RE, Orchard TJ. Cause-specific mortality trends in a large population-based cohort with longstanding childhood-onset type 1 diabetes. Diabetes 2010;59:3216–3222

[16]   Swedish National Diabetes Register.Annual Report 2012 (https:/ / www .ndr .nu/ pdf/Annual_Report_NDR_2012 .pdf).

[17]   Lind M, Svensson AM, Kosiborod M, et al. Glycemic control and excess mortality in type 1 diabetes. N Engl J Med. 2014;371(21):1972–82.

[18]   Livingstone SJ, Looker HC, Hothersall EJ, et al. Risk of cardiovascular disease and total mortality in adults withtype 1 diabetes: Scottish registry linkage study. PLoS Med 2012;9(10):e1001321

[19]   Mameli C, Mazzantini S, Ben nasr M, Fiorina P, Scaramuzza AE, Zuccotti GV. Explaining the increased mortality in type 1 diabetes. World J Diabetes. 2015;6(7):889–95.

[20]   Writing Team for the Diabetes Control and Complications Trial/Epidemiology of Diabetes Interventions and Complications Research Group 2002 Effect of intensive therapy on the microvascular complications of type 1 diabetes mellitus. *JAMA* 287:2563–2569

[21]   Writing Team for the Diabetes Control and Complications Trial/Epidemiology of
       Diabetes Interventions and Complications Research Group 2003 Sustained effect of
       intensive treatment of type 1 diabetes mellitus on development and progression of
       diabetic nephropathy: the Epidemiology of Diabetes Interventions and Complica-
       tions (EDIC) study. *JAMA* 290:2159–2167

[22]   Ceriello A, Ihnat MA, Thorpe JE. Clinical review 2: The "metabolic memory": is more
       than just tight glucose control necessary to prevent diabetic complications?. J ClinEn-
       docrinolMetab. 2009;94(2):410–5.

[23]   Fullerton B, Jeitler K, Seitz M, Horvath K, Berghold A, Siebenhofer A. Intensive glu-
       cose control versus conventional glucose control for type 1 diabetes mellitus. Co-
       chrane Database Syst Rev. 2014;2:CD009122.

[24]   The Diabetes Control and Complications Trial (DCCT)/Epidemiology of DiabetesIn-
       terventions and Complications (EDIC) Research Group. Beneficial effects ofintensive
       therapy of diabetes during adolescence: outcomes after the conclusionof the diabetes
       control and complications trial (DCCT). J Pediatr 2001;139:804–12.

[25]   Diabetes Control and Complications Trial/Epidemiology of Diabetes Intervention-
       sand Complications Research Group. Prolonged effect of intensive therapyon the risk
       of retinopathy complications in patient with type 1 diabetes mellitus:10 years after
       the Diabetes Control and Complications Trial. Arch Ophthalmol2008;126(12):1707–
       15.

[26]   White NH, Sun W, Cleary PA, et al, for the DCCT-EDIC Research Group. Effect ofp-
       rior intensive therapy in type 1 diabetes on 10-year progression of retinopathyin the
       DCCT/EDIC: comparison of adults and adolescents. Diabetes 2010;59(5):1244–53.

[27]   UK Prospective Diabetes Study (UKPDS) Group. Intensive blood-glucose control
       with sulphonylureas or insulin compared with conventional treatment and risk of
       complicationsin patients with type 2 diabetes (UKPDS 33). Lancet 1998;352:837–53.

[28]   Tight blood pressure control and risk of macrovascular and microvascular complica-
       tions in type 2 diabetes: UKPDS 38. BMJ 1998;317:703–13.

[29]   Pyörälä K, Pedersen TR, Kjekshus J, Færgeman O, Olsson AG, Thorgeirsson G. Cho-
       lesterol lowering with simvastatin improves prognosis of diabetic patients with coro-
       nary heart disease: a subgroup analysis of the Scandinavian Simvastatin Survival
       Study (4S). Diabetes Care 1997;20:614–20.

[30]   Ravid M, Lang R, Rachmani R, Lishner M. Long-term renoprotective effect of angio-
       tensin-converting enzyme inhibition in non-insulin-dependent diabetes mellitus: a 7-
       year follow-up study. Arch Intern Med 1996;156:286–9.

[31]   The Heart Outcomes Prevention Evaluation Study Investigators. Effects of an angio-
       tensin- converting–enzyme inhibitor, ramipril, on cardiovascular events in high-risk
       patients. N Engl J Med 2000;342:145–53.

[32] Gaede P, Vedel P, Larsen N, Jensen GV, Parving HH, Pedersen O. Multifactorial intervention and cardiovascular disease in patients with type 2 diabetes. N Engl J Med. 2003;348(5):383–93.

[33] Gaede P, Lund-andersen H, Parving HH, Pedersen O. Effect of a multifactorial intervention on mortality in type 2 diabetes. N Engl J Med. 2008;358(6):580–91.

[34] Wu WX, Ren M, Cheng H, et al. Prevention of macrovascular disease in patients with short-duration type 2 diabetes by multifactorial target control: an 8-year prospective study. Endocrine. 2014;47(2):485–92.

[35] Gaede P, Lund-andersen H, Parving HH, Pedersen O. Effect of a multifactorial intervention on mortality in type 2 diabetes. N Engl J Med. 2008;358(6):580–91.

[36] Franz, Marion J., et al. "Evidence-based nutrition principles and recommendations for the treatment and prevention of diabetes and related complications." *Diabetes care* 25.1 (2002): 148–198.

[37] Bantle, John P., et al. "Nutrition recommendations and interventions for diabetes: a position statement of the American Diabetes Association." *Diabetes care* 31 (2008): S61-S78.

[38] Franz MJ, Monk A, Barry B, et al. Effectiveness of medical nutrition therapy provided by dietitians in the management of non-insulin-dependent diabetes mellitus: a randomized, controlled clinical trial. J Am Diet Assoc. 1995;95(9):1009–17.

[39] MJ Garcia, PM McNamara, T Gordon, WB KannellMorbidity and mortality in diabetics in the Framingham population: sixteen year follow-up study. Diabetes, 23 (1974), pp. 105–111

[40] Pyörälä, M Laakso, M Uusitupa. Diabetes and atherosclerosis: an epidemiologic view. Diabetes Metab, 3 (1987), pp. 464. 46

[41] Stamler, O Vaccaro, JD Neaton, D Wentworth. Diabetes, other risk factors, and 12-yr cardiovascular mortality for men screened in the multiple risk factor intervention trial.Diabetes Care, 16 (1993), pp. 434 pp.

[42] Mihaylova B, Emberson J, Blackwell L, et al. The effects of lowering LDL cholesterol with statin therapy in people at low risk of vascular disease: meta-analysis of individual data from 27 randomised trials. Lancet. 2012;380(9841):581–90.

[43] Baigent C, Keech A, Kearney PM, et al. Efficacy and safety of cholesterol-lowering treatment: prospective meta-analysis of data from 90,056 participants in 14 randomised trials of statins. Lancet. 2005;366(9493):1267–78.

[44] Taylor F, Huffman MD, Macedo AF, et al. Statins for the primary prevention of cardiovascular disease. Cochrane Database Syst Rev 2013;1:CD004816

[45] Carter AA, Gomes T, Camacho X, Juurlink DN, Shah BR, Mamdani MM. Risk of incident diabetes among patients treated with statins: population based study. BMJ 2013;346:f2610

[46] Antiplatelet Trialists' Collaboration Collaborative overview of randomised trials of antiplatelet therapy—I: prevention of death, myocardial infarction, and stroke by prolonged antiplatelet therapy in various categories of patients. BMJ. 1994;308:81–106.

[47] Antithrombotic Trialists' Collaboration Collaborative meta-analysis of randomised trials of antiplatelet therapy for prevention of death, myocardial infarction, and stroke in high risk patients. BMJ. 2002;324:71–86.

[48] Baigent C, Blackwell L, Collins R, et al. Aspirin in the primary and secondary prevention of vascular disease: collaborative meta-analysis of individual participant data from randomised trials. Lancet. 2009;373(9678):1849 60.

[49] Pignone M, Alberts MJ, Colwell JA, et al. Aspirin for primary prevention of cardiovascular events in people with diabetes. J Am CollCardiol. 2010;55(25):2878–86.

[50] Xie M, Shan Z, Zhang Y, et al. Aspirin for primary prevention of cardiovascular events: meta-analysis of randomized controlled trials and subgroup analysis by sex and diabetes status. PLoS ONE. 2014;9(10):e90286.

2

Medical and Surgical Management and Outcomes for Coronary Artery Disease

Allan Mattia and Frank Manetta

Abstract

Coronary artery disease (CAD) is a major cause of death and disability in developed countries. Although coronary artery disease mortality rates worldwide have declined over the past decades, CAD remains responsible for about one third or more of all deaths in individuals over the age of 35 years. Various methods of treatment have been proposed including medical therapy, catheter-based interventions, and lastly, coronary artery bypass grafting. The purpose of this chapter is to outline those treatment regimens and examine the literature detailing their outcomes in hopes of guiding treatment.

Keywords: coronary artery disease, management, outcomes, coronary artery bypass grafting, PCI

1. Introduction: coronary artery disease, an overview and disease burden

Coronary artery disease (CAD) represents a spectrum of clinical syndromes caused by insufficient coronary blood flow to the myocardium. It is almost always due to subintimal atheroma deposition leading to arterial luminal stenosis or occlusion and wall thickening. Coronary atherosclerosis usually involves the proximal portions of larger coronary arteries, especially at or just beyond branching sites. Myocardial ischemia and necrosis occur when coronary blood flow is impaired by atherosclerotic stenosis, resulting in increased oxygen demand. In the setting of symptomatic CAD, compensatory physiologic processes are insufficient to provide adequate myocardial perfusion. The effect is either supply ischemia, responsible for myocardial infarction (MI) and most episodes of unstable angina, or demand ischemia, where coronary blood flow is insufficient during period of increased myocardial demands from exercise, tachycardia, fever, hypertension, or emotional distress [1]. Because the heart has virtually no stores of oxygen and relies entirely on aerobic metabolism, within seconds of coronary occlusion, its high rate of energy expenditures results in a sudden decline of oxygen tension and left ventricular function impairment. The subendocardium is most vulnerable to myocardial ischemia as its collateral flow is lowest; thus, myocardial necrosis progresses toward the epicardium with continued ischemia.

Coronary artery disease is a major cause of death and disability in developed countries. Although coronary artery disease mortality rates worldwide have declined over the past decades, CAD remains responsible for about one third or more of all deaths in individuals over the age of 35 years. In 2017, the Heart Disease and Stroke Statistics update of the American Heart Association reported that 16.5 million persons aged 20 years or older in the United States have coronary artery disease, with a slight male predominance of 55%. In 2013, The Global Burden of Disease estimated that 17.3 million deaths worldwide were related to cardiovascular disease, a 41% increase since 1990 [2–6]. Significant risk factors include but are not limited to age, male sex, hypertension, hyperlipidemia, diabetes mellitus, obesity, tobacco use, family history, and peripheral vascular disease. As one can see, the incidence and prevalence of coronary artery disease are staggering; thus, managing and treating these patients is of utmost concern.

2. Treatment goals of coronary artery disease

The goal of treatment for coronary artery disease is to decrease the frequency and severity of angina symptoms and to increase the duration of one's functional capacity (duration of angina-free exercise). Furthermore, one hopes to prolong life and reduce the incidence of acute coronary syndromes. Such goals are accomplished by increasing myocardial oxygen supply or decreasing myocardial oxygen consumption or both. The reduction in cardiac mortality and incidents of myocardial infarction is achieved by pharmacotherapy and stabilization of atherosclerotic plaques. Comorbid conditions that are treatable could aggravate

Goal	How to Achieve the Goal
Abolish or reduce anginal episodes	Trial of antianginal drugs
	Coronary revascularization
Increase angina-free walking or exercise	Antianginal drugs
	Coronary revascularization
Prolong life and reduce acute coronary events (unstable angina, myocardial infarction, coronary death)	Lifestyle modification
	Modify or correct risk factors
	Daily aspirin
	Pharmacotherapy of dyslipidemia
	Control of hypertension
	Beta blockers, ACE inhibitors, and CABG surgery in special situations

Figure 1. Management of chronic stable angina.

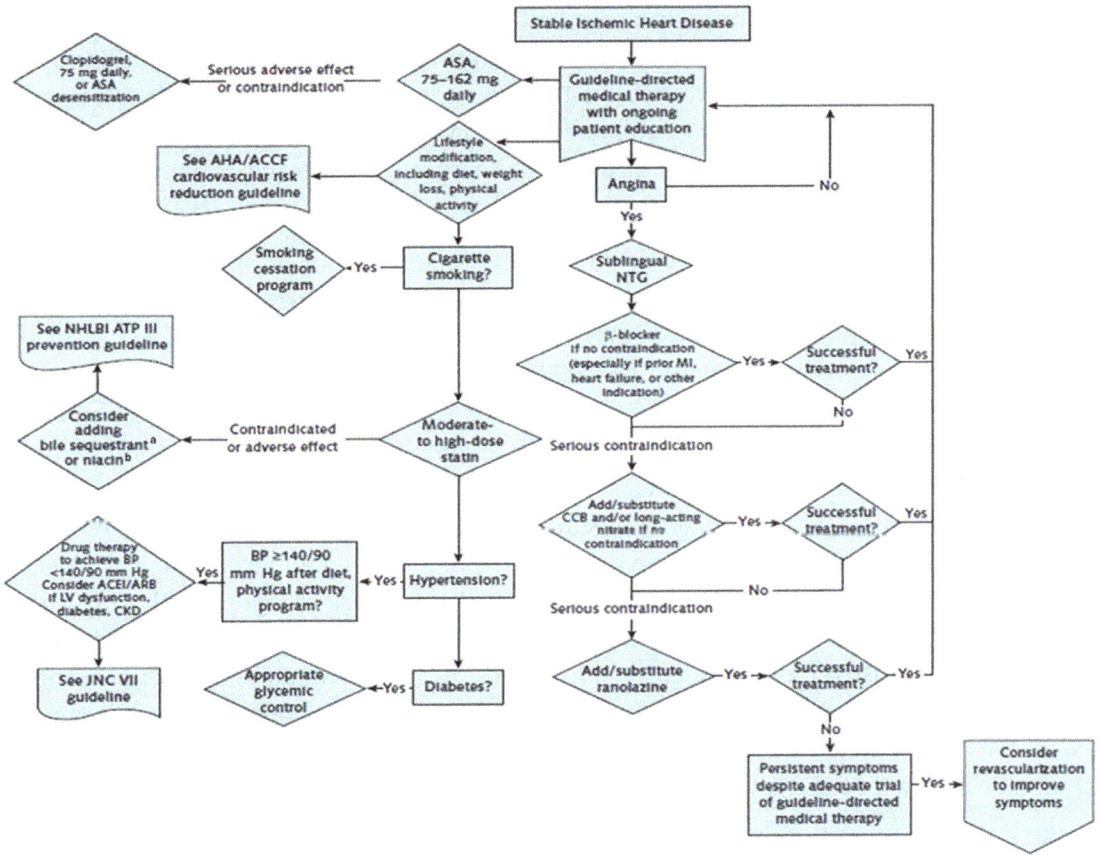

Figure 2. Treatment algorithm for stable ischemic heart disease. *From Ref. [11].

angina, and these conditions must be sought and treated in all patients who have chronic stable angina. There are three options for treatment of stable angina-drug therapy, coronary balloon angioplasty, and coronary artery bypass graft surgery [7–10].

As no two patients are the same, therapy should be individualized and consideration should be given to the risks and benefits of each therapeutic option with regard to symptom relief and longevity. **Figure 1** shows the treatment goals for chronic stable angina and how to achieve them [7–10], and **Figure 2** shows the treatment algorithm for chronic stable angina [11].

3. Medical management of coronary artery disease

From the above treatment algorithm, one can see that there is a large armamentarium at one's disposal for the treatment of coronary artery disease. The uses of these drugs and their mechanisms of action will be outlined below.

Beta blockers have been shown to be very effective in the treatment and management of stable angina. These agents decrease myocardial work and improve exercise tolerance. The primary mechanism of this benefit is through a competitive blockade of β-adrenergic receptors that reduces heart rate and contractility and therefore myocardial O_2 demand. In addition, beta blockers decrease exercise-induced vasoconstriction and blunt the rise in systolic blood pressure during exercise. Beta blockers also increase coronary perfusion by prolonging diastolic perfusion time. Such drugs should be titrated to a heart rate of 50–60 beats per minute at rest and less than 100 beats per minute with exercise.

Calcium channel blockers act mainly by vasodilatation and reduction of peripheral vascular resistance. The nondihydropyridine agents (verapamil and diltiazem), a T-channel blocker (mibefradil), and bepridil inhibit the sinoatrial and atrioventricular nodes and thus also reduce myocardial oxygen demand. The dihydropyridine agents (e.g., nifedipine, amlodipine, felodipine, and nisoldipine) do not affect the sinoatrial or atrioventricular nodes in humans; their mechanism of action is primarily by dilating the coronary arteries and reducing peripheral vascular resistance (and thus reducing myocardial O_2 demand) and by increasing coronary blood flow. Calcium channel blockers block the entry of calcium into the calcium channels in both smooth muscle and myocardium so that less calcium is available to the contractile apparatus. The net result is vasodilatation and a decrease in myocardial contractility. All calcium channel blockers inhibit L-type calcium current in arterial smooth muscle at low concentration and therefore dilate coronary arteries. A major antianginal effect is coronary vessel dilatation and prevention of exercise-induced vessel constriction. Afterload reduction and, in the case of nondihydropyridine channel blockers, the suppressant effects on the sinoatrial node and myocardium also contribute to antianginal efficacy.

Nitrates are coronary vasodilators, and they are anti-ischemic, although the antianginal effects are more far-reaching. Nitrates produce venodilatation, thereby reducing preload, and high doses of nitrates also reduce afterload through arterial vasodilatation. The reduction of preload is secondary to reduced venous return, which in turn reduces ventricular volume and intracavitary pressure and ventricular wall stress. Nitrates can produce dilatation of the site of stenotic coronary lesions and thus increase perfusion to the ischemic myocardium. Nitrates also increase collateral blood flow to ischemic areas. These drugs have not been shown to have an impact on cardiac death from coronary artery disease; however, they have been shown to reduce the rate of angina frequency and increase time to ischemia ECG findings on stress test.

Ranolazine is a selective inhibitor of late sodium influx into myocytes, reducing myocardial contractility. This drug is usually used in combination with beta blockers significantly reducing the frequency of angina and increases exercise duration and time to onset of angina.

Statins are lipid-lowering drugs that work by inhibiting HMG-CoA Reductase. Improvement of myocardial ischemia during ambulatory monitoring has been shown in several studies; however, it is not known whether these agents improve exercise performance [12]. Lipid-lowering agents are recommended for patients with stable angina who have dyslipidemia because these agents have an important influence on prognosis for these patients. High intensive therapy targets an LDL reduction of greater than 50% in high-risk patients and a reduction of 30–50% in those patients who cannot tolerate a high-intensity treatment regimen.

ACE inhibitors (captopril, enalapril, and lisinopril) work by inhibiting the angiotensin-converting enzyme. These drugs are a class I recommendation for patients with chronic CAD with LV dysfunction LVEF <40% or diabetes and a class II recommendation for CAD patients without these features [13, 14].

Daily use of aspirin has been shown to reduce the incidence of sudden death and acute myocardial infarction in stable angina. In the Swedish Angina Pectoris Aspirin Trial (SAPAT), daily use of aspirin was associated with a 34% reduction in the incidence of sudden death and acute myocardial infarction, with an absolute reduction of 12 sudden deaths for every 1000 patients treated during the 15-month period [15]. The relative reduction in secondary endpoints (vascular events, vascular death, all-cause mortality, and stroke) ranged from 22 to 32%. There was no difference in major bleeding episodes, including hemorrhagic strokes, between the aspirin and placebo groups. On the basis of these data and available data of the usefulness of aspirin in acute myocardial infarction and unstable angina, it is mandatory that aspirin be used in all patients with stable angina, unless they are unable to tolerate the medication because of either an allergic reaction or intolerable gastrointestinal side effects [8, 16].

Clopidogrel works by selectively inhibiting the binding of adenosine diphosphate (ADP) to its platelet P2Y12 receptor and the subsequent ADP-mediated activation of the glycoprotein GPIIb/IIIa complex, thereby inhibiting platelet aggregation. Patients who are intolerant to aspirin therapy may be treated with clopidogrel. Long-term treatment with a combination of aspirin plus clopidogrel is not superior to aspirin treatment alone and increases the risk of bleeding [17], and it is not recommended for treatment of patients with stable angina. However, combination of aspirin plus clopidogrel for up to 3–12 months after coronary artery stenting reduces adverse clinical outcomes and is indicated in this group of patients.

4. Percutaneous coronary intervention (PCI)

PCI has become one of the most commonly performed medical procedures in the United States, with more than 600,000 procedures performed annually. Over the past decade, the use of drug-eluting stents (DESs) has supplanted the use of older stents, referred to as bare-metal stents (BMSs). Almost all percutaneous coronary interventions (PCIs) performed currently involve stent placement. Thus, although the term percutaneous coronary intervention refers to any therapeutic coronary intervention, it has become essentially synonymous with coronary stent implantation. PCI is performed for coronary revascularization in patients with stable coronary disease as well as, in the appropriate clinical settings, in those with acute coronary syndromes. In **Figures 3** and **4**, one can see a schematic diagram of a PCI [18].

Indications for PCI include:

1. Moderate-to-severe stable angina with evidence of reversible ischemia

2. High-risk unstable angina or non-ST segment elevation myocardial infarction

3. Acute ST segment elevation myocardial infarction

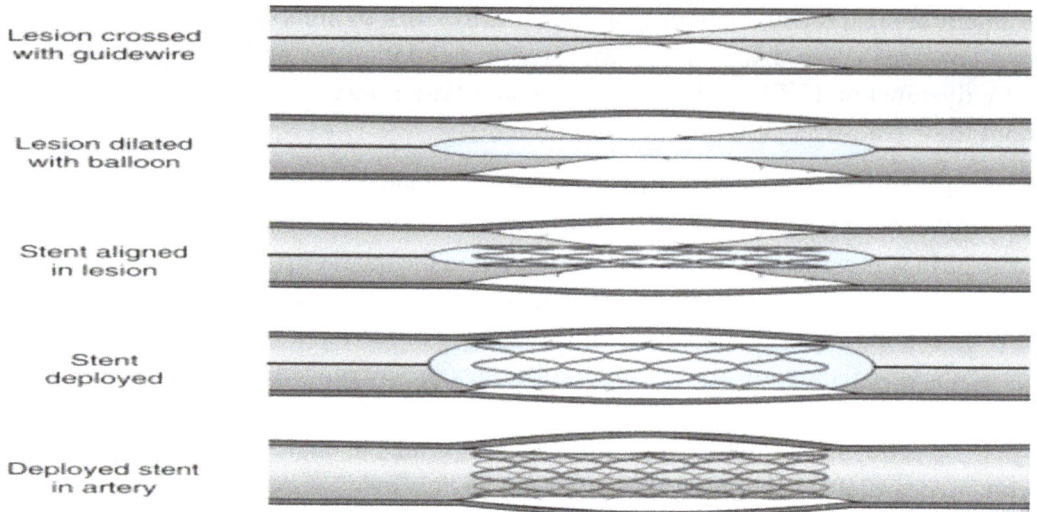

Figure 3. Schematic diagram of a PCI.

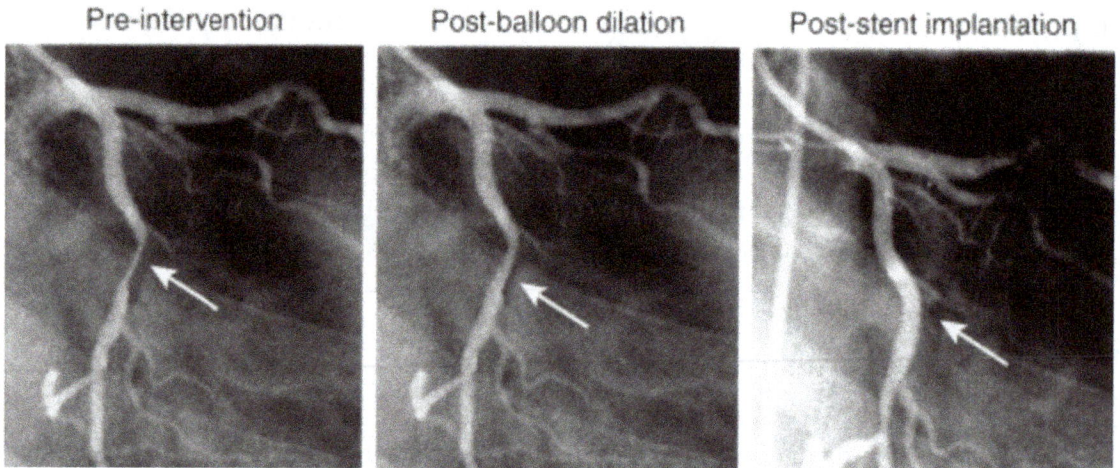

Figure 4. Percutaneous intervention of the circumflex artery seen angiographically [17]. Images from [18].

4. Rescue percutaneous coronary intervention after failed thrombolysis

5. Cardiogenic shock after myocardial infarction

6. Revascularization after successful resuscitation

7. Patients with diabetes mellitus

The only absolute contraindication to PCI is the lack of vascular access or active untreatable severe bleeding, which precludes the use of anticoagulation and antiplatelet agents. Relative contraindications include the following:

• A bleeding diathesis or other conditions that predispose to bleeding during antiplatelet therapy.

- Severe renal insufficiency unless the patient is on hemodialysis or has severe electrolyte abnormalities.

- Sepsis.

- Poor patient compliance with medications.

- A terminal condition, such as advanced or metastatic malignancy, that indicates a short life expectancy.

- Other indications for open-heart surgery.

- Anatomic features of poor success.

- Failure of previous PCI or not amenable to PCI based on previous angiograms.

- Severe cognitive dysfunction or advanced physical limitations.

Patients generally should not undergo PCI if the following conditions are present:

- Only a very small area of myocardium is at risk.

- There is no objective evidence of ischemia (unless the patient has clear anginal symptoms and has not had a stress test) with either noninvasive or invasive testing (e.g., fractional flow reserve). One should also beware of false-negative stress tests in patients with left-main CAD.

- There is a low likelihood of technical success.

- The patient has left main or multivessel CAD with a high SYNTAX score and is a candidate for coronary artery bypass grafting (CABG).

- There is insignificant stenosis (less than 50% luminal narrowing).

- The patient has end-stage cirrhosis with portal hypertension resulting in encephalopathy or visceral bleeding.

Following PCI, the patient should be placed on antiplatelet therapy. Patients who are already on aspirin therapy should continue with 81 mg of aspirin daily. Those who are not on aspirin should receive 325 mg of non–enteric-coated aspirin preferably 24 hours prior to PCI, after which aspirin should be continued indefinitely at a dose of 81 mg daily. A loading dose of a P2Y12 inhibitor should be given prior to PCI with stent placement. Following a loading dose of a P2Y12 inhibitor, a maintenance dose is continued. The recommendations for dose and duration are as follows:

- In patients undergoing elective BMS implantation, the duration of P2Y12 inhibitor therapy should be a minimum of 1 month.

- For patient undergoing elective DES implantation (with a second-generation DES) for stable ischemic heart disease, the duration of P2Y12 inhibitor therapy should be at least 6 months.

- For patients undergoing stent BMS or DES implantation in the setting of ACS, clopidogrel 75 mg daily, prasugrel 10 mg daily, or ticagrelor 90 mg twice daily should be continued for at least 12 months. In this setting, ticagrelor and prasugrel are preferred over clopidogrel.

- Shorter duration therapy may be reasonable in patients at high risk for bleeding. Conversely, longer duration therapy may be reasonable in those at higher risk for ischemia but not for bleeding.

5. Coronary artery bypass grafting (CABG)

The decision for surgery is made based on the comprehensive evaluation of the patient. Anatomic considerations that favor recommendation for CABG include presence of significant LM or proximal LAD CAD, multivessel CAD, and presence of lesions not amenable to stenting. The presence of diabetes also favors surgical revascularization over stenting in operable patients. Depressed ejection fraction has been recognized as an additional indication for CABG.

Although the coronary anatomy may be suitable for bypass, each patient's comorbidities should be considered in the overall risk-benefit analysis. Preoperative renal insufficiency, peripheral vascular disease, recent myocardial infarction, or recent stroke, as well as emergency operation and cardiogenic shock, has been identified as factors that increase mortality. The decision to offer CABG or PCI should be determined by a multidisciplinary heart team that evaluates the appropriate therapy on a case-by-case basis.

The current American Heart Association Guidelines for coronary artery bypass grafting can be found in **Figure 5**.

6. A review of the literature: which treatment is best?

Three early prospective randomized trials comparing CABG with medical therapy were conducted in the late 1970s and were reported in the early 1980s. The Veterans' Affairs (VA) cooperative trial, European Coronary Surgery Study (ECSS), and Coronary Artery Surgery Study (CASS) showed long-term superiority of surgery over medical therapy in patients with left main (LM) coronary artery disease, significant coronary artery disease involving the LAD artery, and multivessel disease.

The first study was reported in 1982 in the European Coronary Surgery Study [19]. This study randomized 768 men to medical or surgical treatment. In follow-up extending to 8 years, survival was significantly improved by surgery in patients with significant three-vessel disease and in patients with significant stenosis in the proximal LAD coronary artery who had two- or three-vessel disease. Compared with medically treated patients, late mortality was reduced by 53% at 5 years in surgically treated patients, and among those with three-vessel disease, the 5-year mortality rate was lowered by 66%. In the subgroup of patients with significant narrowing of the proximal LAD coronary artery, the 5-year mortality rate was lowered 60% by surgery.

The second study reporting the efficacy of coronary revascularization was the 1984 Veterans Administration study [20]. This study evaluated the long-term survival after CABG in 686 patients with stable angina, and patients were observed for an average of 11.2 years. The 7-year survival curves for the total population of patients showed a statistically significant survival benefit of 77% with surgical therapy compared with 70% survival with medical

AHA/ACC Guidelines for CABG

Asymptomatic/Mild Angina
Class I
    1. Left main stenosis
    2. Left main equivalent (proximal LAD and proximal circumflex)
    3. Three-vessel disease
Class IIa
    1. Proximal LAD stenosis and one- or two-vessel disease
Class IIb
    1. One- or two-vessel disease not involving proximal LAD
      If a large territory at risk on noninvasive studies or LVEF<50%, IIa and IIb become
class I indications

Stable Angina
Class I
    1. Left main stenosis
    2. Left main equivalent (proximal LAD and proximal circumflex)
    3. Three-vessel disease
    4. Two-vessel disease with proximal LAD stenosis and EF <50% or demonstrable ischemia
    5. One- or two-vessel disease without proximal LAD stenosis b ut with a large territory at
risk and high-risk criteria on noninvasive testing
    6. Disabling angina refractory to medical therapy
Class IIa
    1. Proximal LAD stenosis with one-vessel disease
    2. One- or two-vessel disease without proximal LAD stenosis, but with a moderate territory
at risk and demonstrable ischemia

Unstable Angina/Non–ST-Segment Elevation MI (NSTEMI)
Class I
    1. Left main
    2. Left main equivalent
    3. Ongoing ischemia not responsive to maximal nonsurgical the rapy
Class IIa
    1. Proximal LAD stenosis with one- or two-vessel disease
Class IIb
    1. One- or two-vessel disease without proximal LAD stenosis w hen PCI not possible
(becomes class I if high-risk criteria on noninvasive testing)

ST-Segment Elevation (Q wave) MI
Class I
    1. Failed PCI with persistent pain or shock and anatomically feasible
    2. Persistent or recurrent ischemia refractory to medical treatment with acceptable anatomy
who have a significant territory at risk and not a candidate fo r PCI
    3. Requires surgical repair of post-infarct ventricular septa l rupture or mitral valve
insufficiency
    4. Cardiogenic shock in patients <75 years of age who have ST elevation, LBBB, or a
posterior MI within 18 hours of onset
    5. Life-threatening ventricular arrhythmias in the presence o f ≥50% left main stenosis or
three-vessel disease
Class IIa
    1. Primary reperfusion in patients who have failed fibrinolyt ics or PCI and are in the early
stages (6–12 h) of an evolving STEMI
    2. Mortality with CABG is elevated the first 3–7 days after STEMI/NSTEMI. After 7 days,
criteria for revascularization in previous sections apply.

Poor LV Function
Class I
    1. Left main stenosis
    2. Left main equivalent
    3. Proximal LAD stenosis and two- to three-vessel disease
Class IIa
    1. Significant viable territory and noncontractile myocardium

Life-Threatening Ventricular Arrhythmias
Class I
    1. Left main disease
    2. Three-vessel disease
Class IIa
    1. Bypassable one- or two-vessel disease
    2. Proximal LAD disease and one- or two-vessel disease.
      These become class I indications if arrhythmia is resuscita ted cardiac death or
sustained ventricular tachycardia.

Failed PCI
Class I
    1. Ongoing ischemia with significant territory at risk
    2. Shock
Class IIa
    1. Foreign body in critical position
    2. Shock with coagulopathy and no previous sternotomy
Class IIb
    1. Shock with coagulopathy and previous sternotomy

Previous CABG
Class I
    1. Disabling angina refractory to medical therapy
    2. Nonpatent previous bypass grafts, but with class I indicat ions for native CAD
Class IIa
1. Large territory at risk
2. Vein grafts supplying LAD or large territory are >50% stenos ed

Figure 5. AHA/ACC guidelines for CABG.

treatment. This benefit diminished by 11 years of observation, but a survival advantage persisted 11 years in surgical patients with three-vessel disease and impaired left ventricular function and in those at high clinical risk defined by preoperative ST-segment depression, history of myocardial infarction, or hypertension (**Figure 6**).

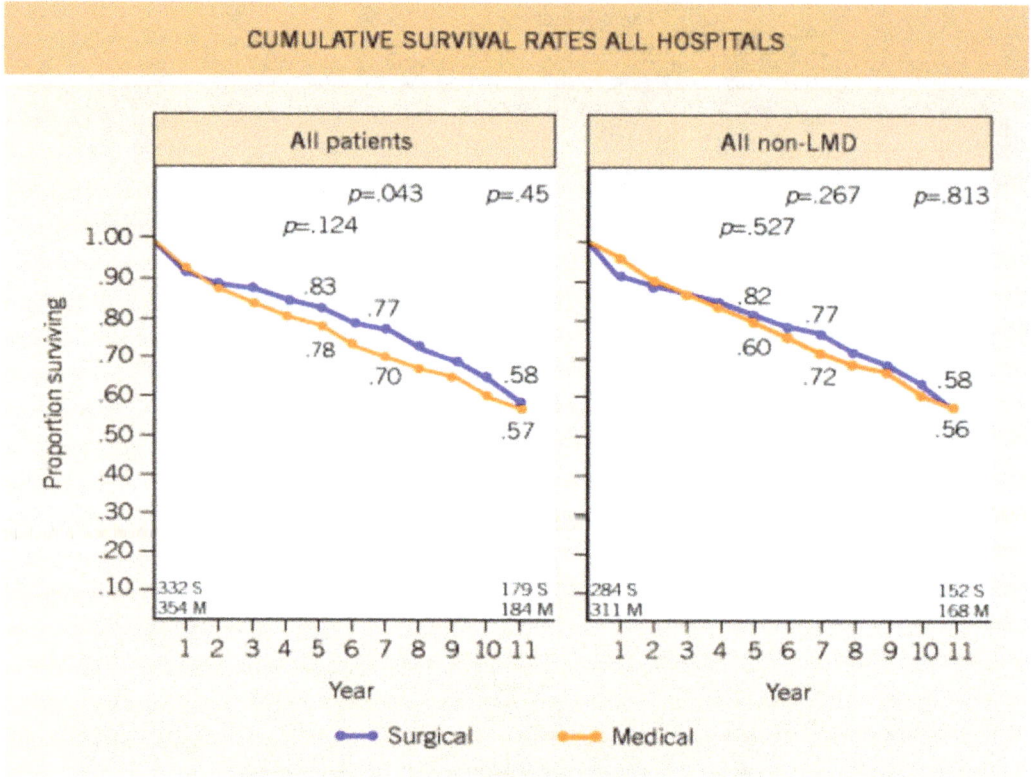

Figure 6. VA study results. Eleven-year cumulative survival for all patients according to treatment assignment. Survival curve for randomized medical (M) and surgical (S) groups in all patients and all patients without left main disease (non-LMD). From Veterans Administration Coronary Artery Bypass Surgery Cooperative Study Group [20].

Finally, the Coronary Artery Surgery Study (CASS) [21] reported survival data of 780 patients with stable angina and ejection fractions greater than 35% who were assigned to receive medical or surgical therapy. At 8 years of follow-up, 87% of surgically treated patients were alive compared with 84% of those receiving medical therapy. Although not statistically significant, the trend favored surgical therapy. Of note, the subgroup with three-vessel disease and a reduced ejection fraction of less than 50% but greater than 35% had a significant survival benefit in the surgical group at 7 years of 88% compared with 65% in the medical therapy group (**Figure 7**).

While the above studies showed the impact coronary revascularization has on patient long-term outcomes compared to medical therapy alone, there remained much debate in regard to efficacy and patient survival when comparing coronary artery bypass grafting and percutaneous coronary interventions. Perhaps, the single most important trial comparing the two interventions was the SYNTAX trial. This trial involved 85 treatment centers and 1800 patients with multivessel or left main coronary artery disease. These showed worse outcomes in the PCI group as compared to the CABG group, with increased composite major adverse cardiac and cerebrovascular events (MACCE: death, stroke, MI, or repeat revascularization). Although there was no significant difference in all-cause mortality and stroke at 5 years, MI and repeat revascularization were both increased in the PCI group. Of note, in patients with three-vessel coronary artery disease (CAD), CABG in comparison with PCI was associated with a significantly reduced rate of MI-related death, which was the leading cause of death

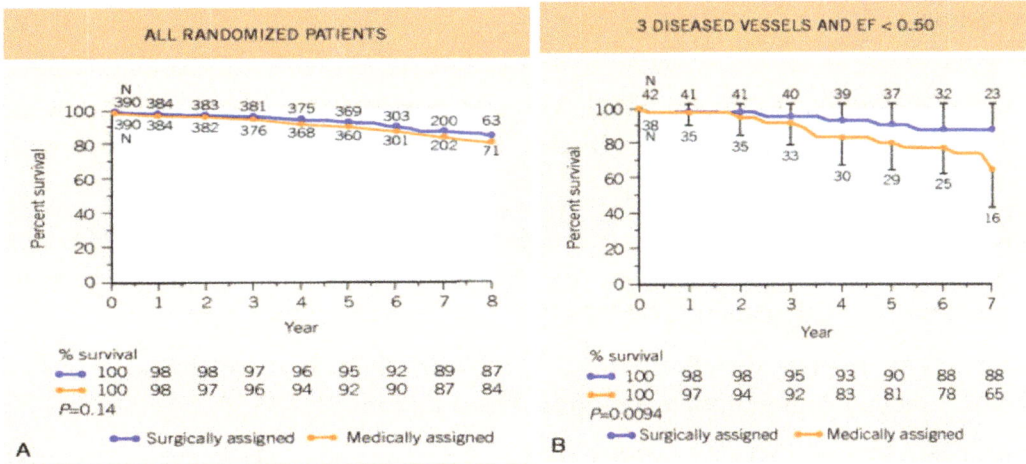

Figure 7. CASS results. Cumulative survival for patients participating in the CASS randomized trial. (A) Survival curve for all patients assigned to medical or surgical therapy and (B) survival curve for patients with three diseased vessels and ejection fractions (EF) less than 0.50 assigned to medical or surgical therapy. From Killip et al. [21].

after PCI. The study concluded that patients with more complex disease (3VD with intermediate-high SYNTAX scores and LM with high SYNTAX score) have an increased risk of a MACCE event with PCI, and CABG is the preferred treatment option.

The syntax score is a scoring system developed by the SYNTAX trial investigators to quantify the extent and complexity of CAD based on findings at cardiac catheterization. Scores are divided into terciles: low (0–22), intermediate (23–32), and high (≥33), with higher scores representing more extensive and complex CAD. The SYNTAX score was found to correlate with PCI risk and outcome but not with CABG risk and outcome. Patients with higher SYNTAX scores generally benefited from a revascularization strategy of CABG in preference to PCI. This is reflected in current guidelines, which state that it is reasonable to choose CABG over PCI as a revascularization strategy in patients with complex three-vessel disease and high SYNTAX score.

It must be noted that for patients with complicated coronary artery disease, coronary artery bypass surgery has been shown to be superior to that of PCI. From the studies above, it can be noted that this difference can be seen after a 5 year follow up period. Thus, for patients with triple vessel disease, diabetes and reduced ejection fraction, coronary artery bypass surgery should be the standard of care.

Author details

Allan Mattia and Frank Manetta*

*Address all correspondence to: fmanetta@northwell.edu

Department of Cardiovascular and Thoracic Surgery, Hofstra Northwell School of Medicine, Manhasset, NY, USA

References

[1] Ganz P, Ganz W. Coronary blood flow and myocardial ischemia. In: Braunwald E, Zipes DP, Libby P, editors. Heart Disease. Philadelphia: W.B. Saunders Company; 2001. pp. 1087-1113

[2] Rosamond W, Flegal K, Furie K, et al. Heart disease and stroke statistics—2008 update: A report from the American Heart Association statistics committee and stroke statistics subcommittee. Circulation. 2008;**117**:e25

[3] Nichols M, Townsend N, Scarborough P, Rayner M. Cardiovascular disease in Europe 2014: Epidemiological update. European Heart Journal. 2014;**35**:2950

[4] Benjamin EJ, Blaha MJ, Chiuve SE, et al. Heart disease and stroke Statistics-2017 update: A report from the American Heart Association. Circulation. 2017;**135**:e146

[5] Lloyd-Jones DM, Larson MG, Beiser A, Levy D. Lifetime risk of developing coronary heart disease. Lancet. 1999;**353**:89

[6] GBD 2013 Mortality and Causes of Death Collaborators. Global, regional, and national age-sex specific all-cause and cause-specific mortality for 240 causes of death, 1990-2013: A systematic analysis for the global burden of disease study 2013. Lancet. 2015;**385**:117

[7] Thadani U. Current medical management of chronic stable angina. Journal of Cardiovascular Pharmacology and Therapeutics. 2004;**9**:S11-S29

[8] Asirvatham S, Sebastian C, Thadani U. Choosing the most appropriate treatment for stable angina: Safety considerations. Drug Safety. 1998;**19**:23-44

[9] Thadani U. Management of stable angina pectoris. Current Opinion in Cardiology. 1999;**14**:349-358

[10] Thadani U. Management of patients with chronic stable angina at low risk for serious cardiac events. The American Journal of Cardiology. 1997;**79**:24-30

[11] Fihn SD, Gardin JM, Abrams J, et al. ACCF/AHA/ACP/AATS/PCNA/SCAI/STS guideline for the diagnosis and management of patients with stable ischemic heart disease: A report of the American College of Cardiology Foundation/American Heart Association Task Force on Practice Guidelines, and the American College of Physicians, American Association for Thoracic Surgery, Preventive Cardiovascular Nurses Association, Society for Cardiovascular Angiography and Interventions, and Society of Thoracic Surgeons. Journal of the American College of Cardiology. 2012;**60**:e44-e164

[12] Tzivoni D, Klein J. Improvement of myocardial ischaemia by lipid lowering drugs. European Heart Journal. 1998;**19**:230-234

[13] Yusuf S, Pitt B, Davis CE, et al. Effect of enalapril on survival in patients with reduced left ventricular ejection fraction and congestive heart failure. The New England Journal of Medicine. 1991;**325**:293-302

[14] Pfeffer MA, Braunwald E, Moye LA, et al. Effect of captopril on mortality and morbidity in patients with left ventricular dysfunction after myocardial infarction. The New England Journal of Medicine. 1992;**527**:669-677

[15] Juul-Moller S, Edvardson N, Jahnmatz B, et al. Double blind trial of aspirin in primary prevention of myocardial infarction in patients with stable chronic angina pectoris. Lancet. 1992;**340**:1421-1425

[16] Food and Drug Administration. Acetylsalicylic acid and the heart. JAMA. 1993;**270**:2669

[17] Bhatt DL, Fox KA, Hacke W, et al. Clopidogrel and aspirin versus aspirin alone for the prevention of atherothrombotic events. The New England Journal of Medicine. 2006;**354**:1706-1717

[18] Levine GN. Color Atlas of Cardiovascular Disease. New Delhi, India: Jaypee Brothers Medical Publishers; 2014

[19] European Coronary Surgery Study Group. Long-term results of prospective randomized study of coronary artery bypass surgery in stable angina pectoris. European Coronary Surgery Study Group. Lancet. 1982;**2**:1173-1180

[20] The Veterans Administration Coronary Artery Bypass Surgery Cooperative Study Group. Eleven-year survival in the Veterans Administration randomized trial of coronary bypass surgery for stable angina. The New England Journal of Medicine. 1984;**311**:1333-1339

[21] Killip T, Passamani E, Davis K. Coronary artery surgery study (CASS): A randomized trial of coronary bypass surgery. Circulation. 1985;**72**:V102-V109

3

Coronary Artery Bypass Grafting in Patients with Diabetes Mellitus: A Cardiologist's View

Bezdenezhnykh Natalia Alexandrovna,
Sumin Alexei Nikolaevich,
Bezdenezhnykh Andrey Viktorovich and
Barbarash Olga Leonidovna

Abstract

The review presents current data on the prevalence of diabetes in the cohort of patients undergoing coronary artery bypass grafting. The relevance of active approach to the identification of diabetes and prediabetes in patients with coronary artery disease (CAD) before coronary revascularization is reviewed. Recent information about the negative impact of diabetes on the prognosis of myocardial revascularization is reported as well as the main mechanisms responsible to the development of adverse outcomes of interventions in these patients. Target perioperative values of glycemia recommended by the leading associations of the study of diabetes have been compared. Beneficial potential of other carbohydrate metabolism markers (glycated hemoglobin, fructosamine, 1,5-anhydroglucitol) in patients with diabetes mellitus (DM) in terms of their impact on cardiovascular prognosis, including coronary intervention. The results of studies comparing different management strategies for these patients are reviewed. The significance of carbohydrate metabolism compensation during myocardial revascularization is reported; thus, a too stringent glycemic control has no benefits neither for percutaneous nor for open coronary intervention. Recent trials suggest the groups of antidiabetic drugs and evidence of their impact on the cardiovascular system. The importance of comprehensive monitoring of major risk factors in diabetic patients with coronary intervention has been proved.

Keywords: diabetes mellitus, prediabetes, early diagnosis of diabetes, ischemic heart disease, coronary artery bypass surgery, percutaneous coronary intervention, myocardial revascularization, target levels of glycemic control, glycated hemoglobin, perioperative antihyperglycemic therapy, perioperative management

1. Introduction

Diabetes mellitus (DM) is one of the most common comorbid conditions in patients with coronary artery disease (CAD), which is important in determining the severity of the disease, treatment strategy, and the prognosis of patients [1].

The increasing prevalence of diabetes has led to a situation where over 380 million people had diabetes mellitus globally in 2013, of whom 99% suffered from type 2 diabetes [2]. According to the population statistics, the number of people present with diabetes is increasing annually. By 2030, this number is expected to rise to more than 550 million people with diabetes and up to 300 million people with prediabetes [2]. This dramatic rise is fuelled mainly by the aging of the population and continuing changes in eating habits and lifestyle with predominant sedentary behavior. In 2014, an estimated 4.9 million deaths were caused by diabetes, of which 60% had the underlying cardiovascular diseases (CVDs) [2].

Therefore, teamwork of cardiologists and endocrinologists is needed to optimally manage diabetes. The efforts of cardiology and diabetes communities have been recently targeted at developing joint guidelines and statements on diabetes management. All current guidelines on management of patients with stable and acute CAD, including guidelines on myocardial revascularization, contain a separate section on diabetes mellitus [3–6], whereas, the guidelines of the International Diabetes Federation, Canadian and American Diabetes Association devote separate sections on cardiovascular diseases (CVD) [7–10]. In 2013, the European Society of Cardiology developed the guidelines on diabetes, prediabetes, and cardiovascular diseases in collaboration with the European Association for the Study of Diabetes [11]. According to the updated guidelines, the search for approaches to optimize the negative impact of diabetes on the results of surgical management remains relevant and includes the study of optimal targets for carbohydrate metabolism, the improvements in the preoperative and perioperative management strategies [7–10]. This review covers the known and insufficiently studied issues of treating patients with diabetes mellitus undergoing myocardial revascularization from the perspective of evidence-based medicine.

2. Prevalence of diabetes in coronary revascularization

The management of CAD patients with concomitant diabetes who need myocardial revascularization is a great challenge. Recent studies demonstrated that a large proportion of CAD patients are present with diabetes [12–15]. The prevalence of diabetes among patients who have undergone percutaneous coronary intervention (PCI) varies greatly from 25 to 30%, according to the DES LATE, ISAR SAFE, RESET, SECURITY trials up to 35–39% in the EXCELLENT, OPTIMIZE, ITALIC, ARCTIC-Interruption trials, and CathPCI Registry [12–14]. The proportion of diabetic patients suffering from CAD undergoing coronary artery bypass grafting accounts for 22–48% of cases [16–20]. In a large Swedish Registry, comprising of 39,235 patients undergoing isolated CABG, 22.8% of patients had diabetes mellitus [18]. The prevalence of diabetes among patients undergoing coronary artery bypass grafting (CABG) is 20–23% according to the results of the Russian studies [20, 21], whereas the US CABG registry suggested the diabetes prevalence to be of 46.9% [19]. A recent Japanese study reported that the proportion of patients with diabetes undergoing direct myocardial revascularization reaches 48% [16].

Differences in diabetes prevalence rates are mainly caused by different diagnostic approaches and racial/ethnic disparities. A large-scale multi-ethnic registry study CREDO-Kyoto comprised 15,580 patients undergoing either CABG or PCI [29]. The lowest rate of diabetes was found in the Caucasian group, whereas the highest ones in the African Americans and the Hispanic group (26.9 vs. 44 vs. 49.5%, respectively). The prevalence rate in the Japanese group was 39% [29].

In addition, several studies confirmed a steady increase in the proportion of diabetic patients undergoing coronary revascularization. In the period from 1999 to 2008, in the Chinese cohort of patients who have undergone CABG, the proportion of diabetic patients increased from 20 to 32% [17], whereas in the American—from 26 to 46% [19]. Moreover, a recent study demonstrated that the rate of diabetes increased by 32% among the patients undergoing CABG [22].

3. Early diagnosis of diabetes in CAD patients undergoing myocardial revascularization

The sharp increase in the prevalence of diabetes among interventional cardiology and cardiac surgery patients is caused by the aging of the population, expanding clinical indications for myocardial revascularization, and recent advances in diagnostic strategies for diabetes and other glycemic disorders [11]. The leading medical associations and communities use the same cut-offs to establish the diagnosis of diabetes mellitus: a fasting plasma glucose concentration ≥ 7.0 and/or 11.1 mmol/l after postglucose load and meal, and/or glycated hemoglobin (HbA1c) >6.5% [7, 8, 10]. However, there are some differences in diagnostic criteria for prediabetes based on fasting glucose and HbA1c. According to the American Diabetes Association (ADA), prediabetes is diagnosed if one or more of the following criteria are met: glycemia of 5.6 mmol/l or HbA1c of 5.7%; whereas the World Health Organization (WHO) implements the following criteria: glucose level of 6.1 mmol/l, or glycated hemoglobin of 6.0% [7, 10].

More rigorous approaches to the diagnosis of carbohydrate metabolism disorders are evident. Type 2 diabetes develops after a long period of euglycemia, but with the existing insulin resistance, which gradually turns into a deficit of beta cells with severe hyperglycemia. The development of CVD in individuals with insulin resistance is a long progressive process. When patients develop hyperglycemia and diagnose type 2 diabetes, 60% of them already have CVD [11, 23, 24].

The guidelines of the American Diabetes Association recommend to assess the glycemic state in adults of any age who are overweight or obese and who have one or more additional risk factors for diabetes (including cardiovascular diseases) and in all people aged >45 years [10]. The European Society of Cardiology and the European Association for the Study of Diabetes recommend if HbA1c and/or fasting plasma glucose (FPG) are inconclusive in individuals with CAD, no diabetes risk score is needed, but an oral glucose tolerance test (OGTT) is indicated [11]. Thus, all patients without previously diagnosed diabetes referred to elective coronary artery bypass grafting should be screened for diabetes or prediabetes.

The rationale for detecting disorders of carbohydrate metabolism has been demonstrated in several studies in patients with CAD, including those undergoing myocardial revascularization. Over 50% of myocardial infarction (MI) patients without known disorders of carbohydrate metabolism had positive OGTT in the in-hospital period [25].

The Spanish trial reported a high prevalence of diabetes up to 45% in patients undergoing PCI, based on continuous OGTT and glycated hemoglobin measurement. Importantly, a third of patients with positive testing were patients who had newly detected diabetes [26]. In their series, 28.8% had known diabetes, 16.2% newly detected diabetes, 25.5% prediabetes, and 29.5% were normoglycemics [26].

Balakrishnan et al. reported 39% of patients with diabetes out of 740 patients admitted to the hospital for PCI. Periprocedural measurement of glycated hemoglobin in patients without known disorders of glucose metabolism allowed to diagnose diabetes and prediabetes in 8.3 and 58.5% of patients, respectively [27].

A prospective Swedish study assessing the prevalence and prognostic impact of the different states of abnormal glucose regulation (AGR) after CABG reported the prevalence of known diabetes of 29.5% [28]. Out of the rest, 11.4% of patients had newly diagnosed diabetes based on oral glucose tolerance test. Thus, the proportion of patients with diabetes increased up to 41%. Another 24% of patients had prediabetes according to the postglucose load. A total of 65% of patients had disorders of carbohydrate metabolism [28].

Why do physicians need to perform active screening for undiagnosed diabetes in patients undergoing cardiac surgeries, and is there any rationale for it? Undiagnosed diabetes may affect the prognosis in this group of patients, similarly to previously diagnosed diabetes [25, 28, 29].

In the EARLY ACS trial of 8795 patients with non-ST-segment elevation ACS, newly diagnosed diabetes was a predictor of 30-day mortality or myocardial infarction [odds ratio (OR) 1.65; confidence interval (CI) 95%; 1.09–2.48] [29]. Previously diagnosed diabetes correlated with a 30-day mortality rate, but not with the MI rate [29].

Similarly, to known disorders of carbohydrate metabolism, newly diagnosed disorders affect the in-hospital and long-term prognosis of patients with myocardial infarction [25]. There was a successive increase in the risk of unfavorable cardiovascular events in the long-term period from normoglycemia through prediabetes to diabetes [28].

4. Benefits of coronary artery bypass grafting over percutaneous coronary intervention and medical therapy in diabetic patients with multivessel coronary artery disease

A sufficient number of studies aimed at choosing an optimal method for myocardial revascularization in patients with diabetes have been performed [30–37]. A large BARI-2D trial focused at assessing myocardial revascularization in patients with diabetes with stable coronary artery disease [30, 31]. Patients selected for the CABG stratum had more extensive coronary artery disease. Nevertheless, the rate of major cardiovascular events was significantly lower in the revascularization group, compared with the medical therapy group [30, 31].

The revascularization group patients demonstrated fewer cases of angina progression (8 vs. 13%, respectively, p < 0.001), recurrent angina (37 vs. 51%, respectively, p < 0.001), and subsequent coronary revascularization, compared to the intensive medical management group (18 vs. 33%, respectively, p < 0.001) [31]. The revascularization group patients exhibited a trend toward being angina-free at 3-year follow-up than the intensive medical management group (66 vs. 58%, respectively, p < 0.003). The superiority of revascularization strategy over medical therapy is believed to be caused by preferring CABG over PCI in patients with more severe coronary artery disease [31].

The FREEDOM (future revascularization evaluation in patients with diabetes mellitus) study is a single, well-powered, randomized trial, comparing CABG and PCI with first-generation drug-eluting stent (DES) (94%) in diabetic patients undergoing elective revascularization for multivessel coronary disease without left main coronary artery stenosis [33]. The rate of the primary outcome was lower in the CABG group than in the PCI group, with divergence of the curves starting at 2 years. This difference was due to a relative reduction in death from any cause (p = 0.049) and a significantly lower incidence of MI in the CABG group (p < 0.001) [33].

A review of 13 RCTs and 5 meta-analyses agreed that CABG surgery should be recommended in patients with diabetes and multivessel CAD, regardless of the severity of coronary anatomy: CABG improved the long-term prognosis. Thus, the 5-year risk of major cardiovascular events was 18.7% in the CABG group vs. 26.6% in the PCI group, p = 0.005) [34].

A recent meta-analysis of six RCTs showed similar results, confirming the benefits of direct revascularization over PCI in patients with diabetes. CABG was associated with a significantly lower mortality, compared with PCI (RR: 0.59, 95% CI 0.42–0.85; p = 0.004). The rates of major cardiovascular and cerebrovascular events, as well as repeat revascularization, were significantly lower in the CABG group (OR 0.51, 95% CI 0.27–0.99, p = 0.03 vs. OR 0.34, 95% CI 0.24–0.49; p < 0.00001, respectively) [35].

Since available data suggesting beneficial effects of myocardial revascularization in patients with diabetes were obtained in the period of advancements in pharmacotherapy and technology of both PCI and surgical revascularization, it is difficult to compare them directly. Nevertheless, many studies have shown that CABG appears to be a better option compared to PCI with DES in diabetic patients, particularly, if the patient has multivessel CAD [33–37]. The superiority of coronary artery bypass grafting over percutaneous coronary intervention in diabetic patients with multivessel coronary disease is currently stated in the international guidelines with the class of recommendation IA [5].

5. Diabetes mellitus and outcomes of myocardial revascularization

Although diabetic patients constitute an increasing number of individuals undergoing PCI and surgical revascularization, they have worse outcomes, than non-diabetic patients [14,

37–39]. The meta-analysis of several randomized clinical trials of coronary angioplasty using bare-metal stents has proved diabetes to be the strongest predictor of restenosis, with a high risk of repeat revascularization of the target lesion [37]. In multivariable analyses of 6081 patients undergoing PCI with the implantation of DES, diabetic vs. non-diabetic patients had higher risks of major adverse cardiac events (odds ratio (OR), 1.25; 95% confidence interval (CI), 1.03–1.53; $p = 0.026$), but similar risks of cardiac death (OR, 1.41; 95% CI, 0.96–2.07; $p = 0.08$) and myocardial infarction (OR, 0.89; 95% CI, 0.64–1.22; $p = 0.45$) [38].

The two major causes of stent failure are stent thrombosis and in-stent restenosis. The incidence of both has reduced considerably in recent years [14]. Current clinical registries and randomized trials with broad inclusion criteria show rates of stent thrombosis at or <1% after 1 year; rates of clinical in-stent restenosis are 5%, respectively [12–14]. Angiographic surveillance studies in large cohorts show rates of angiographic in-stent restenosis of ~10% with new-generation DES [14]. However, the contribution of diabetes to the development of restenosis remains significant. One of the largest analysis, comprising of 10,004 patients with completed angiographic follow-up after PCI found that diabetes mellitus was an independent predictor of restenosis (OR 1.32, 95% CI 1.19–1.46), as well as previous CABG, complex lesion morphology, smaller vessel reference diameter before the procedure, and greater stented length of the vessel [14]. Angiographic follow-up of 123 patients after PCI demonstrated that DM was associated with a 3-fold increased risk of plaque neovascularization. Importantly, more than half of the patients (56.5%) failed to reach the target range of glycated hemoglobin [40].

There is a strong association between diabetes and high rates of complications after CABG. Despite the fact that in-hospital mortality rates among diabetic patients significantly decreased from 3% in the period 1998–2002 to 1.3% in the period 2003–2005 [35], postoperative complication rates remain high. Thus, a retrospective analysis, comprising 667 CAD patients, who have undergone CABG, showed that diabetes did not affect in-hospital mortality, but was an independent predictor of sternal wound infection [41]. Similar findings were obtained in another retrospective study, suggesting the absence of any correlations between diabetes and the risk of cardiovascular complications and mortality. However, the obtained findings revealed a significant association between diabetes and renal complication after CABG [42]. Diabetic patients have poor immediate outcomes after CABG and unfavorable long-term prognosis, compared to non-diabetic patients. Moreover, patients with diabetes had higher rates of the hospitalization and major cardiovascular events [18, 28, 43]. A recent Russian study with the 5-year follow-up period reported that 14.2% of patients with diabetes had one of the major cardiovascular events (myocardial infarction, stroke, or cardiovascular death) vs. 6.3% patients without diabetes ($p = 0.028$) [39]. Despite new insights into pathophysiology of diabetes and recent improvements in the perioperative management, DM remains a challenging issue for coronary procedures and interventions.

6. Diabetes-specific risk factors for adverse prognosis in coronary procedures and interventions

Adverse prognosis in this group of patients is partially explained by initial characteristics of diabetic patients referred to elective revascularization. These patients commonly have higher perioperative risk due to advanced age, obesity, female gender, previous cardiovascular events and revascularization procedures, multivessel coronary disease, severe heart failure, chronic kidney disease, and chronic obstructive pulmonary disease. These conditions are known to independently affect the prognosis of patients with CAD [5, 23]. In addition, diabetic patients are more likely to have multivessel coronary disease, diffuse coronary lesions, poor distal vascular bed, and calcification [5].

However, there are diabetes-specific factors, namely hyperglycemia, insulin resistance, and hyperinsulinemia, which cause a cascade of pathogenetic reactions [44]. Thus, diabetic patients have more intense intravascular inflammation than non-diabetic ones. Excess pro-inflammatory cytokines and other biologically active substances lead to the destabilization of an atherosclerotic plaque, the progression of coronary atherosclerosis to unaffected segments of the vascular wall [44, 45]. Moreover, the analysis reported a diminished numerical density of mast cells and a significantly higher volume density of the mononuclear cells [46]. Hyperglycemia can lead to the development of endothelial dysfunction, associated with reduced nitric oxide, a key signaling regulator of vascular tone, and increased oxidative stress. In addition, acute hyperglycemia worsens insulin activity in endothelial cells even at physiologically adequate levels [23].

A prospective study, comprising of 1035 patients with myocardial infarction, who have undergone primary PCI in one of the Chinese hospitals, found a relationship between acute hyperglycemia at the time of admission and poor short- and long-term prognosis [47]. Pre- and postoperative hyperglycemia is the main risk factor for developing infectious complications after CABG in both diabetic and non-diabetic patients [41]. Hyperglycemia is associated with impaired leukocyte function, including diminished chemotaxis, decreased phagocytosis, impaired bacterial killing, and abnormal adhesive properties [44]. Diabetic patients showed higher endothelial activation and lower antiinflammatory response to CPB compared to non-diabetics [46]. Chronic hyperglycemia can lead to the central nervous system injury, resulting in diabetic encephalopathy with the onset of mild and moderate cognitive disorders [48]. Bruce et al. found that 64% of diabetic patients with coronary artery disease had cognitive or emotional disorders [49].

In addition, diabetes mellitus is a predictor of increased aggregation potential. SP-selectin, intercellular adhesion molecules, and platelet aggregation were significantly higher in diabetic patients, than in non-diabetics [44]. Despite receiving the same dose of aspirin and clopidogrel, patients with diabetes had higher values of platelet reactivity according to the findings of the recent study evaluating the effects of double antiplatelet therapy in diabetic patients with stable coronary artery disease [46]. Periprocedural control of glycemia in patients undergoing coronary interventions is pivotal for both endocrinologists and cardiologists. The current guidelines of the Canadian Diabetes Association (CDA) state that patients with diabetes do not receive the necessary glycemic control when they are admitted to non-profile hospitals [8].

7. Perioperative target glycemic range for myocardial revascularization and the risk of hypoglycemia

The current national guidelines, based on evidence-based medicine, have regulated the perioperative target range of glycemia [7–10]. The target range of glycemia for the majority of ICU patients, defined by the International Diabetes Federation, the American and Canadian Diabetes Associations, are the following: 140–180 mg/dL without hypoglycemia and 80–180 mg/dL for the perioperative period [8, 10].

All guidelines strictly recommend to avoid hypoglycemia. The risk of developing hypoglycemia inevitably increases with the attempts to achieve compensation for carbohydrate metabolism. Therefore, many studies, suggesting beneficial effects of perioperative glucose control, did not confirm their hypothesis [50–53]. A tighter control did not show its superiority neither for the immediate outcomes after CABG [50, 51], nor for the long-term outcomes [52]. Intensive insulin therapy with the achievement of perioperative target glucose levels of 100–140 (5.5–7.7 mmol/l) after CABG does not significantly reduce the number of postoperative complications, compared with the target glucose level of 140–170 (7.8–9.2 mmol/l) [51, 53].

A scientific statement from the American Diabetes Association and the American Heart Association Society suggests that severe hypoglycemia is the most likely cause of increased cardiovascular mortality in diabetic patients with intensive control of glycemia [54]. Unfortunately, hypoglycemia is more likely to happen when blood glucose decrease up to physiological values.

Hypoglycemia commonly develops with intensive insulin therapy, and is a well-known risk factor for MI, stroke, and death from any causes [53]. The relative risk for developing MI, associated with severe hypoglycemia 1 year before the index event, was 12%, 5.5 months before MI—20%, and 2 weeks before—65% [55].

Hypoglycemia triggers a powerful stimulation of the autonomic nervous system and the excess release of catecholamines, which promote vasospasm, tachycardia, arterial hypertension, and increased blood viscosity and coagulation [56]. These processes may cause changes in the regional blood flow and provoke myocardial or cerebral ischemia, resulting in myocardial infarction, heart failure, or stroke. Unfortunately, similar to fatal events, it is very difficult to demonstrate any relationship between severe hypoglycemia and serious vascular events, since clinical evidence of the impact of hypoglycemia are mainly random [55]. Death caused by hypoglycemia can be mistaken for death from acute coronary syndrome, because no one measures glycemia before. There are no anatomical and morphological postmortem signs of hypoglycemia [55, 56].

Withholding glucose in the target range without hypoglycemia and its impact on the prognosis are highly relevant issues for further research, as well as the use of integrated glucose metabolism indicators, such as glycated hemoglobin, which may improve the comprehensive risk assessment of surgical intervention.

8. Glycated hemoglobin and outcomes of coronary procedures and interventions

Glycated hemoglobin (HbA1c) is used for monitoring blood glucose levels in diabetic patients; it should be measured in all diabetic patients once in 3 months, and before any surgical interventions, including coronary revascularization. A systematic review of 11 studies addressing the relationship between glycated hemoglobin levels and the results of CABG in diabetic and non-diabetic patients was performed [57]. Four studies found significant increase in early and late mortality at higher HbA1c levels, regardless of a preoperative diagnosis of diabetes. In particular, the mortality risk for CABG is quadrupled at HbA1c levels >8.6% [57]. However, four studies of early mortality outcomes in diabetic patients only showed no significant differences between patients with normal and those with deranged HbA1c levels (p = 0.99). Three studies identified a significant increase in infectious complications in patients with poorly controlled HbA1c: superficial sternal wound infection (p = 0.014 and 0.007, respectively) and minor infections (p = 0.006) [57].

Unexpected data were obtained in one of the Japanese surgical clinics. Elevated HbA1c was associated with a lower incidence of arrhythmias after CABG. The incidence of postoperative atrial fibrillation was 28.3% in the lower tertile, 17.4% in the middle tertile, and 12.5% in the upper tertile [58]. Thus, the mean and high levels of glycated hemoglobin were associated with a lower incidence of atrial arrhythmias. One possible explanation is that patients with elevated HbA1c require more insulin, which has been reported to reduce the risk of postoperative atrial fibrillation [58]. Similar results were obtained in the recent American study. The incidence of atrial fibrillation after CABG was 20.9% in patients with HbA1c < 7.0% and 15.1% in patients with HbA1c ≥ 7.0% (p = 0.007), adjusted OR 0.73; 95% CI 0.55–0.96 [57]. However, elevated HbA1c was associated with higher rates of postoperative stroke, renal failure, and deep wound infection [57].

Some studies have called into question the predictive potential of HbA1c for short-term outcomes in well-controlled diabetics. However, poor control and elevated HbA1c may result in high rate of adverse events in the short- and long-term postoperative periods [57, 59].

Maintaining a level of glycemia close to the physiological level is an achievable goal of hypoglycemic therapy in type 2 diabetes. Its significance is evident and is associated with the risk of developing specific chronic complications induced by hyperglycemia. However, appropriate glycemic control with glucose levels closer to normal is associated with a high risk of hypoglycemia, which is known to affect the prognosis in diabetic patients with CVD [56]. Therefore, the search and development of optimal and safe tools to manage high glucose levels are pivotal for modern medical research.

9. The degree of compensation of carbohydrate metabolism and long-term prognosis in patients with diabetes and coronary artery disease

The UKPDS study was the first one to demonstrate the significance of the compensation of carbohydrate metabolism for the progression of complications [60]. The obtained results stimulated other researches in this area addressed to the assessment of the control intensity in patients with CVD, but the obtained data did not show the superiority of the tight strategy [61–63].

Three major studies (ACCORD, ADVANCE, and VADT) evaluated the impact of attaining euglycemia (ACCORD) or near-euglycemia (ADVANCE, VADT) in older patients with diabetes and high cardiovascular risk [61–63]. None of these studies, either individually or on pooled analysis, demonstrated any reduction in cardiovascular or all-cause mortality with tight glucose control [60]. A higher mortality was observed in the intensive glucose control arm of ACCORD, resulting in the premature termination of the glucose-lowering component of this study. Also, the occurrence of hypoglycemic episodes (total and major) was significantly higher in the intensive glucose control arms of all three studies [60].

The Diabetes Control and Complications Trial (DCCT) and the Epidemiology of Diabetes Interventions and Complications (EDIC) study, DCCT's long-term follow-up study, were aimed at assessing the rate of micro- and macrovascular complications in diabetic patients and their relationships with hypoglycemic therapy. In the DCCT study, the incidence of cardiovascular events was not significantly associated with intensive insulin therapy. 93% of the original cohort of the DCCT study agreed to join the EDIC study with an 11-year follow-up period. The obtained results proved that intensive treatment was associated with reduced risk of any cardiovascular events by 42% during the 17-year follow-up ($p < 0.01$). Thus, DCCT (EDIC), and UKPDS showed that glycemic control in diabetic patients is important for the prevention of microvascular complications, but long-term follow-up is needed to demonstrate these effects [11].

In 2015, the American Diabetes Association and The European Association for the Study of Diabetes updated the positioned statement on the management of hyperglycemia of 2012, suggesting the need for strengthening the patient-centered approach to the management of diabetic patients [64]. They highlighted the necessity to individualize the range for glycemic control. They recommend to use the HbA1c range of 7.5–8% for elderly patients with diabetes and patients with a positive history of cardiovascular events, depending on their life expectancy, age, and social status [64]. A more tight target range (HbA1c 6.5–7.0%) may be used in patients with slow-onset diabetes, long life expectancy, and those without significant cardiovascular disease (CVD), if it can be achieved without hypoglycemia [64].

What tools may be used to control glycemia in patients undergoing myocardial revascularization?

10. Hypoglycemic therapy in patients undergoing myocardial revascularization—the lack of evidence

A number of new classes of drugs for the treatment of diabetes and their effects on cardiovascular system have been studied well. However, there are limited data regarding in-hospital hypoglycemic therapy in patients undergoing myocardial revascularization. The concerns of medical community on this issue may be found directly in the headlines of recently published manuscripts. Hoogwerf addressed this issue in his article entitled "Perioperative management of diabetes mellitus: how should we act on the limited evidence?" [65]. Despite the fact that this article was published 10 years ago, and during this period new knowledge and evidence have been obtained, the question regarding optimal medical management of glycemia in patients undergoing coronary revascularization remains crucial. Recent guidelines on the management of diabetes [7–10] state the lack of evidence for using non-insulin hypoglycemic drugs in the perioperative period in diabetic patients.

Insulin remains the only approved perioperative method of hypoglycemic therapy. The current guidelines recommend use of basal insulin or basal-bolus regimen, and strongly discourage use of sliding-scale while a sliding schedule is strongly discouraged [8, 10].

Continuous intravenous insulin infusion is recognized as the preferred method for achieving and maintaining the glycemic control in critically ill patients [8–10]. The protocols for insulin infusion have been already developed and approved by diabetic communities [8–10]. They allow to adjust the rate of insulin infusion according to the glycemic levels. Insulin therapy should be initiated to treat persistent hyperglycemia, starting at a threshold of 180 mg/dL (10 mmol/L). Episodes of hypoglycemia should be noted in medical records and strictly monitored, since glucose level of 70 mg/dL require the changing of treatment regimen [8–10].

The multicenter DIGAMI, DIGAMI 2, HI-5 trials studied the intensity of the glucose control in ACS patients, including those undergoing PCI. Initially, DIGAMI reported low mortality in MI patients enrolled in the insulin therapy group [66]. However, the follow-up DIGAMI 2 trial with a double sample size and a more careful design did not show any advantages in the group of patients receiving intensive insulin therapy. Moreover, there were no significant differences in the rate of the composite endpoint (cardiovascular death/nonfatal myocardial infarction/stroke) between the intensive control group and the standard therapy group. The HI-5 study received similar results [66]. Since neither the DIGAMI 2, nor the HI-5 achieved differences in the control of glucose between the intensive management group and the control group, the effectiveness of insulin therapy for lowering glucose levels in ACS patients remains controversial. Combined data from these three studies confirmed that glucose-insulin-potassium infusion did not reduce mortality without the glucose control in diabetic patients with ACS (OR 1.07, 95% CI 0.85–1.36, p = 0.547) [66]. None of the protocols noted the improvements of the outcomes in patients with ST-segment elevation ACS after PCI, who received insulin or the intravenous glucose-insulin-potassium infusions [66].

The Japanese study, comprising 2148 patients who underwent PCI in the period from 2003 to 2012, showed an association between insulin use and increased rates of myocardial infarction and stent thrombosis [67]. The subgroup analysis of the FREEDOM trial, aimed at assessing outcomes of diabetic patients undergoing either CABG or PCI, reported that patients receiving insulin had a higher rate of major cardiovascular events [68]. Nevertheless, the use of insulin may be regarded as a marker of the severity and duration of diabetes, and does not reflect the true effects of therapy on the outcomes.

Currently, the discontinuation of long-acting drugs before surgical procedures is preferable, but there is no consensus on PCI, since the management of patients is commonly regulated by the local protocol [69]. There are available data suggesting safe and beneficial effects of long-acting oral hypoglycemic agents in PCI patients, resulting in better glycemic control and lower platelet activity [66].

The American and Canadian Diabetes Associations recommend to withhold metformin 24–48 h prior to CAG or PCI, and restart it 48 h after the procedure in the absence of significantly decreased GFR or later after the normalization of renal function [8, 10]. Although, recent studies showed the safety of continuing metformin therapy during the procedure, their statistical capacity is insufficient to change the current guidelines [10, 70, 71].

The recent study of patients with metabolic syndrome who received metformin for 7 days before PCI vs. the placebo group reported a lower rate of perioperative myocardial damage, estimated by elevated creatine phosphokinase-MB (p = 0.008) and troponin I (p = 0.005). According to the assessment of the 1-year prognosis, the incidence of major cardiovascular events (heart attack/stroke/cardiovascular death) was significantly lower in the metformin group (7.9 and 28.9%, respectively, p = 0.001) [72].

A randomized trial of 100 patients who received either 1000 mg of metformin or placebo after CABG in addition to standard insulin therapy, the metformin therapy was initiated 3 h after extubation and lasted for 3 days [70]. Based on the results, the mean dose of insulin, as well as the mean number of episodes of both hyper- and hypoglycemia, were significantly lower in the metformin group (p < 0.05). At the same time, the risk of acidosis in the metformin group did not increase [70].

There were some attempts to use metformin in non-diabetic patients undergoing coronary artery bypass grafting. The researchers concluded that the short-term use of metformin prior to CABG was relatively safe, but ineffective strategy for reducing periprocedural myocardial damage in non-diabetic patients [71].

The updated ADA 2017 guidelines noted that the SGLT2 inhibitors, despite their proven cardiovascular effects, cannot yet be recommended for the hospital use, and, therefore, should be avoided before surgical interventions [10].

11. Comprehensive risk factor control in diabetic patients in coronary procedures and interventions

In addition to the compensation of carbohydrate metabolism, multiple monitoring of risk factors in diabetic patients undergoing revascularization should be implemented and include achieving target levels of blood pressure (BP) and lipids, smoking cessation. The BARI-2D trial, focused at assessing coronary revascularization in diabetic patients, reported that both, the tight control over the main risk factors and intensive treatment management in diabetic patients according to the current guidelines, were associated with improved cardiovascular outcomes [23]. Based on the results of the study with a 20-year follow-up after CABG, long-term survival, and freedom from major cardiovascular events in diabetic patients followed CABG was lower. However, the monitoring of carbohydrate metabolism and other risk factors (target levels of lipids and arterial blood pressure, smoking cessation) appears to be significant for the prognosis in this group of patients [43]. Despite the improvements in achieving the goals of treatment for diabetes, it requires further control and monitoring, as only 14.3% of adult Americans with type 2 diabetes have target levels of HbA1c, blood pressure, and low-density lipoprotein cholesterol (LDL-C) [73].

To date, the evidence-based results of randomized clinical trials suggest that statin therapy reduces the incidence of cardiovascular events in diabetic patients [74, 75]. The protective cardiovascular effects of statins significantly outweigh the associated risk of developing diabetes mellitus [75]. The recent joint guidelines of the American Society of Cardiology and the Heart Association recognize diabetic patients aged 40–75 years as one of the four main groups of patients who would most likely benefit from statin therapy [23]. The guidelines of the American and European Society of Cardiologists recommend to initiate statin therapy in all patients who had myocardial infarction, regardless of the cholesterol level [76]. However, there are several studies reporting that low levels of low-density lipoprotein cholesterol (LDL cholesterol), regardless of hypolipidemic therapy, are associated with increased in-hospital mortality in ACS patients, including those undergoing PCI. The results of a study, comprising of 9032 patients with myocardial infarction who underwent primary PCI in 68 centers in Tokyo, convincingly showed that statin therapy significantly reduced in-hospital mortality, even in patients with low LDL cholesterol and those with diabetes [77].

A large retrospective analysis, including 16,192 patients undergoing CABG, demonstrated that the use of statins, regardless of diabetes and other risk factors, was associated with a significant reduction of in-hospital mortality in five logistic regression models [78]. Importantly, angiotensin-converting enzyme (ACE) inhibitors, beta-blockers, and calcium antagonists did not show any significant correlations with the outcomes followed CABG [78]. However, there are available data on beneficial effects of statins on reducing the incidence of atrial fibrillation and cognitive impairment after CABG, including patients with diabetes mellitus [48, 78].

Undoubtedly, patients with diabetes, undergoing revascularization, need to achieve the target levels of systolic blood pressure < 140 mm Hg and diastolic blood pressure < 90 mm Hg. These target levels are required to reduce cardiovascular risk according to the recent statement of the American Heart Association and American Diabetics Association. Moreover, the AHA/ADA guidelines recommend to use ACE inhibitors and angiotensin II receptor antagonists for treating arterial hypertension in diabetic patients [54].

Thus, we may conclude that the negative impact of diabetes on the prognosis after myocardial revascularization and the need to achieve the target ranges of carbohydrate metabolism, as well as the comprehensive cardiovascular control are evident in treating diabetic patients. However, the benefits of the intensive glycemic management remain controversial. Other treatment strategies, such as continuing prescribed hypoglycemic drugs, including long-acting ones, should be considered only in patients undergoing PCI, but not in those who are referred to elective open-heart surgeries. Currently, the issues that require further research have been highlighted in our review and, in a few years, new clinical trials will provide new insights for medical community dealing with diabetes and coronary artery diseases.

Author details

Bezdenezhnykh Natalia Alexandrovna[1]*, Sumin Alexei Nikolaevich[1],
Bezdenezhnykh Andrey Viktorovich[1] and Barbarash Olga Leonidovna[1,2]

*Address all correspondence to: n_bez@mail.ru

1 Federal State Budgetary Institution, Research Institute for Complex Issues of Cardiovascular Diseases, Kemerovo, Russian Federation

2 Federal State Budgetary Institution of Higher Professional Education, Kemerovo State Medical Institution, Kemerovo, Russian Federation

References

[1] Inohara T, Kohsaka S, Goto M, et al. Hypothesis of long-term outcome after coronary revascularization in Japanese patients compared to multiethnic groups in the US. PLoS One. 2015;**10**(5):e0128252. DOI: 10.1371/journal.pone.0128252

[2] Guariguata L, Whiting DR, Hambleton I, et al. Global estimates of diabetes prevalence for 2013 and projections for 2035. Diabetes Research and Clinical Practice. 2014;**103**:137-149

[3] Task Force Members, Montalescot G, Sechtem U, Achenbach S, et al. 2013 ESC guidelines on the management of stable coronary artery disease. European Heart Journal. 2013;**34**:2949-3003. DOI: 10.1093/eurheartj/eht296

[4] Task Force on the management of ST-segment elevation acute myocardial infarction of the European Society of Cardiology (ESC), Steg PG, James SK, Atar D, et al. ESC Guidelines for the management of acute myocardial infarction in patients presenting with ST-segment elevation. European Heart Journal. 2012;**33**:2569-2619. DOI: 10.1093/eurheartj/ehs215

[5] Authors/Task Force members, Windecker S, Kolh P, Alfonso F, et al. Guidelines on myocardial revascularization: The task force on myocardial revascularization of the European Society of Cardiology (ESC) and the European Association for Cardio-Thoracic Surgery (EACTS) developed with the special contribution of the European Association of Percutaneous Cardiovascular Interventions (EAPCI). European Heart Journal. 2014;**35**:2541-2619

[6] Patel MR, Calhoon JH, Dehmer GJ, Grantham JA, Maddox TM, Maron DJ, Smith PK. ACC/AATS/AHA/ASE/ASNC/SCAI/SCCT/STS 2017 appropriate use criteria for coronary revascularization in patients with stable ischemic heart disease. Coronary Revascularization Writing Group. Journal of the American College of Cardiology. 2017;**69**:2212-2241. DOI: 10.1016/j.jacc.2017.02.001

[7] International Diabetes Federation. Global Guideline for Type 2 Diabetes [Internet]. 2012. Available from: http://www.idf.org

[8] Canadian Diabetes Association. 2013 clinical practice guidelines for the prevention and management of diabetes in Canada. Canadian Journal of Diabetes. 2013;**37**(1):1-216

[9] Dedov II, Shestakova MV. Standards of specialized diabetes care. 7th edition (Russian). Diabetes mellitus. 2017;**20**(1S):1-112. DOI: 10.14341/DM20171S8

[10] Standards of medical care in diabetes 2017: Summary of revisions. Diabetes Care. 2017;**40**(Suppl. 1):S1-S2. DOI: 10.2337/dc17-S001

[11] Authors/Task Force Members, Rydén L, Grant PJ, Anker SD, et al. ESC Guidelines on diabetes, pre-diabetes, and cardiovascular diseases developed in collaboration with the EASD: The task force on diabetes, pre-diabetes, and cardiovascular diseases of the European Society of Cardiology (ESC) and developed in collaboration with the European Association for the Study of Diabetes (EASD). European Heart Journal. 2013;**34**(39):3035-3087

[12] Schulz-Schüpke S, Byrne RA, ten Berg JM, et al. ISAR-SAFE: A randomized, double-blind, placebo-controlled trial of 6 versus 12 months of clopidogrel therapy after drug-eluting stenting. European Heart Journal. 2015;**36**:1252-1263

[13] Colombo A, Chieffo A, Frasheri A, Garbo R, et al. Second-generation drug-eluting stent implantation followed by 6- versus 12-month dual antiplatelet therapy: The SECURITY randomized clinical trial. Journal of the American College of Cardiology. 2014;**64**:2086-2097

[14] Byrne RA, Joner M, Kastrati A. Stent thrombosis and restenosis: What have we learned and where are we going? The Andreas Grüntzig Lecture ESC 2014. European Heart Journal. 2015;**36**:3320-3331. DOI: 10.1093/eurheartj/ehv511

[15] Tarasov RS, Kochergin AM, Ganiukov VI, et al. The results of endovascular revascu-larization in elderly patients with myocardial infarction and ST-segment elevation in multivessel lesion depending on the severity of coronary atherosclerosis (Russian). Terapevticheskij Arkhiv. 2016;**88**(1):23-29

[16] Shimizu T, Miura S, Takeuchi K, et al. Effects of gender and aging in patients who undergo coronary artery bypass grafting: From the FU-Registry. Cardiology Journal. 2012;**19**(6):618-624. DOI: 10.5603/CJ.2012.0114

[17] Zhang H, Yuan X, Osnabrugge RL, et al. Influence of diabetes mellitus on long-term clinical and economic outcomes after coronary artery bypass grafting. The Annals of Thoracic Surgery. 2014;**97**(6):2073-2079

[18] Holzmann MJ, Rathsman B, Eliasson B, et al. Long-term prognosis in patients with type 1 and 2 diabetes mellitus after coronary artery bypass grafting. Journal of the American College of Cardiology. 2015;**65**(16):1644-1652. DOI: 10.1016/j.jacc.2015.02.052

[19] D'Agostino RS, Jacobs JP, Badhwar V, et al. The Society of Thoracic Surgeons Adult Cardiac Surgery Database: 2016 update on outcomes and quality. The Annals of Thoracic Surgery. 2016;**101**(1):24-32. DOI: 10.1016/j.athoracsur.2015.11.032

[20] Akchurin RS, Vlasova EE, Mershin KV. Diabetus mellitus and surgical treatment of coronary heart disease (Russian). Annals of the Russian Academy of Medical Sciences. 2012;**1**:14-19

[21] Borodashkina SY, Podkamenny VA, Protasov KV. Cardiovascular complications and carbohydrate metabolism in coronary shunting "off-pump" according to the regimen of glucose lowering treatment in ischemic heart disease and diabetes (Russian). Russian Journal of Cardiology. 2016;**2**:19-24. DOI: 10.15829/1560-4071-2016-2-19-24

[22] Kindo M, Hoang Minh T, Perrier S, Bentz J, Mommerot A, Billaud P, Mazzucotelli JP. Trends in isolated coronary artery bypass grafting over the last decade. Interactive Cardiovascular and Thoracic Surgery. 2017;**24**(1):71-76. DOI: 10.1093/icvts/ivw319 Epub 2016 Sept. 22

[23] Wang CL, Hess CN, Hiatt WR, et al. Clinical update: Cardiovascular disease in diabetes mellitus: Atherosclerotic cardiovascular disease and heart failure in type 2 diabetes mellitus—Mechanisms, management, and clinical considerations. Circulation. 2016;**133**:2459-2502

[24] Romeo GR, Lee J, Shoelson SE, et al. Metabolic syndrome, insulin resistance and roles of inflammation: Mechanisms and therapeutic targets. Arteriosclerosis, Thrombosis, and Vascular Biology. 2012;**32**:1771-1776

[25] Belenkova YA, Karetnikova VN, Dyachenko AO, et al. Inflammation's role in the development of poor prognosis in patients with myocardial infarction-segment elevation ST, undergoing percutaneous coronary intervention, against the background of impaired glucose tolerance and diabetes mellitus (Russian). Russian Cardiology Journal. 2014;**8**(112):84-91

[26] de la Hera JM, Delgado E, Hernández E, et al. Prevalence and outcome of newly detected diabetes in patients who undergo percutaneous coronary intervention. European Heart Journal 2009;**30**(21):2614-2621. DOI: 10.1093/eurheartj/ehp278

[27] Balakrishnan R, Berger JS, Tully L, et al. Prevalence of unrecognized diabetes, prediabetes and metabolic syndrome in patients undergoing elective percutaneous coronary intervention. Diabetes/Metabolism Research and Reviews. 2015;**31**(6):603-609. DOI: 10.1002/dmrr.264

[28] Petursson P, Herlitz J, Lindqvist J, et al. Prevalence and severity of abnormal glucose regulation and its relation to long-term prognosis after coronary artery bypass grafting. Coronary Artery Disease. 2013;**24**(7):577-582

[29] Giraldez RR, Clare RM, Lopes RD, et al. Prevalence and clinical outcomes of undiagnosed diabetes mellitus and prediabetes among patients with high-risk non-ST-segment elevation acute coronary syndrome. American Heart Journal. 2013;**165**(6):918.e2-925.e2. DOI: 10.1016/j.ahj.2013.01.005

[30] Frye RL, August P, Brooks MM, et al. A randomized trial of therapies for type 2 diabetes and coronary artery disease. The New England Journal of Medicine. 2009;**360**(24):2503-2515

[31] Shaw LJ, Cerqueira MD, Brooks MM, et al. Impact of left ventricular function and the extent of ischemia and scar by stress myocardial perfusion imaging on prognosis and therapeutic risk reduction in diabetic patients with coronary artery disease: Results from the bypass angioplasty revascularization investigation 2 diabetes (BARI 2D) trial. Journal of Nuclear Cardiology. 2012;**19**(4):658-669

[32] Brooks MM, Chaitman BR, Nesto RW, et al. Clinical, angiographic risk stratification differential impact on treatment outcomes in the bypass angioplasty revascularization investigation 2 diabetes (BARI 2D) trial. Circulation. 2012;**126**(17):2115-2124

[33] Farkouh ME, Domanski M, Sleeper LA, et al. Strategies for multivessel revascularization in patients with diabetes. The New England Journal of Medicine. 2012;**367**:2375-2384

[34] Deb S, Wijeysundera HC, Ko DT, et al. Coronary artery bypass graft surgery vs. percutaneous interventions in coronary revascularization: A systematic review. Journal of the American Medical Association. 2013;**310**(19):2086-2095. DOI: 10.1001/jama.2013.281718

[35] Bundhun PK, Wu ZJ, Chen M-H. Coronary artery bypass surgery compared with percutaneous coronary interventions in patients with insulin-treated type 2 diabetes mellitus: A systematic review and meta-analysis of 6 randomized controlled trials. Cardiovascular Diabetology. 2016;**15**:2. DOI: 10.1186/s12933-015-0323-z

[36] Bangalore S. Outcomes with coronary artery bypass graft surgery versus percutaneous coronary intervention for patients with diabetes mellitus: Can newer generation drug-eluting stents bridge the gap? Circulation. Cardiovascular Interventions. 2014;**7**(4):518-525

[37] Luthra S, Leiva-Juárez MM, Taggart DP. Systematic review of therapies for stable coronary artery disease in diabetic patients. The Annals of Thoracic Surgery. 2015;**100**(6):2383-2397. DOI: 10.1016/j.athoracsur.2015.07.005 Epub 2015 Oct. 31

[38] Koskinas KC, Siontis GC, Piccolo R, et al. Impact of diabetic status on outcomes after revascularization with drug eluting stents in relation to coronary artery disease complexity: Patient-level pooled analysis of 6081 patients. Circulation. Cardiovascular Interventions. 2016;**9**(2):e003255. DOI: 10.1161/CIRCINTERVENTIONS.115.003255

[39] Sumin AN, Bezdenezhnykh NA, Bezdenezhnyh AV, et al. Risk factors major cardiovascular events in the long term coronary artery bypass grafting in patients with coronary heart disease in the presence of type 2 diabetes (Russian). Russian Journal of Cardiology. 2015;**6**(122):30-37

[40] Gao L, Park SJ, Jang Y, Lee S, et al. Comparison of neoatherosclerosis and neovascularization between patients with and without diabetes: An optical coherence tomography study. JACC. Cardiovascular Interventions. 2015;**8**(8):1044-1052. DOI: 10.1016/j.jcin.2015.02.020

[41] Sumin AN, Bezdenezhnyh NA, Ivanov SV, et al. Factors associated with in-hospital mortality in coronary bypass surgery in patients with coronary artery disease combined with type 2 diabetes. (Russian). Diabetes Mellitus.2014;**4**:25-34

[42] Koochemeshki V, Salmanzadeh HR, Sayyadi H, et al. The effect of diabetes mellitus on short term mortality and morbidity after isolated coronary artery bypass grafting surgery. International Cardiovascular Research Journal. 2013;**7**(2):41-45

[43] Pang PY, Lim YP, Ong KK, et al. 2015 young surgeon's award winner: Long-term prognosis in patients with diabetes mellitus after coronary artery bypass grafting: A propensity-matched study. Annals of the Academy of Medicine, Singapore. 2016;**45**(3):83-90

[44] Lontchi-Yimagou E, Sobngwi E, Matsha TE, et al. Diabetes mellitus and inflammation. Current Diabetes Reports. 2013;**13**:435-444

[45] Tavlueva EV, Yarkovskaya AP, Barbarash OL. The relationship of diabetes with proinflammatory status in STEMI females and males. Complex Issues of Cardiovascular Diseases. 2014;**1**:42-46. DOI: 10.17802/2306-1278-2014-1

[46] Ujueta F, Weiss EN, Sedlis SP, et al. Glycemic control in coronary revascularization. Current Treatment Options in Cardiovascular Medicine. 2016;**18**(2):12. DOI: 10.1007/s11936-015-0434-6

[47] Chen PC, Chua SK, Hung HF, et al. Admission hyperglycemia predicts poorer short- and long-term outcomes after primary percutaneous coronary intervention for ST-elevation myocardial infarction. Journal of Diabetes Investigation. 2014;**5**:80-86. DOI: 10.1111/jdi.12113

[48] Trubnikova OA, Mamontova AS, Maleva OV, et al. Predictors of persistant post-operation cognitive dysfunction in 2 type diabetes patients after coronary bypass grafting (Russian). Russian Journal of Cardiology. 2016;**2**:12-18. DOI: 10.15829/1560-4071-2016-2-12-18

[49] Bruce DG. Type 2 diabetes and cognitive function: Many questions, few answers. Lancet Neurology. 2015;**14**(3):241-242. DOI: 10.1016/S1474-4422(14)70299-6

[50] Sathya B, Davis R, Taveira T, et al. Intensity of perioperative glycemic control and post-operative outcomes in patients with diabetes: A meta-analysis. Diabetes Research and Clinical Practice. 2013;**102**(1):8-15. DOI: 10.1016/j.diabres.2013.05.003

[51] Masoumi G, Frasatkhish R, Bigdelian H, et al. Insulin infusion on postoperative complications of coronary artery bypass graft in patients with diabetes mellitus. Research in Cardiovascular Medicine. 2014;**3**(2):e17861. DOI: 10.5812/cardiovascmed.17861

[52] Pezzella T, Holmes SD, Pritchard G, et al. Impact of perioperative glycemic control strategy on patient survival after coronary bypass surgery. The Annals of Thoracic Surgery. 2014;**98**:1281-1285. DOI: 10.1016/j.athoracsur.2014.05.067

[53] Umpierrez G, Cardona S, Pasquel F, et al. Randomized controlled trial of intensive versus conservative glucose control in patients undergoing coronary artery bypass graft surgery: GLUCO-CABG trial. Diabetes Care. 2015;**38**(9):1665-1672. DOI: 10.2337/dc15-0303

[54] Fox CS, Golden SH, Anderson C, et al. Update on prevention of cardiovascular disease in adults with type 2 diabetes mellitus in light of recent evidence: A scientific statement from the American Heart Association and the American Diabetes Association. Diabetes Care. 2015;**38**(9):1777-1803. DOI: 10.2337/dci15-0012

[55] Skyler JS, Bergenstal R, Bonow RO, et al. American Diabetes Association, American College of Cardiology Foundation, American Heart Association. Intensive glycemic control and the prevention of cardiovascular events: Implications of the ACCORD, ADVANCE, and VA Diabetes Trials: A position statement of the American Diabetes Association and a Scientific Statement of the American College of Cardiology Foundation and the American Heart Association. Journal of the American College of Cardiology. 2009;**53**(3):298-304. DOI: 10.1161/CIRCULATIONAHA.108.191305

[56] Pankov V. Clinical aspects of hypoglycemia as a risk factor for cardiovascular complications in type 2 diabetes. International Journal of Endocrinology. 2011;**5**(37): [Russian]

[57] Tennyson C, Lee R, Attia R, et al. Is there a role for HbA1c in predicting mortality and morbidity outcomes after coronary artery bypass graft surgery? Interactive Cardiovascular and Thoracic Surgery. 2013;**17**(6):1000-1008. DOI: 10.1093/icvts/ivt351

[58] Kinoshita T, Asai T, Suzuki T, et al. Preoperative hemoglobin A1c predicts atrial fibrillation after off-pump coronary bypass surgery. European Journal of Cardio-Thoracic Surgery. 2012;**41**(1):102-107. DOI: 10.1016/j.ejcts.2011.04.011

[59] Sumin AN, Bezdenezhnyh NA, Bezdenezhnyh AV, Ivanov SV, Barbarash OL. Factors associated with immediate results of coronary artery bypass grafting in patients with ischemic heart disease in the presence of type 2 diabetes. Kardiologiia. 2016;**10**:13-21. DOI: 10.18565/cardio.2016.10.13-21

[60] Schernthaner G. Diabetes and cardiovascular disease: Is intensive glucose control beneficial or deadly? Lessons from aCCORD, aDVaNCE, VaDT, UKPDS, PROactive, and NICE-SUGaR. Wiener Medizinische Wochenschrift (1946). 2010;**160**:8-19. DOI: 10.1007/s10354-010-0748-7

[61] Gerstein HC, Miller ME, Byington RP, et al. Action to control cardiovascular risk in diabetes study group. Effects of intensive glucose lowering in type 2 diabetes. The New England Journal of Medicine. 2008;**358**:2545-2559. DOI: 10.1056/NEJMoa0802743

[62] Patel A, MacMahon S, Chalmers J, et al., ADVANCE Collaborative Group. Intensive blood glucose control and vascular outcomes in patients with type 2 diabetes. The New England Journal of Medicine. 2008;**358**:2560-2572. DOI: 10.1056/NEJMicm066227

[63] Duckworth W, Abraira C, Moritz T, et al. Intensive glucose control and complications in American veterans with type 2 diabetes. The New England Journal of Medicine. 2009;**360**:129-139. DOI: 10.1056/NEJMoa0808431

[64] Inzucchi SE, Bergenstal RM, Buse JB, et al. Management of hyperglycemia in type 2 diabetes, 2015. Update to a position statement of the American Diabetes Association and the European Association for the Study of Diabetes. Diabetes Care. 2015;**38**:140-149. DOI: 10.2337/dc14-2441

[65] Hoogwerf BJ. Perioperative management of diabetes mellitus: How should we act on the limited evidence? Cleveland Clinic Journal of Medicine. 2006;**73**:95-99

[66] Shah B, Berger JS, Amoroso NS, et al. Periprocedural glycemic control in patients with diabetes mellitus undergoing coronary angiography with possible percutaneous coronary intervention. The American Journal of Cardiology. 2014;**113**:1474-1480. DOI: 10.1016/j.amjcard.2014.01.428

[67] Ike A, Shirai K, Nishikawa H, et al. Associations between different types of hypoglycemic agents and the clinical outcome of percutaneous coronary intervention in diabetic patients—From the FU-Registry. Journal of Cardiology. 2015;**65**:390-396. DOI: 10.1016/j.jjcc.2014.06.012

[68] Dangas GD, Farkouh ME, Sleeper LA, et al. Long-term outcome of PCI versus CABG in insulin and non-insulin-treated diabetic patients: Results from the FREEDOM trial. Journal of the American College of Cardiology. 2014;**64**:1189-1197. DOI: 10.1016/j.jacc.2014.06.1182

[69] Platoshkin NE, Kanus II. Clinical guidelines and evidence-based medicine position on the issue of perioperative management of patients with diabetes mellitus. Health and Environmental Problems. 2012;**3**(33):35-39

[70] Baradari AG, Zeydi AE, Aarabi M, et al. Metformin as an adjunct to insulin for glycemic control in patients with type 2 diabetes after CABG surgery: A randomized double blind clinical trial. Pakistan Journal of Biological Sciences. 2011;**14**(23):1047-1054

[71] Messaoudi SE, Nederlof R, Zuurbier CJ, et al. Effect of metformin pretreatment on myocardial injury during coronary artery bypass surgery in patients without diabetes (MetCAB): A double-blind, randomised controlled trial. The Lancet Diabetes and Endocrinology. 2015;**3**(8):615-623. DOI: 10.1016/S2213-8587(15)00121-7

[72] Li J, JP X, Zhao XZ, et al. Protective effect of metformin on myocardial injury in metabolic syndrome patients following percutaneous coronary intervention. Cardiology. 2014;**127**(2):133-139. DOI: 10.1159/000355574

[73] Ali MK, Bullard KM, Saaddine JB, et al. Achievement of goals in U.S. diabetes care, 1999-2010. The New England Journal of Medicine. 2013;**368**:1613-1624. DOI: 10.1056/NEJMsa1213829

[74] Moutzouri E, Tellis CC, Rousouli K, et al. Effect of simvastatin or its combination with ezetimibe on Toll-like receptor expression and lipopolysaccharide-induced cytokine production in monocytes of hypercholesterolemic patients. Atherosclerosis. 2012;**225**:381-387. DOI: 10.1016/j.atherosclerosis.2012.08.037

[75] Sattar NA, Ginsberg H, Ray K, et al. The use of statins in people at risk of developing diabetes mellitus: Evidence and guidance for clinical practice. Atherosclerosis. Supplements. 2014;**15**:1-15. DOI: 10.1016/j.atherosclerosissup.2014.04.001

[76] Stone NJ, Robinson JG, Lichtenstein AH, et al. 2013 ACC/AHA guideline on the treatment of blood cholesterol to reduce atherosclerotic cardiovascular risk in adults: A report of the American College of Cardiology/American Heart Association Task Force on Practice Guidelines. Circulation. 2014;**129**(25S2):1-45. DOI: 10.1161/01.cir.0000437738.63853.7a

[77] Miura M, Yamasaki M, Uemura Y, et al. Effect of statin treatment and low-density lipoprotein-cholesterol on short-term mortality in acute myocardial infarction patients undergoing primary percutaneous coronary intervention—Multicenter registry from Tokyo CCU Network Database. Circulation Journal. 2016;**80**(2):461-468. DOI: 10.1253/circj.CJ-15-0889

[78] Venkatesan S, Okoli GN, Mozid AM, et al. Effects of five preoperative cardiovascular drugs on mortality after coronary artery bypass surgery: A retrospective analysis of an observational study of 16,192 patients. European Journal of Anaesthesiology. 2016;**33**(1):49-57. DOI: 10.1097/EJA.0000000000000340

4

Surgical Treatment in Diffuse Coronary Artery Disease

Kaan Kırali and Yücel Özen

Abstract

Diffuse coronary artery atherosclerosis can be defined as "consecutive or longitudinal" and "complete or partial" obstruction in coronary vessels. Most of the patients with diabetes, hyperlipidemia, chronic renal insufficiency, connective tissue disease, and multi-stented coronary arteries have diffuse atherosclerotic lesions in the coronary territory. Viable large myocardium without necrosis is the only coronary bypass indication in these patients, because it is very difficult to find any healthy area for anastomosis. This type of coronary occlusion frequently stimulates the formation of collateral vessels that protect against extensive myocardial ischemia. The choice of a surgical method also depends on the nature of the coronary artery, and multisegment plaques and healthy-area intervals simplify complete revascularization. On the other hand, a more aggressive treatment modality should be preferred when no soft site can be identified for arteriotomy or there is an extensively diseased area that is not amenable to grafting. The less invasive techniques are "don't touch the plaque" techniques (jumping multi-bypass, sequential bypass, hybrid interventions). Sometimes an aggressive diffuse plaque formation needs to be treated with "touch the plaque" techniques (long-segment anastomosis, patch-plasty, endarterectomy ± patch-plasty). In simple forms, a limited long-segment anastomosis of conduits eliminates the occlusion of the limited atherosclerotic plaque where the whole lesion is opened and cross-covered by the graft. In the accelerated form of coronary arteriosclerosis, the atherosclerotic plaque appears widespread and the full-length lumen of the coronary artery can get very narrow or occluded totally. The long-segment lesion is usually calcified and it inhibits any kind of stitching; however, the plaque can be separated easily from the arterial wall in order to create an appropriate lumen in the total occluded coronary artery. Because the aggressive endarterectomy increases the operation risk, the arteriotomy should be extended until the normal lumen with normal intima in the distal segment of the coronary artery. In general, severity and distribution of coronary arteriosclerosis tend to increase with time but the rate of increase is highly variable and difficult to predict. Although diffuse atherosclerosis is severe enough, it is uncommon to render any patient unsuitable for surgery.

Keywords: Diffuse atherosclerosis, endarterectomy, patch-plasty, sequential bypass, jumping bypass

1. Introduction

Coronary artery disease usually involves the proximal portion of the larger epicardial coronary arteries, but generally not their intramural branches. In most patients, atherosclerotic lesions in coronary territory are segmental and eccentric, and they affect particularly bifurcations and sharp curvatures, whereas the rest of long segments of coronary arteries are plaque-free. Diffuse coronary artery disease can be defined as the presence of multiple atherosclerotic stenoses or long-segment occlusions in coronary territory. Atheromatous materials spread toward distal and retain a long segment of coronary arteries which can obstruct coronary lumen "consecutive or longitudinal" and "complete or partial".

In general, severity and distribution of coronary arteriosclerosis tend to increase with time but the rate of increase is highly variable and difficult to predict. Diffuse atherosclerosis severe enough to render the patient unsuitable for surgery is uncommon. On the other hand, progression of atherosclerosis in the native coronary arteries after coronary bypass surgery is not rare and accelerated atherosclerosis usually is the main contraindication for reoperation. The early and late results of endarterectomy are inferior to those of routine coronary bypass, but it offers a viable alternative not to leaving a territory ungrafted. Rate of aggressive progression of atherosclerosis cannot as yet be examined directly in multivariable risk factor analyses, but this progression can be slowed by intensive lipid-lowering therapy.

The nature of atherosclerotic coronary artery disease is a chronic inflammation and fibroproliferation of large- and medium-sized epicardial arteries consisting of the progressive deposition or degenerative accumulation of lipid-containing plaques on the innermost layer of the arterial wall. The basic mechanism of atherosclerosis is endothelial dysfunction which is characterized by the reduction of the endothelium-derived vasodilators, especially nitric oxide, and an increase in endothelium-derived contracting factors. The immune-inflammatory response involving macrophages, T-lymphocytes and intimal smooth muscle cells tries healing and repairing injured endothelium, stabilizing plaques, protecting rupture, and avoiding thrombosis. If the atherosclerotic stimuli persist over long time, the reparative response may accelerate and target to the progressive occlusion of the arterial lumen. Progressive diffuse coronary artery stenosis involves the following processes: local atheroma, lipid accumulation, biologic stimuli of vessel wall, chronic inflammation, cellular necrosis, plaque formation and complications, and calcification. Arterial wall injury is most often related to age, diabetes, smoking, dyslipidemia, hypertension, hyperuremia, and immunosuppressive therapy, which trigger and accelerate the inflammatory response aimed at restoring arterial wall integrity. During the progression of atherosclerosis, endothelial and smooth muscle cells die by apoptosis, and an atheromatous plaque covers the defects of the endothelium. A vulnerable plaque is a nonobstructive, silent coronary lesion, which suddenly becomes obstructive and symptomatic. Plaque rupture with/without thrombotic complications is the main reason for this acute coronary syndrome with/without complications. The lesions responsible for acute episodes are generally less calcified than plaques responsible for chronic stable angina, because calcification is the last part of the healing response to atherosclerosis and it appears to have no direct link to thrombosis. Because diffuse type of coronary disease is time-consuming, slowly developing occlusions frequently stimulate the formation of collateral vessels that protect myocardium against extensive ischemia. Viable large myocardium without necrosis is the only indication for coronary revascularization in these patients (without mechanical complications of myocardial infarction), because it is very difficult to find any healthy area for anastomosis. Consequently, the relative severity and associated risk balance between focal stenosis and diffuse disease cannot be easily compared when making revascularization decisions [1]. The physiological anatomy of coronary arteries must be detailed for myocardial revascularization, but quantifying the anatomic severity of diffuse lesions is difficult. Lower coronary flow reserve associated with severe diffuse disease may neutralize or override any potential benefit from eliminating stenosis by stents. On the other hand, more diffusely expanded coronary atherosclerosis can cause higher mortality rate during coronary bypass artery grafting (CABG) than focal lesions because of association of more complicated vessels, which are not appropriate for suturing or distal perfusion after anastomosis. Patients with diffuse coronary artery disease can also face a twofold increased risk of in-hospital mortality or major morbidities, which is independent of reoperation [2].

2. Etiology

Most of the patients with diabetes, hyperlipidemia, chronic renal insufficiency, connective tissue disease, heart transplantation, and multi-stented coronary arteries have diffuse atherosclerotic lesions in the coronary territory. All of these diseases affect and accelerate coronary arteriosclerosis differently [3]. Restenosis after first CABG can also be a reason for the diffuse coronary atherosclerosis, but usually these patients have ungraftable diffuse diseased coronary vasculature and none of the specific revascularization methods can be used.

2.1. Diabetes mellitus

Compared with nondiabetic patients, diabetes mellitus increases the incidence of coronary artery disease two to four times as much and accelerates the nature of the atherosclerosis. The nature of coronary artery disease in diabetic patients is clinically challenging because it causes an extensive and diffuse multivessel involvement. Hyperglycemia is directly related to the atherosclerotic development, progression, and instability due to induced endothelial dysfunction (abnormal nitric oxide biology, increased endothelin and angiotensin II, reduced prostacyclin activity), abnormalities in lipid metabolism (high triglyceride and LDL-cholesterol, low HDL-cholesterol), systemic inflammation (increased oxidative stress, accumulation of advanced glycation and products), and disorders in the proteo-fibrinolytic system and platelet biology (thrombosis). Hyperglycemia can deplete the cellular NADPH pool and induce with high levels of fatty acids to oxidative stress on phospholipids and proteins. Insulin resistance is the main actor to the endothelial dysfunction in type II diabetes, and endothelial dysfunction is closely complicated with microangiopathy and atherosclerosis in diabetic patients. Endothelial dysfunction decreases the capacity of nitric oxide synthase enzyme and depleted nitric oxide, which effects endothelial cell-dependent vasodilatation. Overexpression of growth factors causes endothelial cells and vascular smooth muscle proliferation. All of these negative changes accelerate atherosclerosis in all arterial territories, and the involvement of coronary arteries can be very extensive and diffuse with either serious jumping stenoses or long-segment narrowing with/without occlusion. The optimal strategy of coronary revascularization is controversial, but CABG has better long-term survival and freedom from re-interventions [4]. Diabetic patients have a higher restenosis rate after stent implantation and also progression of diffuse disease after stent implantation forms new lesions in diabetic patients than non-diabetic patients more often. Clinical outcomes in CABG patients are similar for diabetic and non-diabetic patients, while outcomes after stent could be worse for diabetic patients [5]. In diabetic patients with multivessel coronary artery disease, rates of death and myocardial infarction in 5 years are significantly lower in patients treated with CABG due to more complete revascu-larization, which bypasses several lesions and prevents coronary territory against progressive proximal coronary stenosis [6]. On the other hand, the operative risk in patients with diabetes might be a consequence of a preoperatively endothelial dysfunction and an inflammatory response to extracorporeal circulation characterized by an impaired release of interleukin-6 and increased turnover of E-selectin [7]. Simple distal anastomosis for each coronary artery cannot be enough to supply blood along the coronary territory, and most of the diabetic patients with diffuse multivessel coronary artery disease require specific surgical revascula-rization modalities, which can increase perioperative myocardial damage and operative mortality.

2.2. Hypercholesterolemia

Cholesterol is one of the most important risk factors for the development of premature coronary artery disease, which is characterized without any serious intravascular stenosis. Cholesterol levels and coronary artery disease show a strong and linear relationship, whereas cholesterol levels even in the normal range may inhibit endothelium-dependent vasodilatation in all arterial beds. The pathogenesis of atherosclerosis in the obese population can be related to metabolic syndrome associated with insulin intolerance and dyslipidemia, which cause endothelial dysfunction with decreasing nitric oxide production. Lowering of LDL-cholesterol rather than moderate weight loss is more effective to improve endothelial function, because the coronary vasculature is affected by the atherosclerosis process, and the most atherosclerotic lesions are associated with remarkable neovascularization of the vasa vasorum, which can cause intra-plaque rupture and bleeding. Hypercholesterolemia is one of the most important factors to stimulate this process and its role begins in the early atherosclerotic remodeling before plaque formation [8]. Hyperlipidemia-related coronary lesions are very predisposed to spread lengthways coronary territory and cause diffuse stenosis or occlusion, and calcification is usually associated with this type of atherosclerosis.

2.3. End-stage renal disease

A strong relationship subsists between chronic renal failure and coronary artery disease, and atherosclerosis can be accelerated in patients with end-stage renal disease due to multifactorial reasons [9]. Increased oxidative stress, hyperhomocysteinemia, hyperlipidemia, hyperglyce-mia and others are also important comorbidities. The main pathology is the impairment of endothelium-dependent vasodilatation. Dialysis-dependent renal failure patients undergoing CABG can have a greater degree of distal and/or diffuse coronary artery disease burden compared with matched patients with silent renal failure. The diffuseness of coronary atherosclerosis in patients with end-stage renal disease can be severe and the intraluminal lesions are usually calcified. Extensive calcification of all arterial structures in the body can inhibit conventional CABG strategies, which increase surgical outcomes. Impaired distal run-off of the coronary arteries is another strong independent predictor of operative mortality. All kinds of complex anastomotic techniques can be used in these patients, and endarterectomy can be very easy to perform to get adequate distal run-off. Restenosis after CABG is not uncommon in this group of patients, especially if saphenous vein is used.

2.4. Connective tissue disease

Several connective tissue diseases (systemic lupus erythematosus, rheumatoid arthritis, systemic sclerosis, Takayasu disease) are characterized by vascular dysfunction and excessive fibrosis. The presence of coronary microvascular dysfunction is the common pathologic change in various chronic inflammatory diseases [10]. Cardiac manifestation of these chronic diseases can be estimated lower, because most of them are asymptomatic. Diffuse form of these pathologies has a distressed clinical course with severe organ involvement. First, an endothelial injury occurs early in the disease process leading to endothelial dysfunction. Myofibroblasts drawn into the arterial wall by cellular growth factors contribute to the thickening of the intimal layer, compromising regional blood flow by narrowing the arterial lumen. In the absence of epicardial coronary stenosis, the abnormal coronary flow is dependent on the structural remodeling of the small coronary arteries and arterioles. Aggressive surgical interventions are usually ineffective, but multi-anastomoses can be applicable. Because diffuse atherosclerosis shows strict adhesions between arterial wall layers, endarterectomy can never satisfy to load out the intra-arterial lumen for appropriate anastomosis.

2.5. Heart transplantation

The occurrence of coronary artery disease is common in posttransplant patients, and atherosclerotic process is different from normally occurring coronary artery disease. This type of atherosclerosis is specific for heart transplanted patients, and it affects the entire length of the coronary arteries, and diffuse intimal proliferation develops without damage to the internal elastic lamina in contrast to classic atherosclerosis. The intimal proliferation developed by smooth muscle cells and macrophages contains cholesterol crystals and lipid components, but calcification is rare. This lesion affects large epicardial coronary arteries as well as the penetrating intramyocardial branches, and occlusion of these small branches is the first reason for acute coronary syndrome. Coronary endothelial vasodilator dysfunction is a common and early indicator for graft atherosclerosis, which is caused by both immunological and classic risk factors. The immunological response is the first stimulus causing endothelial damage and this injury alters endothelial permeability, with consequent myointimal hyperplasia and extracellular matrix synthesis. Alloimmune injury starts when donor antigens expressed from the donor endothelial cells interact with recipient dendritic cells, and the activated macrophages secrete several factors, which stimulate the proliferation of smooth muscle cells and vascular remodeling [11]. Before microvasculature occlusions, stent or standard CABG can be preferred for the treatment of newly developed epicardial lesions, but endarterectomy may not be usually applicable in most diffuse cases, and retransplantation is the only option under these circumstances.

2.6. Multistented coronary arteries

The problem of restenosis after stenting represents a special case of arterial hyperplastic disease and the in-stent restenosis is made from myxomatous tissue, whereas accelerated intimal hyperplasia occludes the distal segment of the same coronary vessel after stenting. Availability of access to healthy coronary wall for revascularization is usually feasible in patients receiving a single stent implantation in one or each coronary artery. However, the distal vascular bed of multi-stented coronary artery is often influenced by the accelerated atherosclerosis and diffusely diseased where it is impossible to find any healthy area for distal anastomosis. Sometimes, open endarterectomy with removal of stent(s) can remain the last option for surgical revascularization.

3. Surgical treatment techniques

Diffuse atherosclerosis has been highly widespread among patients with coronary artery disease in the last two decades, because simple lesions are usually treated with stent interventions in the early phase of the coronary pathology. Diffuse coronary lesion and reduced coronary flow reserve can be silent due to several collaterals, but it might result in severe functional limitation, chronic low-level ischemia, and myocardial remodeling. Low-level ischemia can be a potential driver of both first coronary vasomotor and myocardial dysfunction, and then remodeling in heart failure with preserved ejection fraction. Diffuse atherosclerosis and microvascular dysfunction-associated coronary artery disease comorbid conditions may guide new, more effective, aggressive, and therapeutic interventions for global cardiovascular risk reduction due to complete revascularization. There is no difference in event-free survival between CABG or stent implantation in patients with high coronary flow reserve; however, CABG is significantly more effective than stent in patients with low coronary flow reserve [12]. Diffuseness of coronary artery disease is a serious risk factor for early and late adverse events after coronary revascularization, but the acceptable strategy should be complete revascularization. Standard bypass method (finding an appropriate lumen and performing anastomosis) is usually not possible in the diffusely diseased coronary arteries, and such a region, which may be found at most distal, cannot be expected to bring any benefit. For this reason, in such cases, it is required to apply a complex method other than standard bypass method. When the atherosclerotic stenosis is local, it is technically possible and easy to revascularize the distal segment directly, but in diffuse coronary artery disease or in the presence of diffuse stenotic regions, different techniques should be implemented for complete revascularization.

The treatment of the diffused-type coronary artery disease has always been an issue; however, this scenario is challenging for cardiac surgeons because diffuse atheromatous lesions frequently render epicardial coronary vessels unsuitable for conventional distal grafting. However, there are some strategies to perform a complete revascularization with increasing complexity and mortality risk sequentially in these patients. Second, to attenuate or prevent perioperative infarction and/or postischemic ventricular dysfunction caused by inadequate myocardial protection, there are many different administrative ways for cardioplegic solutions, but the optimal delivery method of cardioplegia also remains controversial. Off-pump bypass can be another option when coronary artery is totally occluded and retrograde flow supplies the myocardium.

The aggressive involvement type of atherosclerosis is the corner stone for coronary revascularization, and the first choice of the aggressive surgical techniques also depends on this nature (Table 1). A coronary artery with multisegment plaques and healthy-area intervals simplifies complete revascularization, and multiple revascularization of this coronary artery with different methods seems applicable by every cardiac team. On the other hand, a more aggressive treatment modality should be preferred when no soft site can be identified for arteriotomy or there is an extensively diseased area not amenable to grafting or no other methods except transplantation. The routine application for arteriotomy in patients with local stenosis is to perform the anastomotic incision proximal enough to get the larger-sized coronary target but distal enough from atherosclerotic lesion. Arteriotomy should be more complicated or extended to get appropriate coronary lumen and anastomotic area in patients with diffuse coronary lesions. The main goal of CABG is to finish complete revascularization using different surgical approaches during open-heart surgery. Using a single graft or multi-grafts or a hybrid procedure (stent + bypass) is a reliable option to revascularize all segments of each coronary artery: **don't touch the plaque techniques**. Sometimes an aggressive plaque formation needs to be touched using extended arteriotomy with/without endarterectomy and patch-plasty: **touch the plaque techniques**.

Don't Touch the Plaque Techniques

1. Jumping bypass technique

This technique is used for revascularization of the same coronary artery with more than one anastomosis (Figure 1). Most patients with diffuse coronary artery disease have multiple severe stenoses along coronary arteries or diseased coronary artery may have critically important side branches before the last stenosis that could not be bypassed. Jumping bypass is performed via single or multiple conduits on the same coronary artery and is the only solution to supply blood throughout the diseased coronary artery, especially for the left anterior descending (LAD) artery and the right coronary artery (RCA). The circumflex artery (Cx) may have multiple major branches and each one does not need to be revascularized consecutively with this technique; on the contrary, these branches should be revascularized separately with sequential grafting. The jumping bypass technique has several advantages to avoid unexpected adverse complications intraoperatively (Table 2). It is the simpler technique to perform complete revascularization in diffuse coronary disease patients. This technique can be applied via different approaches.

A. No-touch the plaque techniques
1. Jumping bypass (the same coronary artery)
a. with multiple grafts
b. with a single graft
c. with a composite graft
d. with a bifurcated graft
2. Sequential bypass (multiple coronary arteries)
a. with a single graft
b. with a composite graft
c. with a bifurcated graft
3. Hybrid revascularization (different coronary arteries)
B. Touch the plaque techniques
1. long-segment anastomosis
2. patch-plasty
3. endarterectomy ± patch-plasty
a. closed
b. open

Table 1. Aggressive bypass strategies for diffusely diseased coronary territory

1. To achieve complete revascularization of the same major coronary artery
2. To supply blood to the myocardium via grafting major side branches of the same coronary artery
3. To avoid more aggressive surgical procedures ("touch the plaque" techniques)
4. To shorten ischemic and cardiopulmonary bypass times
5. To salvage myocardium from perioperative myocardial infarction caused by graft failure

Table 2. Advantages of the jumping bypass technique

a.   Jumping grafting with multiple conduits

This approach is the easiest approach, and it is usually used for the LAD revascularization, whereas the RCA is seldom preferred. This jumping bypass approach using more than one conduit is usually preferred in emergency situations to salvage myocardium perioperatively, but it can also be used in elective cases. Two arteriotomies are performed on the same coronary

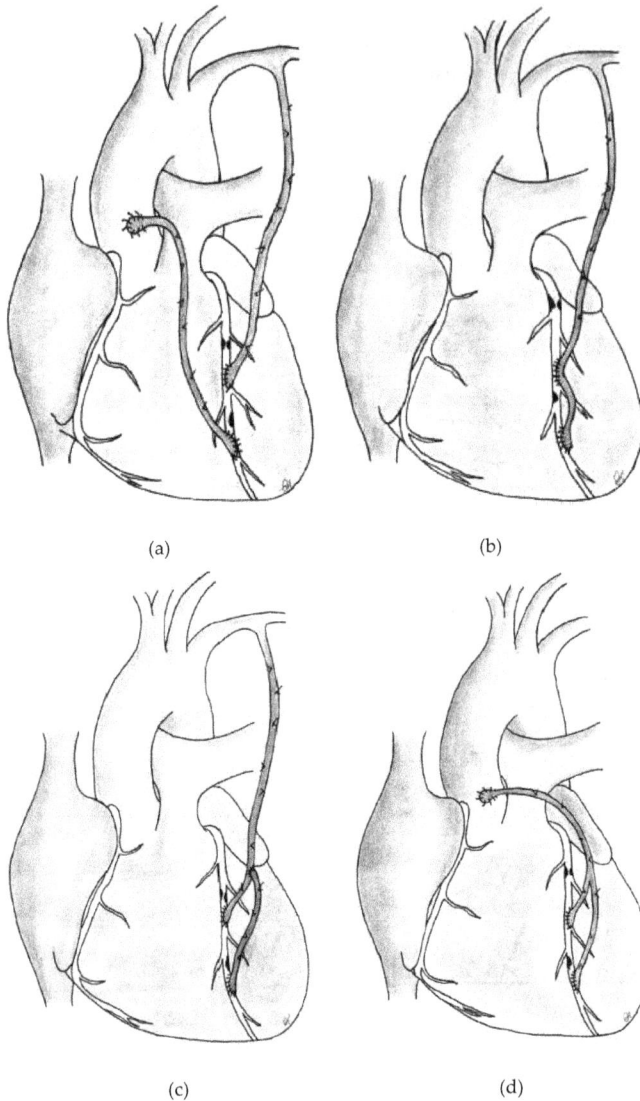

Figure 1. Jumping grafting is an alternative to multi-revascularization of the same coronary artery with multi-segment stenoses. **a)** Jumping grafting with multiple conduits. **b)** Jumping grafting with a single conduit. **c)** Jumping grafting with a composite conduit. **d)** Jumping grafting with a bifurcated conduit.

artery and both are grafted by different conduits (Figure 1a). Two conduits are anastomosed in an end-to-side fashion, and this approach achieves double suppliers with double sources. This approach is usually preferred for the LAD, and the left internal mammarian artery (LIMA) is often anastomosed between the proximal and distal lesions, because the length of LIMA is usually not enough to reach to the distal segment. The distal segment of the coronary artery is revascularized using a second conduit, especially with a vein graft. In elective and planned surgery, the second graft could be an arterial conduit: the right internal thoracic artery (RIMA) or radial artery (RA). In the emergency salvage re-exploration after perioperative myocardial infarction, the saphenous vein graft (SVG) should be chosen for its precipitous harvesting. This approach can be preventative against early graft failure, whereas the second independent conduit can continue to supply blood. This approach is also lifesaving when perioperative myocardial infarction is developed because of the graft failure, and the second graft is anastomosed at the distal part of the affected coronary artery. This alternative procedure is mostly used to salvage myocardium when the LIMA or the other conduit does not work due to any reason perioperatively.

b. Jumping grafting with a single conduit

This approach can be used for the LAD or RCA elective and planned revascularization, but it is not feasible for emergency surgery. This approach is similar to sequential bypass technique, but the only difference is to be a single target vessel requiring multiple anastomoses. If harvesting of a second conduit is not possible due to any reason and the target coronary artery has multiple stenosis, the harvested single graft can be anastomosed on the same coronary artery consecutively (Figure 1b). In situ or free conduits can be used for jumping grafting. The double arteriotomies are made in the direction of the long axis at the mid and distal soft segments of the target coronary artery, and a single proximal arteriotomy is made at the conduit. The two proximal incisions are aligned parallel and the proximal anastomosis is performed in a side-to-side fashion and created kissing anastomosis, which is the critical part of this approach, but "aligned perpendicular and created a diamond-shaped anastomosis" is never used for this anastomosis like the routine sequential bypass technique. The distal end of the graft is anastomosed to the distal arteriotomy on the target coronary artery as the standard end-to-side fashion. Using a larger graft for consecutive anastomoses on the same coronary artery can be performed with a lower technical risk than the LIMA because of its borderline diameter, and the best conduits for this approach are the RA and SVG. This approach is often complication free and consecutive grafting of the same target coronary artery permits efficient use of limited conduits, but it is preferred rarely.

c. Jumping grafting with a composite conduit

This approach can be used for the LAD revascularization. This approach is more time-consuming than the other approaches and needs more attention. A composite conduit can be built as T- or Y-graft with the in situ LIMA. This second graft is usually prepared from a free arterial graft (a short segment of the RA or RIMA), and both free ends of the second arterial conduit are anastomosed on the same coronary artery, whereas the LIMA is anastomosed at the middle part of the second conduit conduit (T-graft) or the LIMA is anastomosed on the LAD, whereas both free ends of the second arterial conduit are anastomosed on the distal segment of the LAD and at the middle part of the LIMA (Y-graft) (Figure 1c). This application arranges uniform distal anastomoses using the same conduit with the same diameter and prevents stealing coronary blood by any larger conduit. In the absence of the second arterial graft, a short SVG can be also used as the composed part.

d. Jumping grafting with a bifurcated conduit

This approach can be used for the LAD or RCA revascularization. This approach is easy to apply, but it is very uncommon to find a bifurcated conduit in the body. The two branches of the LIMA have a smaller diameter and are very vasospastic, which are not suitable for grafting. The only option is to harvest the SVG with its first major bifurcated branches (Figure 1d). The advantages are avoiding the second proximal anastomosis on the ascending aorta or on the other conduit, any handicap caused by anastomosis between both grafts, and technical difficulties and risks of kissing anastomosis.

2.   Sequential bypass technique

This technique is used for revascularization of more than one target coronary arteries or major branches of the same coronary artery with the same conduit. The number of the sequential bypassed vessels depends on the availability of multi-conduits, which allow one or more sequential bypass at the same time. If harvesting adequate conduits is feasible, the true way is bypassing all diseased coronary artery separately as the "one graft-to-one target coronary artery" rule. The main purpose of this technique is the efficient usage of limited conduits to achieve complete revascularization (Table 3). The most distal anastomosis should be to the furthest target coronary artery with an acceptable diameter, and the conduit is anastomosed at several coronary arteries before its proximal anastomosis. The most possible drawback is more than one distal anastomoses with a single proximal source that can cause an aggravated risk of inadequate myocardial perfusion. It cannot be hazardous, if the equal coronary territory is bypassed with the same conduit sequentially. On the other hand, if the distal coronary artery has a small diameter, it would be hazardous, and this smaller distal anastomosis lies under the risk of total occlusion because of preferential graft flow to the larger proximal coronary arteries. All available conduits can be used for sequential grafting, especially the SVG. The RA is usually used for sequential anastomosis during full arterial revascularization [13]. The LIMA should not be used for sequential bypass grafting, if it supplies the LAD flow, but it can be used as a donor for composite T- or Y-grafting of other arterial conduits, especially with the RIMA, in order to achieve complete arterial revascularization. The distal anastomosis is performed with the standard end-to-side technique and all proximal anastomoses with the side-to-side technique. Both the target coronary artery and the conduit are incised longitudinally and aligned perpendicular to each other, and all proximal sequential anastomoses must be constructed in a diamond-shaped fashion to prevent any stenosis, kinking, distortion or tension on the anastomoses and conduit. Both the arteriotomy and the incision on the conduit should not exceed the diameter of the conduit. The distal anastomosis is completed first and the other anastomoses are performed towards the proximal consecutively.

1. To achieve complete revascularization of the different coronary arteries
2. To perform complete revascularization if conduits are inappropriate
3. To supply blood to the myocardium via grafting major side branches of the same or different coronary arteries
4 To avoid more aggressive surgical procedures ("touch the plaque" techniques)
5. To shorten ischemic and cardiopulmonary bypass times
6. To salvage myocardial revascularization intraoperatively when the conduits are shorter for proximal anastomosis on the ascending aorta.

Table 3. Advantages of the sequential bypass technique

a.   Sequential grafting with a single conduit

This approach can be used for all coronary arteries and is the most used approach for complete revascularization. If harvesting of sufficient conduits is not possible due to any reason and there are a large number of target coronary arteries, the harvested single graft can be anastomosed on the different coronary arteries (RCA-Cx-Diagonal-LAD) or on the several branches of a single coronary artery (Cx 1-3) sequentially (Figure 2a). All free grafts are suitable for this sequential bypass approach. The best conduit for this approach is the SVG or RA. Proximal anastomosis is always performed on the ascending aorta without any concern on the long-term patency [14]. In situ arterial grafts should be used alone to the target coronary artery, especially both IMAs. First, the distal end of the graft is anastomosed to the distal target coronary artery in an end-to-side fashion. The other proximal coronary arteries are bypassed consecutively through the anterior surface of the heart. The small arteriotomies are made in the direction of the long axis of the target coronary artery and small incisions are made at the conduit. The two incisions are aligned perpendicularly creating a diamond-shaped anastomosis and the sequential anastomosis is performed in a side-to-side fashion, which is the critical part of this approach; however, "aligned parallel and created a kissing anastomosis" is never used for this anastomoses. This approach is often complication free, and sequential grafting of the different target coronary arteries permits efficient use of limited conduits.

b.   Sequential grafting with a composite conduit

This approach can be performed in two different methods. The first method is usually used if the distal SVGs remain shorter for proximal anastomosis on the ascending aorta intraoperatively, especially for revascularization of the Cx-branches. A composite conduit can be built as Y-graft and the second short graft is usually anastomosed on the main conduit, and the most preferred conduits are the SVG and RA (Figure 2b-1). The main graft is anastomosed to the largest target coronary artery first, and the proximal anastomosis of the other shorter graft(s) is performed on this main graft before or after releasing the aortic cross-clamp. The second method is used for complete arterial revascularization of all coronary arteries, but this method is more time-consuming and needs more competency (Figure 2b-2). This composite conduit is prepared for T- or Y-graft and it can reach all surfaces of the heart. The most preferred conduits are the LIMA as a pedicle graft source and the RIMA as a composed part for grafting all target coronary arteries.

c.   Sequential grafting with a bifurcated conduit

This approach can be used for revascularization of the distal RCA- or Cx-branches (Figure 2c). This approach is easy to apply, but it is very uncommon to find a bifurcated conduit in the body. The advantages are avoiding the second proximal anastomosis on the ascending aorta, any handicap caused by anastomosis between both grafts, and technical difficulties and risks of kissing anastomosis.

3.   Hybrid revascularization

The standard hybrid coronary revascularization combines the benefits of the LIMA-to-LAD grafting and stent implantation to the other coronary territory. The hybrid revascularization

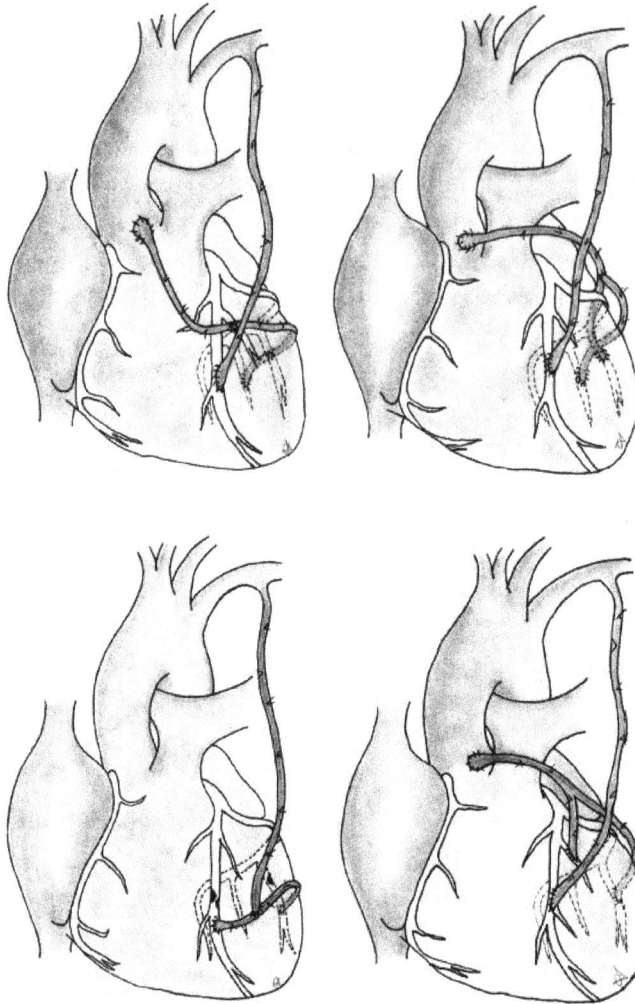

Figure 2. Sequential grafting is the best alternative for the multivessel revascularization in the absence of adequate conduits. **a)** Sequential grafting with a single conduit. **b)** Sequential grafting with a composite conduit: **1-** classic approach with inadequate saphenous vein grafts; **2-** T- or Y- graft for total arterial revascularization. **c)** Sequential grafting with a bifurcated conduit.

technique can be chosen with several indications in patients with diffuse coronary artery disease (Table 4). Patients with severe comorbidities or patients with multiple stenoses may be the best candidates for this procedure. If complete multivessel surgical revascularization increases operative adverse outcomes in high-risk patients, stent implantation in one or more coronary arteries, except the LAD, can be a preventative alternative to complete myocardial revascularization (Table 4). Hybrid revascularization can be performed concomitant or staged. Concomitant hybrid revascularization needs a specific operating room, whereas staged hybrid revascularization can be performed in every clinic. Percutaneous coronary intervention is applied before or after CABG. The decision depends on the severity of proximal lesions which may not be revascularized, and the aim is the avoidance of any perioperative myocardial infarction. Especially proximal or ostial left main or LAD serious stenosis should be treated by stent, if single LIMA-to-LAD grafting cannot achieve complete blood supply to the LAD territory. Ungraftable RCA or Cx vessels with severe stenosis should be treated by percutaneous intervention to achieve complete revascularization.

1. Invisible coronary artery during surgery threatening a huge myocardium
2. Multiple stenosis with a very proximal lesion threatening proximal larger branches
3. To shorten cardiopulmonary and ischemic times
4. Absence of sufficient conduits for complete revascularization
5. Impaired or diseased conduits

Table 4. Indication for hybrid revascularization

Touch the Plaque Techniques

1. Long-segment (1-3 cm) anastomosis

This technique is chosen when the plaque with limited length obstructs the coronary blood flow. This simplest form includes a limited long-segment anastomosis of a conduit to eliminate the occlusion of the limited atherosclerotic plaque (Figure 3). This technique is a prolonged version of the standard anastomosis technique to revascularize proximal and distal segments of the coronary artery and makes jumping grafting with/without a second graft unnecessary. The whole diseased coronary artery segment is opened at full length of the atherosclerotic lesion and the arteriotomy is extended bidirectionally until the healthy coronary artery lumen comes out. The aim of this maneuver is to forward graft blood flow directly into the healthy coronary artery lumen bidirectionally. The distal end of the graft is opened longer than coronary arteriotomy to prevent any tension, tightening, stenosis or inadequately anastomotic length of the conduit, and then the graft is anastomosed on the coronary arteriotomy longitudinally. All attention should be directed to avoid any distal embolization of atherosclerotic debris or to prevent the continuity of the coronary artery.

2. Patch-plasty (> 3 cm) anastomosis

A diffusely diseased coronary artery cannot be grafted by conventional grafting technique and side branches and/or distal segment would not be revascularized. This technique is preferred mostly for the LAD, but the RCA or the Cx artery can be also bypassed with this technique. The patch-plasty technique is necessary if any kind of endarterectomy cannot be applied and the long-segment lesions should be opened in full length. The main principle is to avoid touching the atherosclerotic plaques during the patch reconstruction. The in situ or free conduit can be used alone (Figure 4a) or it can be anastomosed onto the second graft, which is sewn on the long-segment arteriotomy as a hood (Figure 4b). The arteriotomy can be made as long as the length of the attainable epicardial coronary artery, and then a conduit is used to close this arteriotomy without the occlusion of side branches. The graft should also be opened as long as the arteriotomy and anastomosed with a running single suture. In the standard approach, the bites can be taken at the free ends of the arteriotomy to get the largest lumen

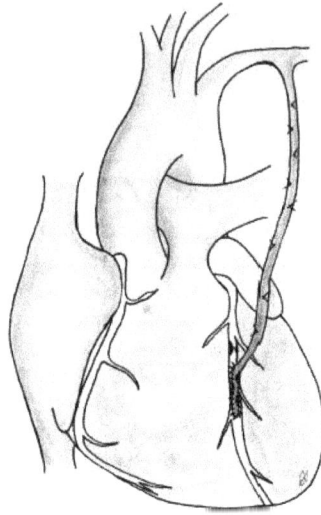

Figure 3. Long-segment anastomosis (1-3 cm) is the simplest alternative to eliminate the distal eccentric lesion.

(Figure 5a). If the lateral walls of the coronary arteriotomy are much calcified, the bites can also be taken very closely to the septal branches, however, this approach needs grafting epicardial side branches separately (Figure 5b). This technique is more useful for the diffusely occluded LAD to perfuse septal branches as far as possible or for the distal major branches of the RCA with septal branches. The Cx artery can be grafted with this technique to make the anastomosis safe.

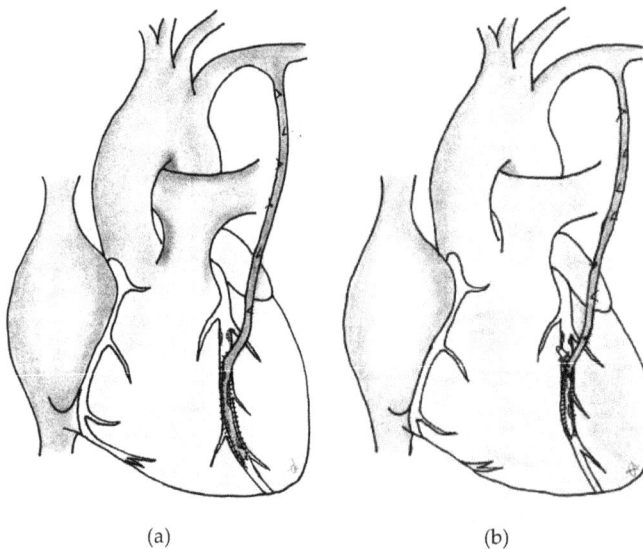

(a)   (b)

Figure 4. Patch-plasty is the best alternative to avoid endarterectomy in the extended long-segment (> 3 cm) diffuse coronary artery disease. **a)** The in situ or free conduit is anastomosed onto the long-segment coronary artery as a patch. **b)** The limited second conduit is anastomosed as a hood and the main conduit is anastomosed onto this conduit.

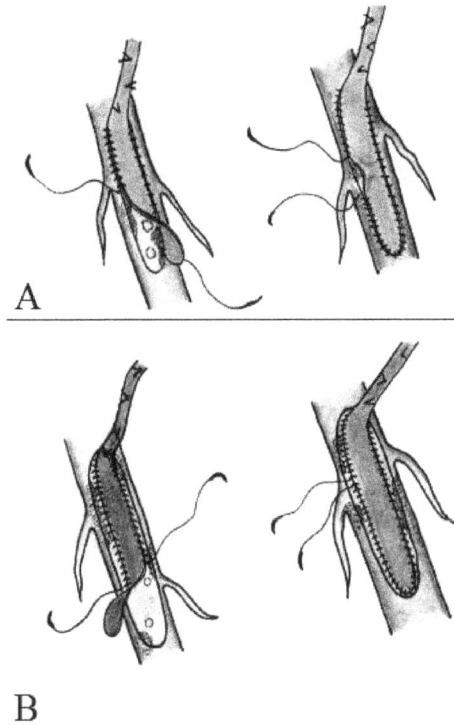

Figure 5. The stitching maneuvers of the patch-plasty technique. **a)** Bites on the free margins of the coronary arteriotomy. **b)** Bites close to the septal branches.

3. Endarterectomy with/without patch-plasty

In the accelerated form of coronary arteriosclerosis, the atherosclerotic plaque appears widespread and the full-length lumen of the coronary artery can be narrowed strictly or occluded totally. Coronary endarterectomy can be applied via off- or on-pump techniques, but the Cx endarterectomy with off-pump technique is used very seldom because it is more difficult and needs more competence [15]. This technique can be often used for every coronary artery, but it is usually preferred for the LAD and RCA [16]. The long-segment lesion is usually calcified and it inhibits any kind of stitching; however, the plaque can be separated easily from the arterial wall. Endarterectomy and graft anastomosis is preferred only to create an appropriate lumen in the total occluded coronary artery due to the removal of the atheromatous material. Long-standing atherosclerosis permits a successful endarterectomy to get adequate distal run-off. All debris and layer until the adventitia should be removed, and then the vessel wall is reconstructed with a conduit. The early occlusion of the endarterected coronary artery is caused by thrombosis or intimal flap formation, but the reason for late occlusion is intimal hyperplasia. The endarterectomy and patch plasty approach has a very satisfactory graft patency compared with the other approaches for the coronary territory [17,18].

a. Closed Endarterectomy

The closed approach is preferred for the LAD or RCA (Figure 6a). Approximately 2 cm arteriotomy is performed and an endarterectomy plane between the medial layer and the adventitia is developed with the coronary scissors. The circumferential plane is performed and the core is pulled out from the distal arterial wall. Distal plaque removal causes usually a better coronary distal bed, but proximal plaque removal via a limited arteriotomy can cause poor outcomes as the native vessel laceration resulting native coronary artery dissection or a native passage of high blood flow from the aorta to the distal coronary resulting competition, and early thrombosis. To optimize the technique, avoiding proximal endarterectomy by the pull-out method and cutting the proximal part without any traction would come along with better results [19]. The core usually is separated cleanly from the distal vessel, but all debris must be cleaned from the septal ostia. If the core branches can be reached, major side branches are endarterectomized separately. The main aim is to get the distal core without any rupture; otherwise the arteriotomy should be extended until the ruptured distal end to continue the closed endarterectomy.

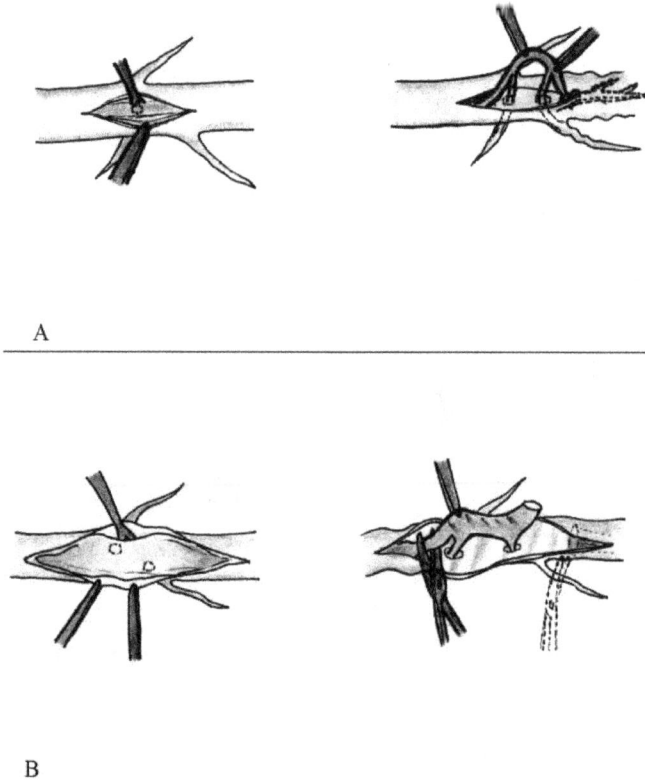

A

B

Figure 6. Endarterectomy is the most aggressive method for coronary bypass surgery. **a)** Closed endarterectomy. **b)** Open endarterectomy.

b.　Open Endarterectomy + Patch-plasty

The open approach is a useful procedure for the total occluded LAD (Figure 6b). The open approach prevents any obstruction of septal branches and inadequate endarterectomy of diagonal branches. The arteriotomy is started at the middle segment of the LAD and extended bidirectionally as proximal and distal as possible. If septal branches are easy to be revascularized with long-segment grafting, anastomosis can be finished without endarterectomy. If the direct anastomosis is impossible because of severe calcified vessel wall or no lumen, a long-segment endarterectomy should be performed to separate the core from the adventitia. The core is removed gently and both ends of the core at the ends of the arteriotomy should be cut without any traction. Because aggressive endarterectomy increases the operation risk, the arteriotomy should be extended until the normal lumen with normal intima in the distal and proximal segments of the coronary artery. All coronary arteries have very small lumen and thin wall at the distal, and the arteriotomy should be stopped 2-3 cm before the last bifurcation. The arteriotomy is reconstructed with a long segment of the conduit or a graft patch into which the in situ conduit is anastomosed.

Author details

Kaan Kırali* and Yücel Özen

*Address all correspondence to: imkbkirali@yahoo.com

Department of Cardiovascular Surgery, Koşuyolu Herat and Research Hospital, Istanbul, Turkey

References

[1] Gould KL, Johnson NP. Physiologic severity of diffuse coronary artery disease: Hidden high risk. (Editorial) Circulation 2015;131(1):4-6.

[2] McNeil M, Buth K, Brydie A, MacLaren A, Baskett R. The impact of diffuseness of coronary artery disease on the outcomes of patients undergoing primary and reoperative coronary artery bypass grafting. Eur J Cardiothorac Surg 2007;31(5):827-833.

[3] Hadi HA, Carr CS, Suwaidi JA. Endothelial dysfunction: Cardiovascular risk factors, therapy, and outcome. Vasc Health Risk Manag 2005;1(3):183-198.

[4] Kurlansky P, Herbert M, Prince S, Mack MJ. Improved long-term survival for diabetic patients with surgical versus interventional revascularization. Ann Thorac Surg 2015;99(4):1298–1305.

[5] Kappetein AP, Head SJ, Morice MC, et al. Treatment of complex coronary artery disease in patients with diabetes: 5-year results comparing outcomes of bypass surgery and percutaneous coronary intervention in the SYNTAX trial. Eur J Cardiothorac Surg 2013;43(5):1006-1013.

[6] Fanari Z, Weiss SA, Zhang W, Sonnad SS, Weintraub WS. Meta-analysis of three randomized controlled trials comparing coronary artery bypass grafting with percu-

taneous coronary intervention using drug-eluting stenting in patients with diabetes. Interactive Cardiovasc Thorac Surg 2014;19(6):1002-1007.

[7]   Lehle K, Preuner JG, Vogt A, et al. Endothelial cell dysfunction after coronary bypass grafting with extracorporeal circulation in patients with type 2 diabetes mellitus. Eur J Cardiothorac Surg 2007;32(4):611-616.

[8]   Galili O, Sattler KJ, Herrmann J, et al. Experimental hypercholesterolemia differentially affects adventitial vasa vasorum and vessel structure of the left internal thoracic and coronary arteries. J Thorac Cardiovasc Surg 2005;129(4):767-772.

[9]   Wong D, Thompson G, Buth K, Sullivan J, Ali I. Angiographic coronary diffuseness and outcomes in dialysis patients undergoing coronary artery bypass grafting surgery. Eur J Cardiothorac Surg 2003;24(3):388-392.

[10] Faccini A, Agricola E, Oppizzi M, et al. Coronary microvascular dysfunction in asymptomatic patients affected by systemic sclerosis. Circ J 2015;79(4):825-829.

[11] Vecchiati A, Tellatin S, Angelini A, Iliceto S, Tona F. Coronary microvasculopathy in heart transplantation: Consequences and therapeutic implications. World J Transplant 2014;4(2):93-101.

[12] Taqueti VR, Hachamovitch R, Murthy VL, et al. Global coronary flow reserve is associated with adverse cardiovascular events independently of luminal angiographic severity and modifies the effect of early revascularization. Circulation 2015;131(1): 19-27.

[13] Kaya E, Mansuroglu D, Göksedef D, et al. Long-term angiographic results of coronary artery bypass surgery with the use of arterial graft combinations. Turkish J Thorac Cardiovasc 2005;13(4):309-313.

[14] Akıncı E, Uzun K, Erentuğ V, et al. The comparison of the early and midterm results of the proximal anastomosis techniques in sequential radial artery grafting. Turkish J Thorac Cardiovasc 2004;12(3):235-240.

[15] Kırali K, Sareyyüpoğlu B, Yıldırım Ö, et al [abstract]. Coronary artery endarterectomy: Off-pump or on-pump? 56th International Congress of the European Society for Cardiovascular Surgery, May 17-20, 2007; Venice, Italy. Interact Cardiovasc Thorac Surg 2007;6(Suppl 1):S52.

[16] Kırali K, Yıldırım Ö, Sareyyüpoğlu B, et al [abstract]. Coronary artery endarterectomy: Impact on morbidity and mortality. 56th International Congress of the European Society for Cardiovascular Surgery, May 17-20, 2007; Venice, Italy. Interact Cardiovasc Thorac Surg 2007;6(Suppl 1):S75.

[17] Kırali K, Sareyyüpoğlu B, Yıldırım Ö, et al [abstract]. Left anterior descending coronary artery endarterectomy: 15-year results. 56th International Congress of the European Society for Cardiovascular Surgery, May 17-20, 2007; Venice, Italy. Interact Cardiovasc Thorac Surg 2007;6(Suppl 1):S103.

[18] Kırali K, Yıldırım Ö, Sareyyüpoğlu B, et al [abstract]. Coronary endarterectomy for diffuse right coronary artery disease: 11 years results. 15th Annual Meeting of Asian Society of Cardiovascular Surgery, May 17-20, 2007; Beijing, China.

[19] Sareyyüpoğlu B, Yıldırım Ö, Kırali K. Different results of proximal coronary endarterectomy via conventional pull-out method. Kosuyolu Heart J 2012;15(2):90-91.

5

Noninvasive Imaging for the Assessment of Coronary Artery Disease

Punitha Arasaratnam and Terrence D. Ruddy

Abstract

Noninvasive cardiac imaging is a cornerstone of the diagnostic work-up in patients with suspected coronary artery disease (CAD), cardiomyopathy, heart failure, and congenital heart disease. It is essential for the assessment of CAD from functional and anatomical perspectives, and is considered the gate-keeper to invasive coronary angiography. Cardiac tests include exercise electrocardiography, single photon emission computed tomography myocardial perfusion imaging, positron emission tomography myocardial perfusion imaging, stress echocardiography, coronary computed tomography angiography, and stress cardiac magnetic resonance. The wide range of imaging techniques is advantageous for the detection and management of cardiac diseases, and the implementation of preventive measures that can affect the long-term prognosis of these diseases. However, clinicians face a challenge when deciding which test is most appropriate for a given patient. Basic knowledge of each modality will facilitate the decision-making process in CAD assessment.

Keywords: Noninvasive, imaging, coronary artery disease, assessment, diagnosis

1. Introduction

Noninvasive cardiac imaging is crucial for coronary artery disease (CAD) assessment. The increasing global burden of CAD is a major contributor to the marked growth in the use of noninvasive imaging [1]. In recent years, the development of state-of-the-art hardware and software technologies has broadened the perspective and dimension of noninvasive imaging. This is advantageous to hybrid imaging in CAD assessment, with the introduction of anatomical, physiological, or combined approaches. These techniques allow clinicians to move beyond the dichotomous concept of the presence or absence of CAD by increasing their understanding of the unique pathophysiologic processes in CAD, including subclinical atherosclerosis, plaque vulnerability, myocardial blood flow (MBF), and scar detection.

Invasive coronary angiography (ICA), an anatomical test, is considered the gold standard method for the diagnosis of CAD. Nevertheless, the risk of complications precludes the routine use of ICA and it is only indicated in patients with a high pre-test probability of the disease [2]. Because most patients have low or intermediate pre-test probabilities of disease, noninvasive testing should be considered first, serving as a selection process for ICA. Clinicians can choose from a wide range of noninvasive tests, including exercise electrocardiography (ECG), single photon emission computed tomography (SPECT) myocardial perfusion imaging (MPI), positron emission tomography (PET) MPI, stress echocardiography (SE), coronary computed tomography angiography (CCTA), and stress cardiac magnetic resonance (CMR). Therefore, clinicians are frequently faced with the apparently difficult clinical question: "What is the right test?" However, there are no right tests! The test to be used should be selected for each patient after considering the patient's characteristics, genetic and environmental factors, predisposition, risk factors, and comorbidities. Cardiac testing is generally unnecessary in asymptomatic patients except in high-risk occupations or before starting antiarrhythmic drugs.

A basic understanding of the principles, diagnostic, and prognostic accuracy, and the strengths and limitations of each imaging technique is essential. The clinician must then adopt a structured approach, which will help choose the appropriate test to use after considering the risk and benefit profile of each test. The establishment of a diagnosis of CAD will influence the perceived likelihood of a future cardiac event and warrant secondary prevention to slow or prevent disease progression. The absence of CAD on imaging will reassure the patient, and encourage the clinician to adopt a primary prevention strategy. Hence the ultimate goal is for the chosen test to address the clinical question with a high level of certainty. The theme of this chapter is to provide a comprehensive guide to selecting the appropriate imaging test in patients with suspected CAD.

2. Basic concepts for choosing cardiac imaging tests

2.1. Classification of chest pain

There can be varied presentation of chest pain, including jaw pain, epigastric pain, indigestion, shortness of breath, or reduced effort tolerance. Atypical presentations are commonly seen among diabetics, female, and the elderly. Chest pain can be classified using the criteria below [3]:

Criteria:

1.   Substernal chest pain or discomfort

2. Provoked by exertion or emotional stress

3. Relieved by rest ± nitroglycerin

Typical angina: (1) + (2) + (3)

Atypical angina: (1) + (2) or (1) + (3)

Nonanginal chest pain: (1) or none.

2.2. Pre-test and post-test probabilities

Bayes' theorem proposes the use of a combined pre-test probability and test result to determine the post-test probability of disease [4]. This will help the clinician to determine whether a positive test result is a "true positive" or a "false positive" and whether a negative test result is a "true negative" or a "false negative". For example, a positive test result is likely to be a "true positive" result in a 70-year-old patient with typical angina or a "false positive" result in a 40-year-old female with nonanginal chest pain. Meanwhile, a negative test result is likely to be a "true negative" result in a 35-year-old man with atypical chest pain or a "false negative" result in a 60-year-old man with prior myocardial infarction (MI) and typical angina. Pretest probability can be estimated using the Diamond and Forrester classification [5] (Table 1).

Age	Gender	Typical	Atypical	Nonanginal
(years)		Angina	Angina	chest pain
≤ 39	Men	Intermediate	Intermediate	Low
	Women	Intermediate	Very low	Very low
40-49	Men	High	Intermediate	Intermediate
	Women	Intermediate	Low	Very low
50-59	Men	High	Intermediate	Intermediate
	Women	Intermediate	Intermediate	Low
≥ 60	Men	High	Intermediate	Intermediate
	Women	High	Intermediate	Intermediate

Table 1. Diamond and Forrester Pre-Test Probability of Coronary Artery Disease by Age, Sex, and Symptoms. High: >90% pre-test probability. Intermediate: between 10% and 90% pre-test probability. Low: between 5 and 10% pre-test probability. Very low: <5% pre-test probability [5].

2.3. Appropriate use criteria

The appropriate use criteria (AUC) defines appropriate imaging for the different clinical indications. The AUC for test selection among symptomatic patients with suspected CAD [2] (Table 2).

Indication for noninvasive testing in	Exercise	Stress	Stress	Stress	CCTA
symptomatic patients	**ECG**	**MPI**	**Echo**	**CMR**	
Low pretest probability of CAD ECG interpretable AND able to exercise	A	R	M	R	R
Low pretest probability of CAD ECG uninterpretable OR unable to exercise		A	A	M	M
Intermediate pretest probability of CAD ECG interpretable AND able to exercise	A	A	A	M	M
Intermediate pretest probability of CAD ECG uninterpretable OR unable to exercise		A	A	A	A
High pretest probability of CAD ECG interpretable AND able to exercise	M	A	A	A	M
High pretest probability of CAD ECG uninterpretable OR unable to exercise		A	A	A	M

Table 2. Appropriate Use Criteria for noninvasive testing in symptomatic patients for CAD assessment. A= appropriate, M= maybe appropriate, R= rarely appropriate. Uninterpretable ECG refers to resting abnormalities such as ST-segment depression (≥ 0.10 mV), complete left bundle branch block (LBBB), pre-excitation, digoxin use, or ventricular paced rhythm [2].

3. Non-invasive imaging tests

This section will focus on the unique principles, diagnostic and prognostic accuracy, strengths, limitations, representative cases and clinical pearls for each imaging modality.

3.1. Exercise electrocardiography

3.1.1. Background

Exercise ECG is a well-established and validated functional test used for CAD assessment. It has been used for more than 50 years, despite the increasing use of other imaging modalities. It is the first-line test in patients with suspected CAD who are able to exercise and who have an interpretable resting ECG [2]. Studies have demonstrated a lower diagnostic accuracy of exercise ECG in women because of their lower prevalence of CAD. However the risk of major adverse cardiac events (MACE) in women with good functional capacity and a normal resting ECG was not different between those who underwent exercise ECG compared with exercise SPECT MPI, and exercise ECG was considered a cost-effective strategy [6].

3.1.2. Principles

Exercise ECG evaluates the physiological response of the heart to a controlled level of exercise. The latter can be prescribed using specific exercise protocols such as Bruce and Naughton. Exercise ECG and hemodynamic-specific variables are shown to have diagnostic and prognostic value in the assessment of CAD. These variables include ST deviation, exercise capacity, percentage of the maximum age-predicted target heart rate (HR), heart rate recovery (HRR), blood pressure (BP) response, and the Duke Treadmill Score (DTS) [7].

Abnormal ST deviation is defined as ≥1 mm (0.1 mV) of downsloping or horizontal ST-segment depression (J point + 80 ms); or ≥1 mm of ST segment elevation in leads without pathological Q waves (except aVR). The J-point is defined as the junction of the QRS complex and the ST-segment. The ST deviation should be seen in three or more consecutive beats in the same lead to be considered significant [8, 9]. An upsloping ST-segment depression is considered an "equivocal" response and is not suggestive of myocardial ischemia [10]. High risk features include ST-segment depression ≥ 2mm at < 5 metabolic equivalents (METs) in ≥5 leads and ≥5 minutes into recovery [11]. ST-segment elevation in two or more contiguous leads can help localize the site of significant ischemia, unlike ST-segment depression [12]. In the presence of prior Q waves, ST-segment elevation of > 1.0 mm (J point +60 ms) is considered abnormal. This could represent reversible ischemia in the peri-infarct zone or ventricular dyskinesis or akinesis of a segment of the left ventricle. This finding has been demonstrated among patients with anterior (~30%) and inferior (~15%) infarctions [13, 14].

Exercise capacity (a marker of cardiorespiratory fitness) is an estimate of the maximal oxygen uptake for a given workload, and is measured in METs [15]. The prevalence of significant ischemia was 0.4% and 7.1%, based on the workload achieved (≥10 METs and < 7 METs), respectively, on exercise SPECT MPI [16]. Hence, patients who are able to achieve a high workload (≥10 METs) on exercise ECG, may not require additional functional imaging.

The maximum age-predicted HR is usually described as "220-age". The inability to achieve 85% of the maximum age-predicted HR was associated with decreased survival [17].

HRR is calculated as the peak HR achieved (HR at 1 min) [18]. An abnormal HRR is defined as a decrease in the HR of < 12 bpm in the first minute of recovery, and is predictive of mortality.

A normal blood pressure (BP) response is defined as an increase in systolic BP and an increase or decrease in diastolic BP during exercise. A decrease in systolic BP of >10 mmHg may suggest the presence of acute left ventricular dysfunction owing to ischemia [7]. An abnormal BP response may be a specific marker for left main (LM) or triple vessel disease (TVD) [19].

The DTS is calculated as exercise time (minutes) – (5 x ST depression in mm) – (4 x angina index) (0= no angina; 1= nonlimiting angina; 2= limiting angina) [20]. DTS can be categorized into low risk (≥ +5), intermediate risk (-10 to +4) and high risk (≤ -11).

The absolute and relative contraindications for undergoing and termination of an exercise ECG, respectively, is illustrated in Table 3 and Table 4 [9].

Absolute	Relative
Acute myocardial infarction (<48 hours)	Obstructive left main stenosis
Unstable angina	Moderate aortic stenosis
Decompensated heart failure	Hypertrophic obstructive cardiomyopathy with severe resting gradient
Active endocarditis	
	Significant tachyarrhythmias or bradyarrhythmias
Uncontrolled cardiac arrhythmias	High degree atrioventricular (AV) block
Severe symptomatic aortic stenosis	Recent stroke or transient ischemic attack
Acute pulmonary embolism	Mental impairment with limited ability to cooperate
Acute myocarditis or pericarditis	Uncontrolled BP >200/100 mmHg
Acute aortic dissection	Uncorrected medical conditions, e.g. significant anemia, important electrolyte imbalance, and hyperthyroidism
Physical disability that precludes safe and adequate testing	

Table 3. Absolute and relative contraindications for undergoing exercise ECG [9]

Absolute	Relative
ST segment elevation (> 1.0 mm) in leads without preexisting Q waves (other than aVR, aVL and V1)	Marked ST displacement (horizontal or downsloping of >2 mm measured 60 to 80 ms after the J point
Drop in systolic BP >10 mmHg, despite an increase in workload, in the presence of ischemia	Drop in systolic BP >10 mmHg, despite an increase in workload, in the absence of ischemia
Moderate to severe angina	Worsening chest pain
Central nervous system symptoms (e.g. ataxia, dizziness)	Fatigue, shortness of breath, wheezing, leg cramps or claudication
Signs of poor perfusion	Tachyarrhythmias, including multifocal ectopy, ventricular triplets, supraventricular tachycardia
Sustained ventricular tachycardia (VT), 2nd or 3rd degree AV block	Bradyarrhythmias that potentially become more complex or result in hemodyamic instability
Technical difficulties in monitoring the ECG or BP	BP >250/115 mmHg
Patient's request to stop	Development of bundle branch block which is indistinguishable from VT

Table 4. Absolute and relative indications for termination of exercise ECG [9]

3.1.3. Diagnostic and prognostic accuracy

A meta-analysis evaluating the accuracy of exercise ECG reported a sensitivity of 68% and specificity of 77% for the detection of CAD [21]. The discriminatory cut-off point of 1 mm (0.1

mV) of horizontal or downsloping ST-segment depression had a sensitivity of 68% and specificity of 77% [22]. The frequency of significant CAD in patients with low, intermediate, and high DTS was 19.1%, 34.9%, and 89.2%, respectively. In patients with LM or TVD, the frequency of significant CAD was 3.5%, 12.4%, and 46% in patients with low, intermediate, and high DTS, respectively [23]. The 5-year survival rates in patients with a DTS of ≤ -11 and ≥ +7, were 67% and 93%, respectively[24]. In a recent study of 58,020 adults without CAD, the peak METs and the percentage of the maximum predicted HR were highly predictive of survival [25].

In relation to other imaging modalities, significant risk predictors for hard cardiac events in asymptomatic or symptomatic low-risk patients without CAD included abnormal SPECT findings (hazard ratio [HR] = 1.83), ischemia detected by exercise ECG (HR = 1.70), decreasing exercise capacity (HR = 1.11), decreasing DTS (HR = 1.07), and increasing severity of the coronary calcium score (CS) (HR = 1.29). The CS improved the long-term risk prediction for CAD when stratified according to the Framingham Risk Score [26].

3.1.4. Strengths and limitations

The strengths and limitations of an exercise ECG are shown in Table 5.

Strengths	Limitations
Cheap	Low sensitivity
Widely available	Low specificity
No radiation exposure	Unable to localise ischemic territory
No injection	
Short procedural time	
Assess exercise capacity	

Table 5. Strengths and limitations of exercise ECG

3.1.5. Case example 1

A 71-year-old man presents with atypical chest pain, able to exercise, and a normal resting ECG. Risk factors include ex-smoker and hypertension. Pretest probability of CAD is inter-mediate. Based on the AUC, exercise ECG is considered an appropriate test. Resting ECG revealed sinus rhythm at a HR of 61 bpm (Figure 1A). He underwent exercise ECG using Bruce protocol. He exercised for 7 minutes 31 seconds and achieved 10.1 METS. At 6 minutes into the exercise and at a HR of 121 bpm, ECG demonstrated 1 mm horizontal ST-segment depression in leads II, III, aVF, V3 to V6 and reached a maximum of 3 mm at peak stress at HR of 151 bpm in leads II, III, and aVF (Figure 1B). The changes resolved at 1 minutes 50 seconds during recovery. Test was terminated due to fatigue. He developed chest pain at recovery. The calculated DTS = -11.5. Conclusion: Abnormal exercise ECG with a high DTS. He was referred for ICA.

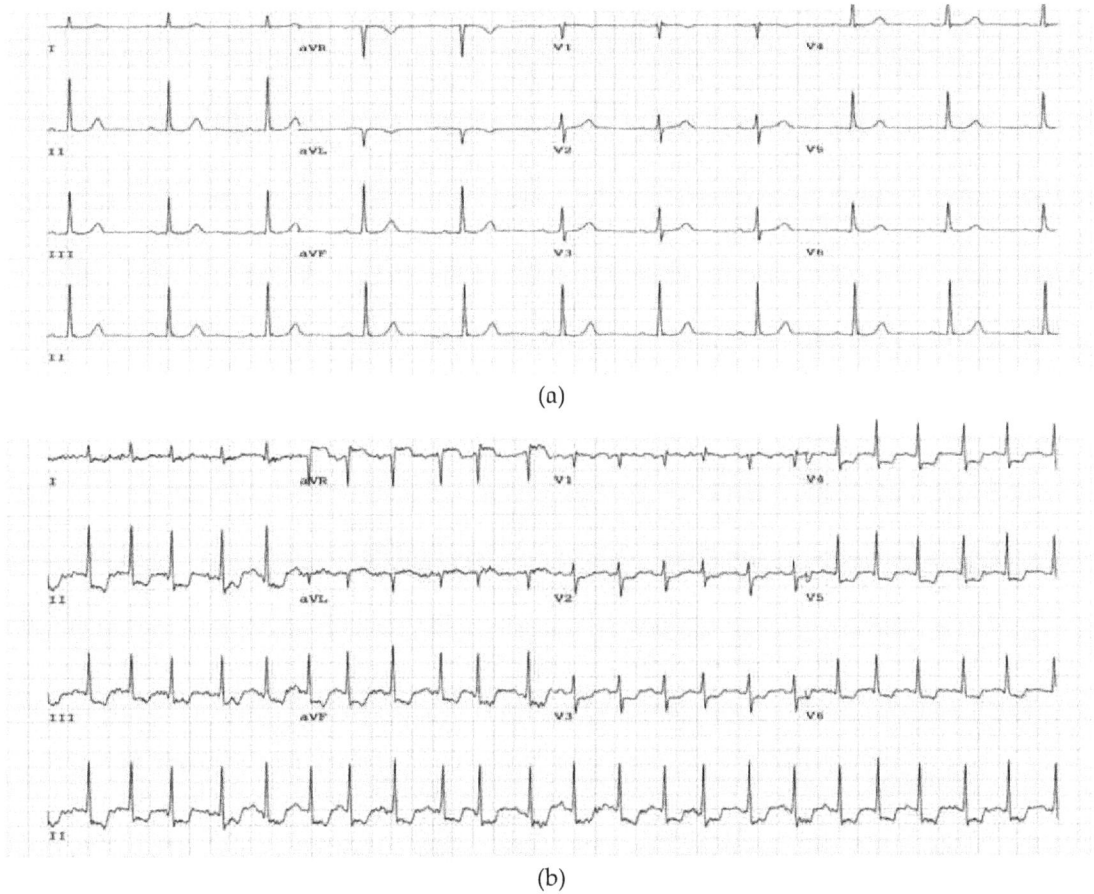

(a)

(b)

Figure 1. (a) Normal resting ECG. (b) Maximum of 3 mm horizontal ST segment depression seen in leads II, III and aVF, 2 mm ST segment depression in leads V3 to V6, at peak stress.

3.1.6. Clinical pearls

1. The J-point is defined as the junction of the QRS complex and the ST segment.

2. Achieving 85% of age predicted HR should not be an indication for test termination.

3. Exercise ECG with a high DTS may warrant ICA.

4. Exercise duration and METs achieved are strong predictors of prognosis.

5. The modification in ECG lead placement during exercise ECG compared to standard ECG may result in shift of the frontal axis to the right, increasing the voltage in the inferior leads, disappearance of Q waves in a patient with prior inferior infarct, or produce artifactual Q waves in normal subjects.

3.2. Single photon emission computed tomography

3.2.1. Background

There is robust evidence supporting the use of SPECT MPI in the workup and risk stratification of patients with suspected or known CAD because of its high diagnostic and prognostic value [27]. The development of solid state detector cameras compared with conventional SPECT (Anger) cameras offer improved signal resolution and shorter image acquisition time, which increases laboratory throughput [28, 29]. The switch from the standard, filtered back projection reconstruction method to iterative algorithms, which include depth independent resolution recovery, noise regularization, and scatter and attenuation correction, has improved the signal-to-noise ratio and image quality. This also allows for low-dose imaging using a standard acquisition time with reduced radiation exposure to the patient and operator,without compromising image quality and accuracy in the detection of CAD [30–32]. This is consistent with the American Society of Nuclear Cardiology's goal to reduce the radiation dose to <9 mSv in 50% of MPI studies by 2014.

3.2.2. Principles

SPECT MPI uses radionuclide-labeled compounds that emit Y ray photons. SPECT perfusion radiotracers include 201-Thallium (Tl-201, half-life $[t_{1/2}]$ = 73 hours), and 99m-Technetium (^{99m}Tc, $t_{1/2}$ = 6 hours)-labeled sestamibi or tetrofosmin. Tl-201 is produced from a cyclotron and ^{99m}Tc is produced by a molybdenum-99-^{99m}Tc generator.

SPECT MPI can be performed using exercise or pharmacological stressors. Exercise is preferred for patients who can exercise at an adequate workload, aiming for a minimum of 85% of the maximal age-predicted HR and 5 METs [33]. A submaximal exercise workload decreases the sensitivity of exercise SPECT MPI for the detection of CAD. Exercise usually increases MBF by 2–3 times of resting flow [24, 34].

A pharmacological stressor should be used in patients who are unable to exercise or those with baseline ECG abnormalities (pre-excitation, paced ventricular rhythm, LBBB). Pharmacological stressors include intravenous vasodilators (adenosine, dipyridamole or regadenoson) or dobutamine, a β-adrenoceptor agonist. Vasodilators activate the adenosine A2A receptor and cause coronary arteriolar vasodilatation. Vasodilators increase MBF by 3–5 times in normal coronary vessels, an increase termed as the coronary flow reserve. Meanwhile, dobutamine increases MBF similar to that induced by exercise. In the presence of flow limiting stenosis, the coronary vessel is maximally vasodilated at baseline. Hence, the administration of a vasodilator is unable to augment coronary flow. MPI assesses the regional flow heterogeneity in normal and diseased coronary vessels [35]. Generally, vasodilators do not cause myocardial ischemia because MBF increases, albeit with some variability in all coronary artery beds with a minimal or no increase in the rate-pressure product, a measure of myocardial oxygen demand. In patients with extensive CAD, ischemia can be induced by the coronary steal phenomenon [33]. Vasodilators may also activate other adenosine receptors (A1, A2B, and A3) resulting in bronchospasm (A2B and, A3) or AV conduction delay (A1). Regadenoson is a selective A2A receptor agonist that is better than other vasodilators in patients with moderate chronic obstructive pulmonary disease (COPD) or asthma [36, 37].

For pharmacological stress SPECT MPI, contraindications include asthma or COPD with active wheezing, 2nd or 3rd degree AV block without a pacemaker or sick sinus syndrome, systolic BP <90 mmHg, use of methylxanthines (e.g., aminophylline or caffeine) <12 hours, known hypersensivity to the vasodilator, acute myocardial infarction (MI) and acute coronary syndrome [33].

3.2.3. Diagnostic and prognostic accuracy

The diagnostic accuracy of all noninvasive tests is subject to the post-test referral bias, also known as the verification bias. This increases the sensitivity and reduces the specificity of the test. A normalcy rate is used as a surrogate for specificity. It is defined as the percentage of normal perfusion scans in patients with a low likelihood (<10%) of CAD based on the results of clinical and ECG stress tests [38–40]. A pooled analysis of 4,480 patients with known or suspected CAD showed that exercise SPECT MPI had a mean sensitivity of 87% and a specificity of 73% for the detection of >50% stenosis [41]. The normalcy rate of SPECT MPI is around 84% [38]. Standard MPI studies include a combination of stress and rest protocols. The use of a stress-only protocol with a "normal" stress study can reduce the radiation dose by 40% and detected similar event rates [42–44]. A "normal" stress-only study is defined as homogenous perfusion, summed stress score (SSS) of <3, normal left ventricular (LV) cavity size, function, and wall motion [43].

The prognostic value of a normal pharmacological stress MPI test is independent of the radiopharmaceutical used [45]. A meta-analysis of 19 SPECT MPI studies comprising 39,000 patients demonstrated a low annual event rate of 0.6%, for hard cardiac events such as cardiac death or nonfatal MI in patients with a normal test result [46]. However, the prognostic value is based on the studied population. For example, the annual event rate among individuals with a normal test result was higher among diabetic patients than in non-diabetic subjects (0.5% vs. 1.7%, respectively, p < 0.005). Diabetic patients with a LV ejection fraction (LVEF) of ≤ 45% had the worst outcome [47]. High-risk MPI variables include large perfusion defect size and extent, transient ischemic dilatation (TID), post stress stunning, increased right ventricular uptake, and increased lung uptake especially with Tl-201. A normal perfusion on exercise SPECT MPI was associated with a low event rate (<1% per year) in subjects with a low or intermediate DTS, compared in subjects with an intermediate DTS and high-risk SPECT variables or those with a high DTS and a normal perfusion [48].

3.2.4. Strengths and limitations

The strengths and limitations of SPECT using ^{99m}Tc-labeled sestamibi or tetrofosmin are shown in Table 6.

3.2.5. Case example 2

A 60-year-old female with hypertension presented with atypical chest pain. Pre-test probability of CAD is intermediate. Pharmacological (dipyridamole) SPECT MPI was performed due to an uninterpretable resting ECG that showed a LBBB. The test is considered appropriate based on the AUC. SPECT MPI demonstrated normal perfusion (Figure 2).

Strengths	Limitations
Widely available	Low specificity
High sensitivity	Lower spatial resolution
Expensive	Prone to attenuation artifacts
Well validated	Long procedural time (≈4 hrs)
Exercise and pharmacological stress	Longer half life of tracers
Improved specificity with gated SPECT	Increase hepatobiliary uptake
	Radiation exposure

Table 6. Strengths and limitations of ^{99m}Tc-labelled sestamibi or tetrofosmin SPECT MPI

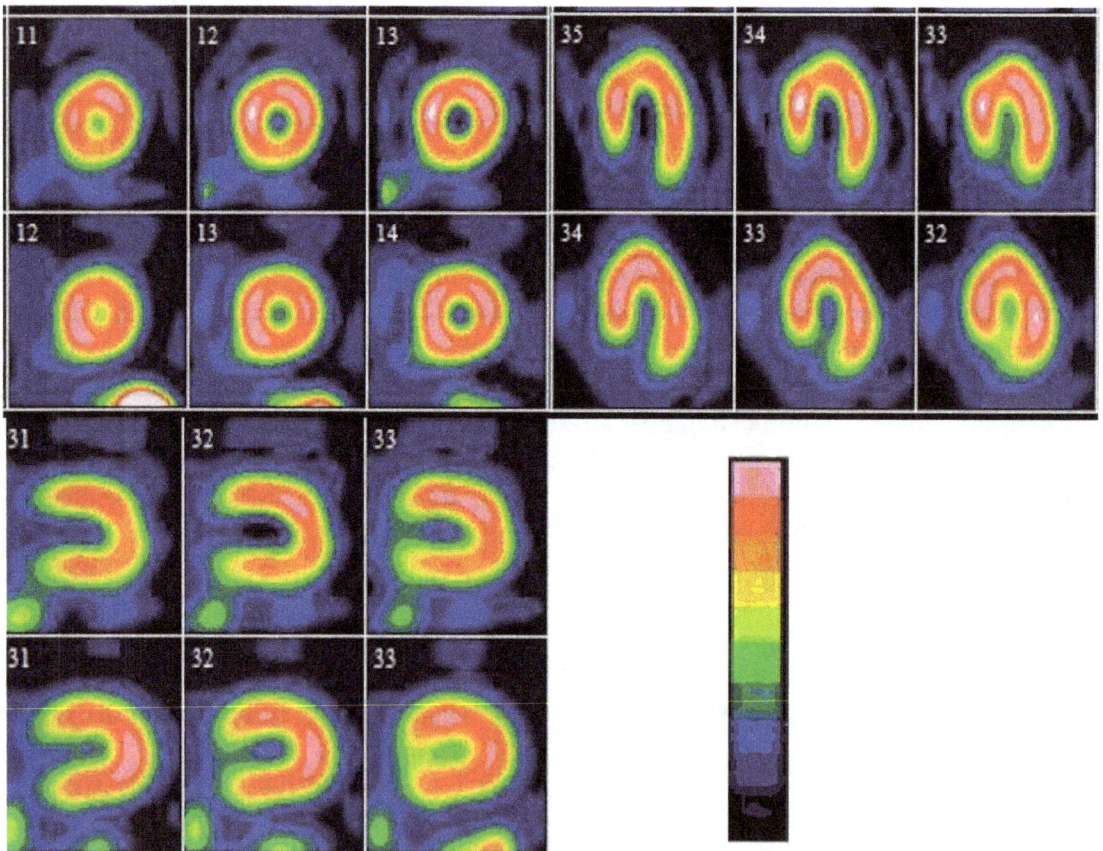

Figure 2. Stress (top row) & Rest (bottom row) images in the short axis (SA), horizontal long axis (HLA) and vertical long axis (VLA) show normal homogenous tracer uptake. Gated images showed normal left ventricular ejection fraction (not shown). This is a normal SPECT MPI study.

3.2.6. Case example 3

A 58-year-old man with a history of hyperlipidemia presented with typical angina (Canadian Cardiovascular Society Class 2). Pre-test probability of CAD: High. He underwent exercise SPECT MPI, which is considered an appropriate test based on the AUC. Baseline ECG showed sinus rhythm (Figure 3A) and resting BP of 140/90 mmHg. At 2 minutes in Bruce protocol, he developed significant ST-segment depression (Figure 3B). A significant BP drop from 140/90 mmHg to 80/60 mmHg during exercise was present and the test was terminated. The ECG changes persisted 5:50 minutes into recovery, and BP gradually returned to baseline. He achieved a total of 5 METS. He remained asymptomatic of chest pain. Calculated DTS was -17 (high risk). SPECT MPI findings as described in Figure 3C. He was referred for ICA (Figure 3D).

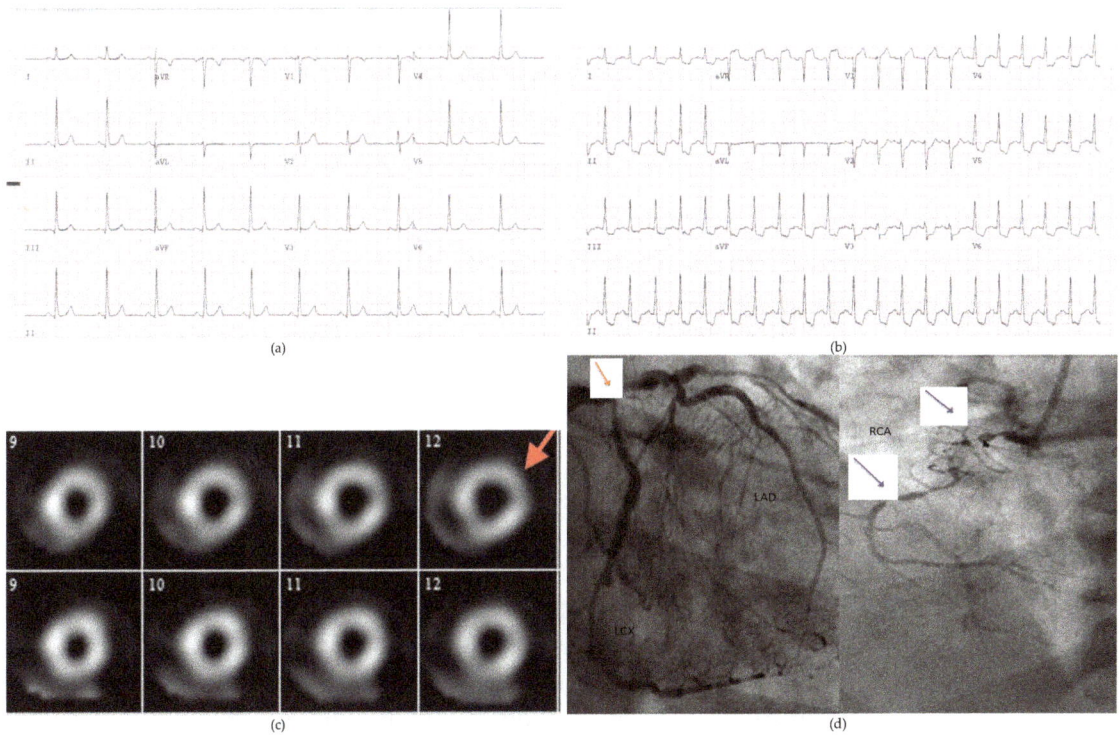

Figure 3. (a) Resting ECG showed normal sinus rhythm (b) ECG showed 3 mm ST segment depression in leads 1, aVF and V3, and a maximum of 4 mm ST segment depression leads II, V4 to V6. (c) Stress (top row), Rest (bottom row) in the SA slices: Mild reduction in tracer uptake in the mid to distal anterolateral walls (arrow) which normalized at rest. This was consistent with mild ischemia in the left circumflex (LCX) artery/ left anterior descending artery territory (LAD). TID is defined as the ratio of ungated LV volumes at stress and rest was present (1.21). TID is due to extensive subendocardial ischemia post stress that resolves on the rest images. ICA showed distal left main 90%, ostial LAD 90%, first diagonal 90%, first obtuse marginal 100%, second obtuse marginal 100%, right coronary artery 100%, and subsequently referred for CABG. This example clearly illustrates, despite a mildly abnormal perfusion (i.e. mild reduction in myocardial tracer uptake), the associated presence of high risk variables such as TID, and a high DTS, identifies a high risk scan. (d) Significant stenosis in the ostial LAD (orange arrow) and occluded proximal RCA with diffuse disease (purple arrows).

4. Clinical pearls

1. Combination of low-level exercise with dipyridamole can improve image quality and reduce symptoms resulting from drug effects.

2. High-risk findings include large defect size and extent, TID, post-stress stunning, increased right ventricular uptake, and increased lung uptake.

3. The prognosis of a normal MPI study is dependent on the study population.

4. A normal SPECT perfusion scan with ischemic ECG changes during vasodilator stress is associated with a significant cardiac event rate (~2% per year) and should be followed up with further cardiac imaging (PET MPI or CCTA).

5. Avoid antianginal medications such as beta-blockers, calcium channel blockers, or nitrates at least 48 hours prior to stress MPI for ischemia detection in suspected CAD.

4.1. Positron emission tomography

4.1.1. Background

PET MPI has superior temporal and spatial resolution, greater count sensitivity, and accurate attenuation correction compared with SPECT. These features translate into greater diagnostic image quality with fewer equivocal results, especially in obese subjects for example [49, 50]. The latest generation of PET cameras are combined with CT usually with ≥16 slices, and provide 3-dimensional imaging. Integrated PET (emission scan)/CT (transmission scan) systems facilitate sequential scanning, faster acquisition of transmission images, and enable functional and anatomic assessments in a single study [51–53]. These features make PET a useful clinical choice, but widespread utilization is limited by cost.

4.1.2. Principles

PET imaging is based on the detection of positron emission from radionuclide decay. After emission, the positron travels a short distance before it collides with an electron, resulting in mutual annihilation. This annihilation results in the production of 2 Y photons of 511 keV that travel in nearly opposite directions. The simultaneous detection of both photons by the detector of a PET camera is called coincidence detection [51–53].

Examples of cardiac PET radiotracers include rubidium-82 (^{82}Rb; $t_{1/2}$ = 76 s), nitrogen-13 ammonia (^{13}N- Ammonia; $t_{1/2}$ = 9.96 min), and oxygen-15 water (^{15}O-H$_2$O; $t_{1/2}$ = 2 min). A shorter $t_{1/2}$ allows a lower radiation dose per test. Radiotracers are produced by a cyclotron, except for ^{82}Rb, which is eluted from a strontium-82 (^{82}Sr)/^{82}Rb generator.

Ischemia is detected in the same way as for SPECT MPI. The fundamental difference in uptake kinetics of radiotracers used in SPECT and PET explain the superior sensitivity of PET for the detection of CAD. The ideal radiotracer is ^{15}O-H$_2$O, which has linear uptake by myocardial tissue with increasing blood flow and "no roll-off" phenomenon. ^{99m}Tc- labeled tracers have a much lower extraction fraction. At high MBF, ^{99m}Tc- labeled tracers are characterized by a roll-off phenomenon to a greater degree, unlike PET radiotracers [54]. At high MBF levels during stress, the relative difference in myocardial tracer uptake may be reduced leading to an underestimation of the regional flow heterogeneity between normal and diseased coronary arteries. With dynamic imaging of the tracer kinetics in PET MPI, it is feasible to measure the myocardial flow reserve (MFR), which is defined as the ratio of absolute MBF during stress compared to MBF at rest. An abnormal global MFR is indicative of diffuse atherosclerosis or microvascular dysfunction.

4.1.3. Diagnostic and prognostic accuracy

PET MPI showed superior sensitivity and diagnostic accuracy, compared to SPECT [55, 56]. A meta-analysis of three different stress perfusion modalities determined the pooled sensitivity, specificity, and area under the curve of SPECT (88%, 61%, and 0.86, respectively), CMR (89%, 76%, and 0.90, respectively) and PET (84%, 81%, and 0.92, respectively) for the detection of CAD [57].

PET MPI can be used to determine prognosis, revealing annual event rates for cardiac death and nonfatal MI of 0.4%, 2.3%, and 7.0% for SSS values of <4 (normal), 4–7, and >8, respectively [58]. A similar trend was noted when subjects were stratified according to the percentage of ischemic LV myocardium, with a relative hazard for cardiac death of 2.3%, 4.2%, and 4.9% for the strata of 0.1–9.9%, 10–19.9%, and $\geq$ 20%, respectively [59]. Parameters that measure the extent of ischemia have been shown to guide the decisions regarding revascularization [60]. An abnormal global MFR (<2.0) was associated with an increased incidence of MACE compared with a normal MFR (1.3% vs. 4.7%, $p = 0.03$), independent of a normal perfusion and a CS of 0 [61].

4.1.4. Strengths and limitations

The strengths and limitations of PET MPI are shown in Table 7.

Strengths	Limitations
High spatial resolution	Expensive
Robust attenuation correction	Not widely available
Improved diagnostic accuracy in the obese	Radiation exposure
Alternative for an equivocal SPECT study	Unable to assess exercise capacity
Short half life of tracers	Pharmacological stress
Absolute MBF	
Assessment of calcium on CT	

Table 7. Strengths and limitations of PET MPI

4.1.5. Case example 4

A 68-year-old female with obesity, hypertension and an ex-smoker presented with chest pain. Noncontrast CT showed a CS of 715. CCTA was not performed. A persantine ^{82}Rb PET MPI was performed (Figure 4A) and gated images were acquired at stress and rest (Figure 4B). Coronary calcium was visualised on CT and MBF was abnormal (Figure 4C).

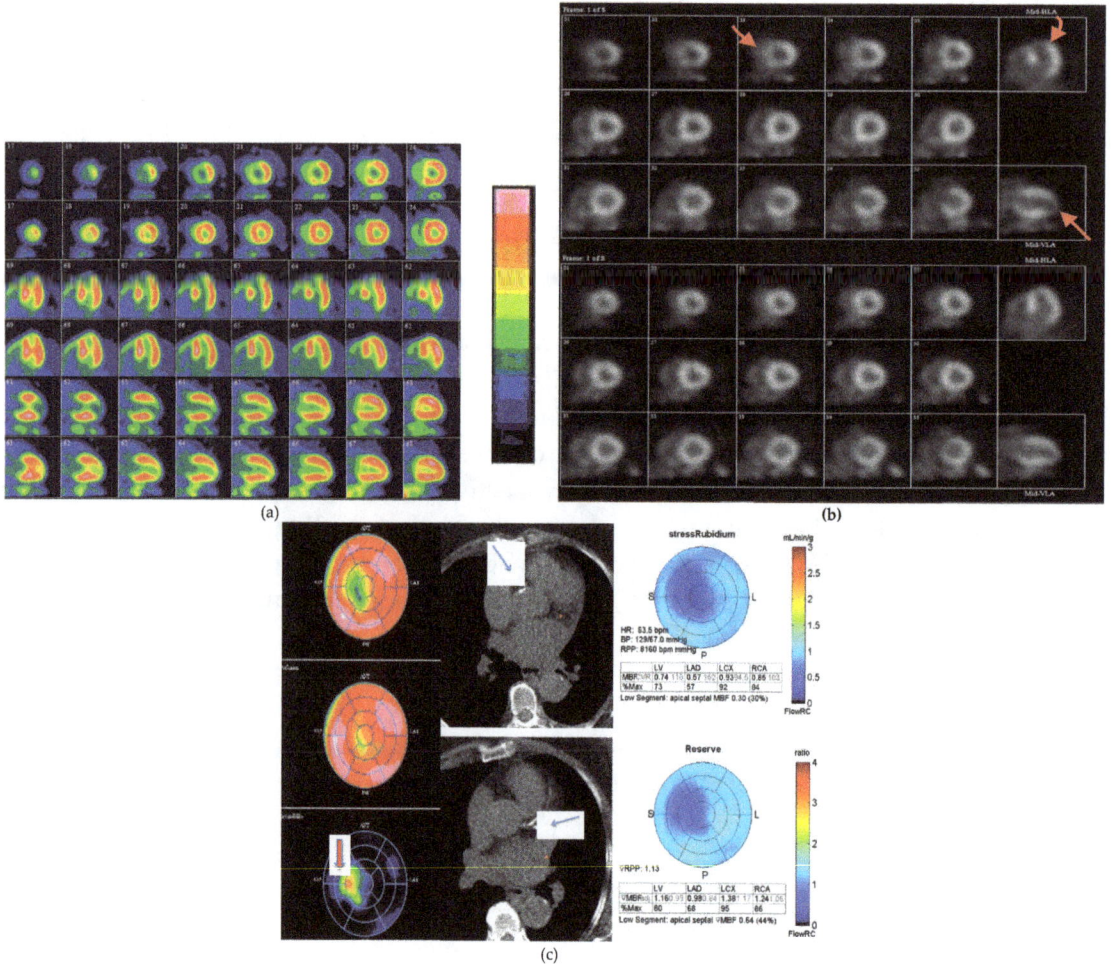

Figure 4. (a) Following stress, there is mild to moderate reduction in tracer uptake in the apical (distal) segments of the septum and anterior wall, and apex, which predominantly improves at the rest. This is consistent with a moderate sized area of moderate ischemia in the distal LAD territory. Stress images (rows 1, 3, and 5) and rest images (rows 2, 4, and 6). (b) Gated stress (top 3 rows) and gated rest (bottom 3 rows) during PET MPI. Normal LVEF and wall motion at rest. Following stress, there is mild hypokinesis in the apical (distal) septum and apex consistent with stress induced ischemia (red arrows). Stress acquisition during PET MPI is acquired at peak stress, and hence presence of regional wall motion is specific for ischemia. This differs from post-stress acquisition during SPECT which is delayed by 30 to 45 minutes. (c) Polar map shows the extent of reversible ischemia in the LAD territory (red arrow). CT shows presence of coronary calcification in the RCA (top, blue arrow), LCX and LAD (bottom, blue arrow). MBF demonstrate marked reduction in stress flow in the areas of reduced perfusion (global MBF= 0.74 ml/min/g), as depicted by the polar map which is labelled as stress Rubidium. Global MFR is reduced at 1.16, and 0.99 (after correction for RPP). There is reduced regional MFR in all three coronary artery territories (LAD= 0.98, LCX= 1.38, and RCA= 1.24), as seen on the polar map labelled as Reserve. The MFR finding is suggestive of underlying triple vessel disease. Measurement of MBF is corrected for rate-pressure product (RPP), and depicted in the shade of gray, next to the uncorrected values.

4.1.6. Clinical pearls

1. PET imaging is based on positron annihilation and coincidence detection of paired 511 keV Y photons.

2. PET has higher diagnostic accuracy compared to SPECT in the assessment of obstructive CAD.

3. PET is an excellent choice for imaging in the obese and those with an equivocal SPECT.

4. Abnormal global MFR suggest diffuse atherosclerosis or microvascular dysfunction.

5. Patient motion can result in significant misregistration artifact between the emission and transmission scans.

6. Normal PET perfusion and MFR confer an excellent prognosis.

4.2. Stress echocardiography

4.2.1. Background

SE is a robust, versatile imaging modality for CAD assessment. Advances in digital image acquisition, strain imaging, tissue harmonics, and contrast agents have increased the use of SE. In particular, the advances in tissue harmonics and contrast agents have greatly improved the visualization of endocardial borders, and diagnostic accuracy of SE for the detection of wall motion abnormalities (WMA) [62–64]. Because SE is highly operator- dependent, those who perform the test should have adequate training and experience to meet the level of competency required for performing and interpreting this test [65].

4.2.2. Principles

The fundamental principle for the detection of myocardial ischemia is the development of new or worsening WMA during stress [65, 66]. Based on the ischemic cascade, WMA appear after perfusion abnormalities and precede the manifestation of ECG changes and symptoms. Thus, SE has decreased sensitivity and superior specificity compared to perfusion-based imaging for the detection of CAD. Images are acquired at rest and stress. The images are compared on a four-screen setup side-by-side for WMA, LV cavity size and LVEF.

The stress component may be exercise (treadmill or bicycle) or pharmacologically (dobutamine or dipyridamole). An adequate level of stress using exercise requires a minimum target of 85% of the age-predicted HR, and is preferably symptom-limiting, considering the additional prognostic value of the subject's exercise capacity. Bicycle SE (supine or upright ergometry) allows simultaneous image acquisition during peak stress, and the measurement of Doppler information. During treadmill exercise SE, the stress images are acquired within 60–90 seconds post stress. The contraindications and indications for terminating an exercise SE are similar to those of exercise ECG.

Pharmacological SE using dobutamine is preferred over dipyridamole for wall motion assessment [65], although either stressor can be used [67]. The dose for dipyridamole in SE is higher at 0.84 mg/kg over 10 minutes, compared to the dose used in nuclear perfusion imaging at 0.14 mg/kg/min over 4 minutes. A typical dobutamine infusion rate is at 5 micrograms/kg/min and increasing at a 3-minute interval to 10, 20, 30, and 40 micrograms/kg/min, aiming to achieve 85% of the age-predicted target HR. Atropine can be used to achieve the desired target HR. The induction of ischemia is due to an increase in myocardial oxygen demand. Deformation analysis using the tissue velocity index (TVI) and two-dimensional speckle tracking (ST)-based strain imaging have been proposed using dobutamine SE [68, 69]. However, TVI- and ST-based analysis conferred no additional diagnostic value over WMA for detection of ischemia [70].

Indications for terminating the test include the de novo or worsening of WMA, significant arrhythmias, hypotension, severe hypertension, and intolerable symptoms. For image interpretation, normal wall motion is defined as normal wall thickening and endocardial excursion. Visual assessment of wall motion can be categorized and scored as follows: 1 = normal, 2 = hypokinetic, 3 = akinetic, 4 = dyskinetic or aneurysmal. Please note that a score of "5" is no longer applicable. Each segment using the 16 segment LV model (i.e., apical cap not included) is scored and the wall motion score index (WMSI) is calculated. A normal WMSI equals to "1". WMSI = Total wall motion score/ Total number segments visualised. Unlike in MPI that utilizes the 17 segment model, for WMA assessment the 16 segment model is preferred. A WMSI of >1.7 corresponds to a perfusion defect of >20% on MPI. If feasible, the right ventricular wall motion should be assessed and presence of WMA suggest greater extent of CAD.

Normal: normal at rest; hyperdynamic at stress

Ischemia: normal at rest; inducible new or worsening WMA (hypokinesis, akinesis or dyskinesis) at stress

Infarction: fixed abnormality at rest and stress

4.2.3. Diagnostic and prognostic accuracy

The development of WMA depends on the extent of stenosis detected by ICA, and occurs at a cut-off relative diameter of 54% for exercise SE, 58% for dobutamine SE, and 60% for dipyridamole SE [71]. The sensitivities and specificities for the detection of CAD were 85% and 77%, respectively, for exercise SE, 80% and 86%, respectively for dobutamine SE, and 78% and 91%, respectively, for dipyridamole SE [71, 72]. SE had a similar diagnostic accuracy to that of SPECT MPI for the detection of CAD [73, 74]. However, because of its greater specificity, SE showed a better discriminatory capacity for the diagnosis of LM and TVD [75]. For patients presenting at an emergency department with chest pain, nondiagnostic ECG, and negative cardiac biomarkers, the overall sensitivity, specificity, positive predictive value (PPV), and negative predictive value (NPV) of SE for the diagnosis of CAD were 90%, 92%, 78% and 97%, respectively. Moreover, exercise SE had a better specificity than dobutamine SE [76].

A normal exercise SE result is associated with an excellent prognosis with an annual event rate of cardiac events of 0.54% [77]. The best discriminator of increased risk of cardiac events was WMSI ≥ 1.25 and ≤ 6 METs in both genders [78]. There was no difference in the prognostic value of dobutamine SE and dipyridamole SE [79, 80]. Therefore, the choice between these techniques may depend on institutional practices. With regards to LV cavity size, an abnormal stress LV end-systolic volume (LVESV) (i.e., no change or an increase) was associated with an increase risk of cardiac events compared with a decrease in the LVESV (2.9% vs. 1.6%) [81].

4.2.4. Strengths and limitations

The strengths and limitations of SE are shown in TABLE 8.

Strengths	Limitations
Cheap	Poor echo window (obese, COPD)
Widely available	Reduced sensitivity in detection of posterior wall ischemia
No radiation	Foreshortened LV apex
Portable	Operator dependent
Contrast echo improves endocardial definition	
Exercise and pharmacological stress	
Medium procedural time	

Table 8. Strengths and limitations of stress echocardiography

4.2.5. Case example 5

65-year-old woman with rheumatoid arthritis and hypertension presented with heartburn and indigestion of increasing severity for 1 month. An exercise SE with contrast was performed at rest. She experienced a similar episode of heartburn and nausea at 2 minutes into exercise. The test was stopped and stress images were acquired immediately (Figure 5A). Rest and stress images are shown as still frames captured at end-systole (Figure 5B i-iv). The patient was admitted in view of a positive SE at low workload. ICA showed ostial LAD 70%, mid LAD 90%, proximal LCX 80%, and mid RCA 100%. She was referred for CABG.

4.2.6. Clinical pearls

1. Normal wall motion at rest does not rule out the presence of obstructive CAD.

2. Abnormal regional wall motion can be seen in the presence of ischemic or nonischemic etiology.

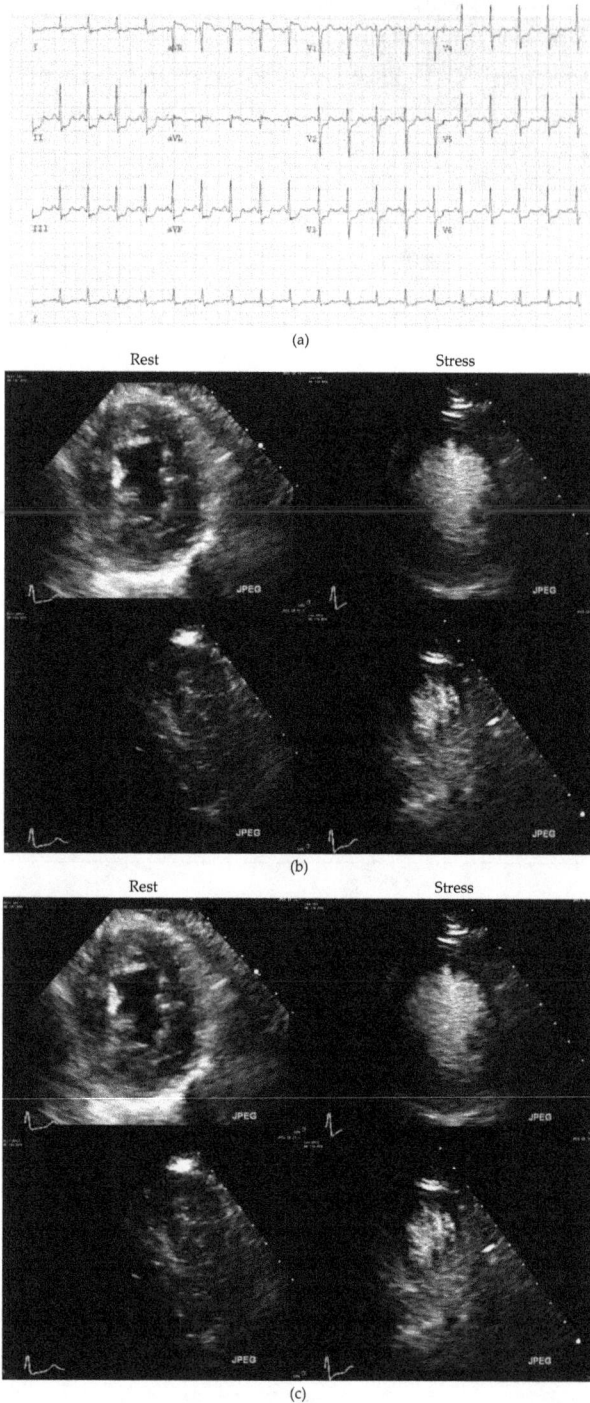

Figure 5. (a) ECG during episode of chest pain demonstrated diffuse 2 mm ST segment depression in leads II, III, aVF, V2 to V6 and ST elevation in aVR. (b) SE using contrast showing images captured at end-systole during rest and stress. The LV in different views are illustrated in the following sequence from top to bottom (i) parasternal long axis, (ii) 2-chamber, (iii) short axis, (iv) apical, demonstrate regional WMA in the anterior, anteroseptum, apex and lateral walls. Note the stress induced LV cavity dilatation, at peak stress which is suggestive of underlying triple vessel disease.

3. The absence of radial motion of the mitral valve annulus can result in a reduction in motion of the basal inferior or inferoseptal segments resulting in a false-positive study.

4. A common cause of a false negative test is a suboptimal stress level.

4.3. Coronary computed tomography angiography

4.3.1. Background

CCTA has come a long way from electron beam CT to the present multidetector CT system, with continually increasing detector rows (i.e., = slices) from 4-slices to 320-slices in some systems. A 64-slice CT system is the minimum requirement for coronary imaging. Other developments include iterative reconstruction, dual-source CT, prospective scanning, tube current modulation, and a z-flying focal spot [82]. These innovations have led to significant improvements in spatial and temporal resolution, radiation dosimetry, and image quality, which are prerequisites for coronary imaging. The ability to visualize subclinical atherosclerosis and characterize plaques has led to techniques for quantifying the extent of the atherosclerotic burden [83].

4.3.2. Principles

CCTA can determine the extent of coronary atherosclerosis and estimate the severity of coronary artery stenosis. The major components of a CT scanner include the table, X-ray tube, detector array and the gantry that rotates the X-ray tube and detector array around the patient. The ability to image a beating heart requires a high temporal resolution, which is defined as the time taken to obtain a complete data set for image reconstruction. The typical temporal resolution of CT is 280–420 ms. Data covering 180° are needed to construct one image, termed "half scan reconstruction". Accordingly, the temporal resolution of a single-source CT system is half the time required for the gantry to rotate 360°. For a dual-source CT (DSCT), the temporal resolution is one-quarter of the gantry rotation time, because data covering 90° are sufficient for image acquisition. A DSCT has a temporal resolution of 75 ms (compared to 20–30 ms for ICA) [84].

The ability for CT to discriminate two structures is called the spatial resolution, which is measured in line pairs per centimeter (lp/cm). The typical spatial resolution of CT is 10 lp/cm, which is equivalent to 0.5 mm (compared to 0.1 mm for ICA). CT data are acquired as isotropic voxels enabling the images to be viewed in multiple planes with similar spatial resolutions [85]. The spatial resolution of CT is less than ideal to accurately quantitate the degree of stenosis, hence a grading method is used [86]:

Normal: 0%; Minimal: <25%; Mild: 25–49%; Moderate: 50–69%; Severe: 70–99%; Occluded: 100%.

ECG gating is essential to minimize cardiac motion by synchronizing image acquisition to the cardiac cycle. There are two types of scanning modes. In prospective ECG-triggered scanning, data acquisition is triggered by the R waves on the ECG. Its advantage is the low radiation dose, typically 3–5 mSv. Disadvantages include image reconstruction limited to the desired phase and functional evaluation is not possible. In retrospective ECG-gated scanning, data acquisition are acquired throughout the cardiac cycle and the ECG signal is simultaneously recorded with the raw data. Advantages include image reconstruction can be performed at any point in the cardiac cycle and it is useful in patients with arrhythmias. Its main disadvantage is the high radiation dose, typically 10–12 mSv because the tube current remains "on" throughout image acquisition. The application of tube current modulation can reduce the radiation dose. The best phase for image acquisition is mid-diastole, when the heart is moving the least.

The images to be acquired are the initial scout image, which defines the scan length, followed by a non-contrast calcium scan and finally the contrast-enhanced CT images. The average scan length for native coronary artery imaging is 12–14 cm. Using a 64-slice scanner, images are acquired over a few cardiac cycles, as opposed to a 320-slice scanner where one cardiac cycle is sufficient because of the larger volume covered. Data can be reconstructed in two or three dimensions, although the two-dimensional axial views should serve as a reference for image interpretation.

Contrast enhancement in the ascending aorta can be tracked using a test bolus or automated bolus tracking. Both methods are acceptable and the choice between them may depend on the institutional protocol. About 80–100 ml of iodinated contrast is typically used. The target HR of 50–65 bpm can be achieved by oral or intravenous β-adrenoceptor blockers. Nitroglycerin spray is recommended to improve image quality by inducing coronary vasodilatation.

Calcium is measured using the Agatston score (i.e., CS), which correlates with the extent of the atherosclerotic plaque burden. Screening for CS are recommended in two groups of asymptomatic patients: (1) patients with low global coronary heart disease (CHD) risk and a family history of premature CAD and (2) patients with intermediate global CHD risk [87]. CT perfusion is still research-based, and will not be discussed in this review.

4.3.3. Diagnostic and prognostic accuracy

There is extensive literature describing the diagnostic and prognostic value of CCTA. The main advantage of CCTA is the ability to exclude disease from the differential diagnosis since CCTA has an excellent NPV. The ACCURACY trial demonstrated sensitivity, specificity, PPV, and NPV of 95%, 83%, 64%, and 99%, respectively, for the detection of ≥ 50% stenosis, and 94%, 83%, 48%, and 99%, respectively, for the detection of ≥70% stenosis. The NPV was high in patient- and vessel-level analyses [88]. The low PPV is due to its tendency to overestimate stenosis, while the presence of artefacts lead may lead to a false positive test. CCTA is considered appropriate for patients with low or intermediate pre-test probabilities of CAD, and a negative scan reliably indicates the absence of significant CAD. However, CCTA is of limited clinical value and functional imaging tests are more appropriate in patients with a high pre-test probability [89]. The presence of severe coronary calcification (CS >400) can reduce the diagnostic accuracy by overestimating the severity of stenosis owing to blooming artefacts [88]. Although there is no specific cut-off level to cancel a CCTA, CS of > 600–1000 is typically used for this purpose, considering the high likelihood of a nondiagnostic study.

The use of CCTA in the emergency department resulted in a shorter hospital stay, increased discharge rate [90, 91], and reduced time to CAD diagnosis [90], while patients with a negative scan had an excellent prognosis [92]. The all-cause mortality rate was 0.65% for normal CCTA, 1.99% for <50% stenosis, 2.9% for ≥50% stenosis, and 4.95% for LM ≥50%, TVD ≥70%, or two vessel disease with proximal LAD disease [93]. The excellent prognosis of a negative CCTA result was seen in other large series of patients [94]. The "warranty period" of a normal CCTA is ~7 years [95]. Coronary calcium has prognostic value beyond traditional risk factors with a hazard ratio of 3.89, 7.08, and 6.84 for CS of 1–100, 101–300, and ≥300, respectively, for coronary events [96].

4.3.4. Strengths and limitations

The strengths and limitations of CCTA are shown in Table 9.

Strengths	Limitations
Excellent negative predictive	High calcium limits accuracy
value	of assessing stenosis
High temporal resolution	Radiation exposure
High spatial resolution	Morbidly obese
Visualize coronary anatomy	Arrhythmias
Short procedural time	Allergy to iodinated contrast
Assessment of calcium score	Heart rate control
	Follow breath hold instruction
	Renal impairment (>2.0 mg/dl)
	No functional assessment

Table 9. Strengths and limitations of CCTA

4.3.5. Case example 6

A 71-year-old female with hypertension, hyperlipidemia, and an ex- smoker presented with atypical chest pain and LBBB. CCTA was performed. Findings included a CS of 269, and ≥70% stenosis (calcified and noncalcified plaque) with positive remodeling in the mid LAD (Figure 6). There was mild disease in ostium of the RCA. She was referred for ICA.

4.3.6. Case example 7

A 57-year-old man with hypertension. CCTA showed a CS of 524 with an occluded proximal RCA. He was referred for ICA and underwent percutaneous coronary intervention to the RCA (Figure 7 A-E).

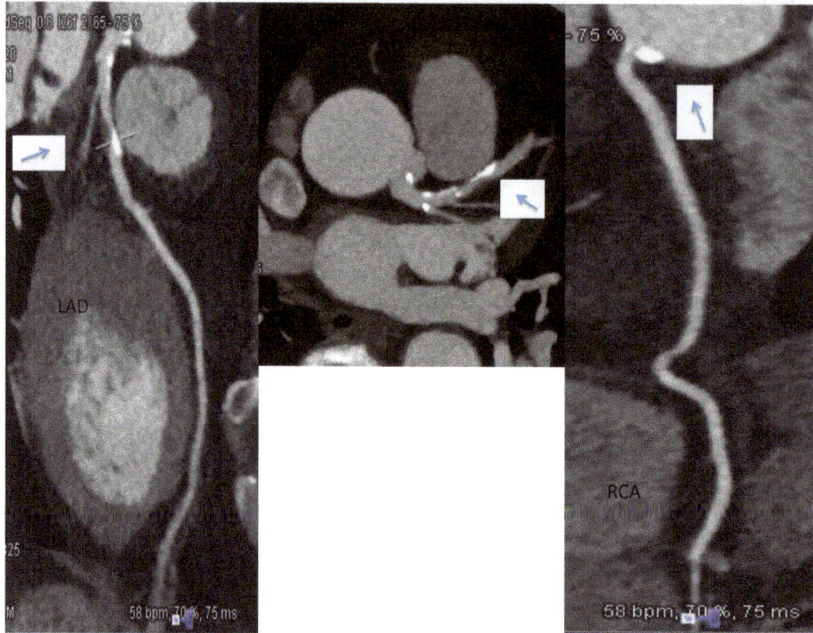

Figure 6. First two images of the curved multiplanar reformatted (MPR) and 2D-axial views demonstrate ≥70% stenosis of the LAD (blue arrows). The third image (curved MPR) of the RCA showing a calcified plaque with minimal stenosis at the ostium (blue arrow).

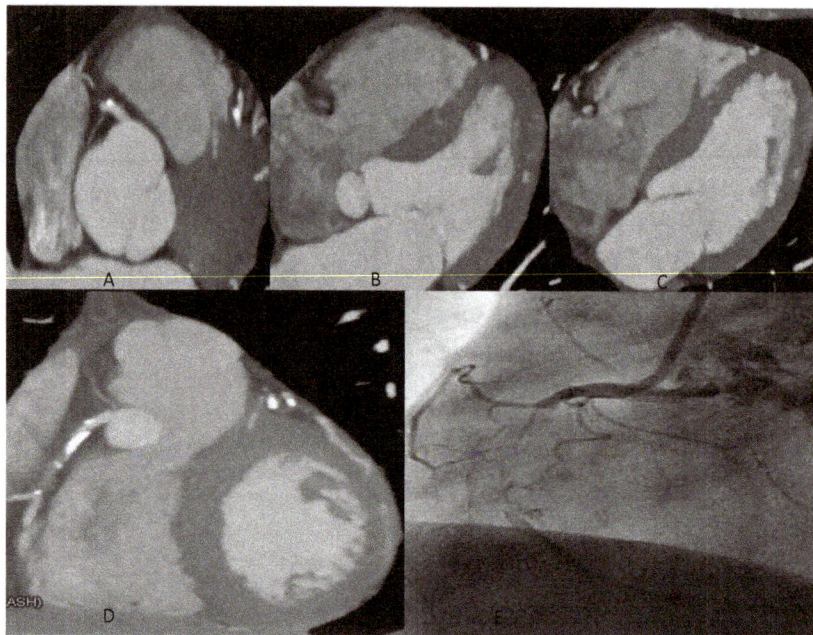

Figure 7. Axial slices from cranial to caudal demonstrate (A) contrast enhanced lumen in the proximal RCA, (B) absent of contrast enhancement and (C) reappearance of the contrast in the RCA. (D) Axial maximum intensity projection of the RCA demonstrate an occluded vessel and correlates with ICA (E).

4.3.7. Clinical pearls

1. An asymptomatic patient with a CS of 0 has a very low event rate of 0.1% per year [97].

2. Prospective ECG-triggered acquisition is preferred in view of the lower radiation dose.

3. Regular, low HR and obeying breath-hold instructions are essential for diagnostic image quality.

4. Appropriate timing of contrast injection is crucial for optimal enhancement as contrast non-uniformity in the distal coronary vessels can simulate stenoses.

5. Volume coverage in the z-axis for a 64-slice CT (0.625 mm detector width) is 4 cm (64 x 0.625), and a 320-slice CT (0.5 mm detector width) is 16 cm.

4.4. Stress cardiac magnetic resonance

4.4.1. Background

CMR has recently emerged clinically as a highly versatile technique with superior spatial and temporal resolution. The development of high field strength magnets (3T) and rapid imaging techniques such as gradient echo, echo-planar, and balanced steady-state free precession, have contributed to the feasibility of MR perfusion. The type of pulse sequence or hybrid sequences affect the contrast-to-noise ratio and the suspectibility to artifacts, which can affect image quality. In the context of MPI, CMR is a promising tool in parallel with well-established and validated modalities such as SPECT and PET MPI. The advantage of MR is its superior sensitivity for the detection of subendocardial perfusion defects without radiation exposure. The paramagnetic property of gadolinium (Gd)-based contrast agents can alter the local magnetic field in the tissue, which enables differentiation between normally and abnormally perfused myocardium. Arterial spin labeling and blood oxygen level-dependent techniques are new advances in perfusion imaging, but are still research-based. The use of coronary magnetic resonance angiography is not well established, except in some highly specialized centers, and will not be discussed here.

4.4.2. Principles

The fundamental basis of CMR perfusion imaging is the first-pass imaging of contrast transit through the LV myocardium. This exploits the effect of Gd on the T1 relaxation time of myocardial tissue [98]. Gd-based contrast agents are paramagnetic, extracellular agents that are rapidly taken up and rapidly washed out of the normal myocardium, but accumulate in damaged tissues with slower washout kinetics. Gd is highly toxic in its native state. Therefore, Gd chelators (e.g., Gd-DTPA) are used clinically. These agents shorten the T1 and T2 relaxation time constants that represent the decay of the MR signal. However, at low doses, T1 shortening is predominant. During first-pass perfusion, the normal myocardium (i.e., normal perfusion) shows substantial Gd uptake, and appears bright (i.e., hyperintense) owing to a short T1.

Ischemic myocardium (i.e., reduced perfusion) shows diminished Gd uptake and appears dark (i.e., hypointense) owing to a long T1 [98].

Similar to pharmacological stress SPECT or PET MPI, stress CMR requires the use of a pharmacological stressor, such as a vasodilator (e.g., adenosine, dipyridamole, and regadenoson) or dobutamine. Diseased coronary arteries, exhibit a lower peak myocardial signal intensity and increases in myocardial contrast transit time (e.g., signal upslope, arrival time, time-to-peak signal, and mean transit time)[99]. The difference in signal intensity can be quantitatively, semiquantitatively, or visually evaluated to identify possible perfusion defects. The use of adenosine and visual interpretation are common, and these approaches are discussed in further detail.

Historically, inducible ischemia was only assessed using stress and rest perfusion cine images. This method demonstrated a sensitivity, specificity, and diagnostic accuracy of 88%, 90%, and 89%, respectively, for the detection of significant CAD [100]. The caveat being, in patients with prior MI, the resultant perfusion deficit may include areas of prior infarct and may not reflect true inducible ischemia. Imaging with late Gd-enhancement (LGE) was used to detect prior infarction. A method combining first-pass stress and rest imaging with LGE demonstrated an overall accuracy of 0.88, or 0.96 for one-vessel disease, 0.75 for two-vessel disease, and 0.9 for prior coronary artery bypass graft, in the detection of significant stenosis [101].

A stress CMR study can be interpreted using the following algorithm [99]:

Step 1. Assess for LGE

Negative: Move to step 2.

Positive: CAD present.

Step 2. Assess stress perfusion

Negative: No CAD

Positive: Move to step 3.

Step 3. Assess rest perfusion

Negative: Inducible ischemia suggestive of CAD.

Positive: Likely artifact*

* Common being the Gibbs artifact, which is more pronounced on a 3T scanner. This usually occurs in the phase encoding direction and tends to be transient. If the segment of perfusion defect is also positive for LGE, then inducible ischemia cannot be assessed in the same segment.

An abbreviated adenosine stress CMR protocol [102]:

1. **LV structure and function module** – scout and cine imaging for cardiac structure and systolic function at rest.

2. **First pass stress perfusion module** – infusion of adenosine (140 mcg/kg/min over 4 minutes), followed by intravenous Gd (0.05 to 0.1 mmol/kg) and saline flush. Once the

contrast bolus has transited the LV myocardium, adenosine is stopped. Stress images are acquired for 40 to 50 heart beats.

3. **Rest perfusion module**– performed after 10 minutes to ensure sufficient clearing of Gd from the blood pool. Reinjection of a second dose of Gd. Rest images are acquired. Slice geometry, scan setting, and Gd dose should be similar to step (2).

4. **LGE module**– performed after 5 minutes of completion of step (3).

5. **Analysis**– visual interpretation using the 17 segment LV model. The stress and rest cine images are viewed side-by-side using equivalent slices, in addition to the LGE images.

(Some centers omit the rest perfusion module, if the first pass stress perfusion study is normal).

Adenosine (t $_{\frac{1}{2}}$ = 10 s) is safe and well-tolerated. The potential adverse effects include flushing, chest pain, palpitations, breathlessness, transient episodes of heart block, hypotension, sinus bradycardia, and bronchospasm [102]. The contraindication to adenosine stress CMR (in addition to the general contraindication of any MR study) include known hypersensitivity to adenosine, known or suspected bronchoconstrictive or bronchospastic disease, 2nd or 3rd degree AV block, sinus bradycardia (HR <45 bpm), and systolic BP <90 mmHg [102].

4.4.3. Diagnostic and prognostic accuracy

Diagnostic accuracy of stress CMR in a population with high prevalence of CAD (57%) showed on an overall sensitivity of 89% and specificity of 80% for the diagnosis of significant obstructive CAD. Adenosine-based stress demonstrated better sensitivity than dipyridamole (90% vs. 86%), but with similar specificity (81% vs. 77%) [103]. Adenosine and dobutamine stress CMR have similar sensitivity and specificity [104]. Stress CMR showed no difference in diagnostic accuracy when compared to SPECT MPI for CAD detection [105]. The concordance and accuracy of stress CMR with 320-detector row CT, showed an excellent agreement (92%, kappa value = 0.81) in an intermediate risk cohort [106]. Adenosine perfusion was the most accurate component of the stress CMR study in predicting which patients had significant CAD, compared with resting WMA and LGE [107].

Negative findings on stress CMR are reassuring and associated with annualized event rates of 0.4% for MI and 0.3% for cardiovascular death. In patients with inducible ischemia, the annual event rates for MI and cardiovascular death were 2.6% and 2.8%, respectively. The concomitant presence of LGE was associated with a worse prognosis [108]. Other predictors of cardiac events were resting WMA, inducible WMA and LGE. Patients with inducible WMA (i.e., ischemia) experienced significant benefits from revascularization, compared with patients without inducible WMA (i.e., without ischemia) [109].

4.4.4. Strengths and limitations

The strengths and limitations of stress CMR are shown in Table 10.

Strengths	Limitations
Good contrast resolution	Expensive
No radiation exposure	Not widely available
Visualization of subendocardial	Cardiac device/metallic
ischemia and scar	implant
Transmurality	Glomerular filtration rate
of scar	<30 mls/min
Procedural time (~45 minutes)	Allergy to gadolinium
	Breath hold instructions
	Pharmacological stress
	Claustrophobia

Table 10. Strengths and limitations of stress CMR

4.4.5. Case example 8

A 65-year-old man with prior coronary artery bypass surgery presents with chest pain. An adenosine stress CMR was performed. For study interpretation, follow the steps as described in the text starting with LGE, stress and rest images. There is inducible inferior wall perfusion defect with no LGE (Figure 8).

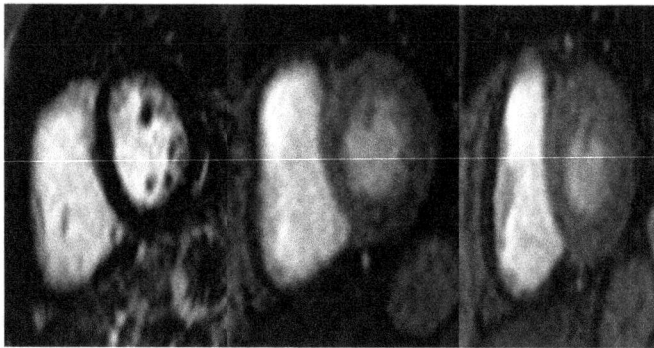

Figure 8. Left to right: 1st image: LV short axis LGE image show no evidence of scar. 2nd image: Stress first pass perfusion image demonstrate an inducible inferior wall perfusion defect. 3rd image: The corresponding rest image demonstrate no perfusion defect in the inferior wall.

4.4.6. Clinical pearls

1. Avoid caffeinated food and beverages, theophylline, and dipyridamole for 24 hours prior to stress CMR.

2.   Stress CMR should be avoided in patients with a glomerular filtration rate (GFR) < 30 mls/min.

3.   The presence of infarction on LGE (subendocardial or transmural in a coronary artery distribution) favors CAD, irrespective of perfusion findings.

4.   Criteria for a perfusion defect is a persistent delay in enhancement pattern during first pass observed in at least 3 consecutive temporal images.

5.   Perfusion defects should be graded according to transmurality.

6.   Dark-rim artifact typically appear as dark lines at the blood pool-myocardium interface, and can mimic a perfusion defect (typically Gibbs artifact).

We have come to the end of our review on the essentials of noninvasive imaging modalities for the assessment of CAD. A proposed algorithm for test selection in suspected CAD is included (Figure 9). The following are four clinical scenarios commonly encountered in clinical practice and the suggested answers:

1.   Would you perform a test in an asymptomatic 35-year-old woman who plans to participate in a marathon next month? She has a normal resting ECG with no cardiovascular risk factor.

Answer: No. Asymptomatic patients generally do not warrant cardiac testing. Her pretest probability of CAD is very low (<5%).

2.   What is the next suitable test in a 60-year-old woman with morbid obesity who presents with chest pain? She completed 4 METs and achieved 70% of the maximum age-predicted HR following an exercise ECG.

Answer: Inability to achieve an adequate stress level reduces the sensitivity of an exercise ECG. Her pretest probability of CAD is intermediate. In the presence of morbid obesity, PET MPI or CCTA would be considered a suitable alternative.

3.   What test would you perform in a 75-year-old man with a sedentary lifestyle who presents with chest pain on exertion that is relieved with nitroglycerin spray? He has underlying COPD, diabetes, and hypertension. Baseline creatinine is 300 micromol/l.

Answer: Pretest probability for CAD is high (≥90%) and the diagnosis of CAD is not in question. He has stable angina. First step would be to inititate medications such as aspirin, beta-blockers, calcium channel blockers, and statin therapy. Pharmacological SPECT or PET MPI for risk stratification is reasonable. Pharmacological SE can be performed if a good echo window can be obtained. In the presence of moderate ischemic burden, high risk variables on MPI, or worsening of symptom despite on optimal medical therapy, ICA is warranted.

4.   Would you repeat another CCTA in a 50-year-old man with an active lifestyle presenting with atypical chest pain? He had a calcium score of 0 and a normal CCTA a year ago.

Answer: No. No testing is required. If symptoms persist, consider an exercise ECG.

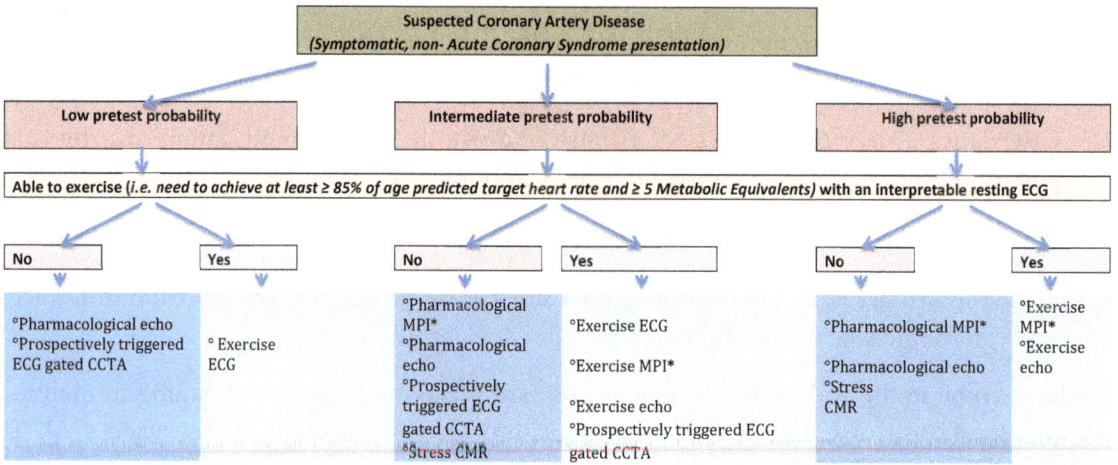

ECG= electrocardiography; CCTA= coronary computed tomography angiography; MPI= myocardial perfusion imaging; CMR= cardiac magnetic resonance; BMI= body mass index. * BMI ≥30 kg/m^2: PET MPI is preferred; BMI <30 kg/m^2: SPECT or PET MPI, depending on resource.

Patients with renal impairment (Creatinine >2.0 mg/dl, avoid CCTA; if GFR <30 mls/min, stress CMR is contraindicated.

For pharmacological MPI, use of low level exercise (1.7 mph, grade 0) is an option, in the absence of LBBB.

Figure 9. Proposed algorithm for test selection in suspected coronary artery disease.

5. Conclusion

Understanding the merits and limitations of each noninvasive imaging modality, together with local expertise and resources, will increase the clinician's confidence in selecting imaging tests for the assessment of CAD. This is crucial to avoid layered testing, unnecessary radiation exposure, and maintain a cost-effective approach. Functional and anatomical noninvasive tests are associated with similar cardiovascular outcomes in patients with low to intermediate risk [110]. The use of stress MPI to serve as a gatekeeper for ICA is well validated [111]. A detailed history and physical examination with sound clinical judgement and the integration of evidence-based guidelines are vital for selecting the right test. In summary, noninvasive tests are the cornerstone of CAD assessment. Although not covered in this chapter, such tests also serve as a guide for ischemia-driven ICA strategies.

6. Conflict of interest

The authors have no conflict of interest to disclose pertaining to the contents of this book chapter.

Acknowledgements

All images used in this chapter were obtained from the University of Ottawa Heart Institute.

Author details

Punitha Arasaratnam[1,2] and Terrence D. Ruddy[1*]

*Address all correspondence to: TRuddy@ottawaheart.ca

1 University of Ottawa Heart Institute, Ottawa, Canada

2 Ng Teng Fong General Hospital, Singapore

References

[1] Shaw L, Marwick T, et al. Why all the focus on cardiac imaging? J Am Coll Cardiol Img. 2010;3(7):789-794.

[2] Wolk, et al. ACCF/AHA/ASE/ASNC/HFSA/HRS/SCAI/ SCCT/ SCMR/ STS, 2013 Multimodality appropriate use criteria for the detection and risk assessment of stable ischemic heart disease. A Report of the American College of Cardiology Foundation Appropriate Use Criteria Task Force, American Heart Association, American Society of Echocardiography, American Society of Nuclear Cardiology, Heart Failure Society of America, Heart Rhythm Society, Society for Cardiovascular Angiography and Interventions, Society of Cardiovascular Computed Tomography, Society for Cardiovascular Magnetic Resonance, and Society of Thoracic Surgeons. JACC 2014; Vol. 63, No. 4, 2014.

[3] Diamond GA. A clinically relevant classification of chest discomfort. J Am Coll Cardiol. 1983;1:574-5.

[4] Weintraub WS, Madeira SW, et al. Critical analysis of the application of Bayes' theorem to sequential testing in the noninvasive diagnosis of coronary artery disease. Am J Cardiol. 1984;54(1):43-9.

[5] Diamond GA, Forrester JS. Analysis of probability as an aid in the clinical diagnosis of coronary artery disease. N Engl J Med. 1979;300:1350-8.

[6] Shaw L, Mieres J, Hendel R, et al. Effectiveness of exercise electrocardiography with or without myocardial perfusion single photon emission computed tomography in women with suspected coronary artery disease. Results form the What Is the Opti-

mal Method for Ischemia Evaluation in Women (WOMEN) trial. Circulation. 2011;124:1239-1249.

[7]   Kohli P, Gulati M. Exercise stress testing in women, going back to the basics. Circulation. 2010;122:2570-2580.

[8]   Okin PM, Bergman G, Kligfield P. Effect of ST segment measurement point on performance of standard and heart rate-adjusted ST segment criteria for the identification of coronary artery disease. Circulation. 1991;84:57-66.

[9]   Fletcher G, Ades P, Kligfield P, et al. Exercise standards for testing and training; A scientific statement from the American Heart Association. Circulation. 2013;128:873-934.

[10] Desai MY, Crugnale S, Mondeau J, Helin K, Mannting F. Slow upsloping ST-segment depression during exercise: Does it really signify a positive stress test? Am Heart J. 2002;143:482-487.

[11] Goldschlager N, Selzer A, Cohn K. Treadmill stress tests as indicators of presence and severity of coronary artery disease. Ann Intern Med. 1976;85:277-286.

[12] Beinart R, Matetzky S, Shechter M, Fefer P, Rozen E, Beinart T, Hod H, Chouraqui P. Stress-induced ST-segment elevation in patients without prior Q-wave myocardial infarction. J Electrocardiol. 2008;41:312-317.

[13] Sullivan ID, Davies DW, Sowton E. Submaximal exercise testing early after myocardial infarction. Difficulty of predicting coronary anatomy and left ventricular performance. Br Heart J. 1985;53:180-185.

[14] Orsini E, Lattanzi F, Reisenhofer B, Tartarini G. Time-domain analysis of exercise-induced ST-segment elevation in Q-wave myocardial infarction: A useful tool for the screening of myocardial viability. Ital Heart J. 2001;2:529-538.

[15] Bruce RA, Kusumi F, Hosmer D. Maximal oxygen intake and nomographic assessment of functional aerobic impairment in cardiovascular disease. Am Heart J. 1973; 85:546-562.

[16] Bourque JM, Holland BH, Watson DD, et al. Achieving an exercise workload of ≥ 10 metabolic equivalents predicts a very low risk of inducible ischemia: Does myocardial perfusion imaging have a role? J Am Coll Cardiol. 2009;54:538-545.

[17] Lauer MS, Francis GS, Okin PM, et al. Impaired chronotropic response to exercise stress testing as a predictor of mortality. JAMA. 1999;281:524-529.

[18] Vivekananthan DP, Blackstone EH, Pothier CE, et. al. Heart rate recovery after exercise is a predictor of mortality, independent of the angiographic severity of coronary disease. J Am Coll Cardiol. 2003;42:83-838.

[19] Sanmarco ME, Pontius S, Selvester RH. Abnormal blood pressure response and marked ischemic ST-segment depression as predictors of severe coronary artery disease. Circulation. 1980;61:572-578.

[20] Mark DB, Shaw L, Harrell FE Jr, et al. Prognostic value of a treadmill exercise score in outpatients with suspected coronary artery disease. N Eng J Med. 1991;325(12): 849-53.

[21] Gianrossi R, Detrano R, Mulvihill D, et al. Exercise-induced ST depression in the diagnosis of coronary artery disease. A meta-analysis. Circulation. 1989;80:87-98.

[22] Gibbons RJ, Balady GJ, Bricker JT, et al. ACC/AHA 2002 guideline update for exercise testing: summary article: A report of the American College of Cardiology/American Heart Association Task Force on Practice Guidelines (Committee to Update the 1997 Exercise Testing Guidelines). Circulation. 2002;106:1883-1892.

[23] Alexander KP, Shaw LJ, Shaw LK, et al. Value of exercise treadmill testing in women. J Am Coll Cardiol. 1998;32:1657-1664.

[24] Mark DB, Hlatky MA, Harrell FE Jr, et al. Exercise treadmill score for predicting prognosis in coronary artery disease. Ann Intern Med. 1987;106(6):793-800.

[25] Ahmed H, Al-Mallah M, McEvoy J, et al. Maximal exercise testing variables and 10-year survival: Fitness risk score derivation from the FIT project. Mayo Clin Proc. 2015;90(3):346-55.

[26] Chang SM, Nabi F, Xu J, et al. Value of CACS compared with ett and myocardial perfusion imaging for predicting long-term cardiac outcome in asymptomatic and symptomatic patients at low risk for coronary disease: Clinical implications in a multimodality imaging world. J Am Coll Cardiol Img. 2015;8(2):134-44.

[27] Klocke FJ, Baird MG, et al. ACC/AHA/ASNC guidelines for the clinical use of cardiac radionuclide imaging- executive summary: A report of the American College of Cardiology/ American Heart Association Task Force on practice guidelines (ACC/AHA/ ASNC Committee to revise the 1995 guidelines for the clinical use of cardiac radionuclide imaging). J Am Coll Cardiol. 2003;42:1318-33.

[28] Patton J, Sandler M, et al. D-SPECT: A new solid state camera for high speed molecular imaging. J Nucl Med. 2006;47:189.

[29] Patton J, Slomka PJ, et al. Recent technologic advances in nuclear cardiology. J Nucl Cardiol. 2007;14:501-13.

[30] Marcassa C, Campini R, et al. Wide beam reconstruction for half-dose or half-time gated SPECT acquisitions: Optimization of resources and reduction in radiation exposure. Eur J Nucl Med Mol Imaging. 2011;38:499-508.

[31] Envoldsen LH, Menashi CAK, et al. Effects of acquisition time and reconstruction algorithm on image quality, quantitative parameters, and clinical interpretation of myocardial perfusion imaging. J Nucl Cardiol 2013. doi:10.1007/s12350-013-97752.

[32] Patil H, Bateman T, et al. Diagnostic accuracy of high-resolution attenuation-corrected Anger camera SPECT in the detection of coronary artery disease. J Nucl Cardiol. 2014;21:127-34.

[33] Henzlova M, Cerqueira M, Christopher L, et al. Stress protocols and tracer. ASNC imaging guidelines for nuclear cardiology procedures. J Nucl Cardiol. 2010;17:646-54.

[34] Loscalzo J, Vita JA. Ischemia, hyperemia, exercise, and nitric oxide: Complex physiology and complex molecular adaptations. Circulation. 1994;90:2556-2559.

[35] Leppo JA. Comparison of pharmacologic stress agents. J Nucl Cardiol. 1996;3:S22-S26.

[36] Thomas GS, Tammelin BR, Schiffman GL, et al. Safety of regadenoson, a selective adenosine A2A agonist, in patients with chronic obstructive pulmonary disease: A randomized, double-blind, placebo-controlled trial (RegCOPD trial). J Nucl Cardiol. 2008 May-Jun;15(3):319-28.

[37] Prenner BM, Bukofzer S, Behm S, et al. A randomized, double-blind, placebo-controlled study assessing the safety and tolerability of regadenoson in subjects with asthma or chronic obstructive pulmonary disease. J Nucl Cardiol. 2012 Aug;19(4):681-92.

[38] Beller G, Zaret B. Contribution of nuclear cardiology to the diagnosis and prognosis of coronary artery disease. Circulation. 2000;101:1465-1478.

[39] Begg CB, Greenes RA. Assessment of diagnostic tests when disease verification is subject to selection bias. Biometrics. 1983;39:207-15.

[40] Iskandrian AE. Exercise MPI. In: Iskandrian AE, Verani MS, eds. Nuclear Cardiac Imaging: Principles and Applications, 3rd ed. New York; Oxford University Press, 2003 pp. 151-163.

[41] Klocke FJ, Baird MG, Lorell BH, et al. ACC/AHA/ASNC guidelines for the clinical use of cardiac radionuclide imaging–executive summary: A report of the American College of Cardiology/American Heart Association Task Force on Practice Guidelines (ACC/AHA/ASNC Committee to Revise the 1995 Guidelines for the Clinical Use of Cardiac Radionuclide Imaging). Circulation. 2003;108:1404 -1418.

[42] Duvall WL, Guma KA, Kamen J, Croft LB, Parides M, George T, et al. Reduction in occupational and patient radiation exposure from myocardial perfusion imaging: impact of stress-only imaging and high-efficiency SPECT camera technology. J Nucl Med. 2013 Aug;54(8):1251-7.

[43] Chang SM, Nabi F, Xu J, Raza U, Mahmarian JJ. Normal stress only versus standard stress/rest myocardial perfusion imaging: Similar patient mortality with reduced radiation exposure. J Am Coll Cardiol. 2010 Jan 19;55(3):221-30.

[44] Duvall WL, Wijetunga MN, Klein TM, Razzouk L, Godbold J, Croft LB, et al. The prognosis of a normal stress-only Tc-99m myocardial perfusion imaging study. J Nucl Cardiol. 2010 Jun;17(3):370-7.

[45] Shaw LJ, Hendel R, Borges-Neto S, et al. Prognostic value of normal exercise and adenosine (99m)Tc-tetrofosmin SPECT imaging: Results from the multicenter registry of 4,728 patients. J Nucl Med. 2003 Feb;44(2):134-9.

[46] Shaw LJ, Iskandrian AE. Prognostic value of gated myocardial perfusion SPECT. J Nucl Cardiol. 2004;11:171-185.

[47] Acampa W, Petretta M, et al. Warranty period of normal stress myocardial perfusion imaging in diabetic patients: A propensity score analysis. J Nucl Cardiol. 2014;21:50-6.

[48] Hachamovitch R, Berman DS, Kiat H, et al. Exercise myocardial perfusion SPECT in patients without known coronary artery disease: Incremental prognostic value and use in risk stratification. Circulation. 1996;93:905-914.

[49] Arasaratnam P, Ayoub C, et al. Positron emission tomography myocardial perfusion imaging for diagnosis and risk stratification in obese patients. Curr Cardiovasc Imaging Re. 2015;8:9304.

[50] Lim SP, Arasaratnam P, et al. Obesity and the challenges of noninvasive imaging for the detection of coronary artery disease. Canadian Journal of Cardiology. 2015;31:223-226.

[51] Machac J. Cardiac positron emission tomography imaging. Sem Nucl Med. 2005;35:17-36.

[52] Machac J, Bacharach S, et al. Quality assurance committee of the american society of nuclear cardiology. Positron emission tomography myocardial perfusion and glucose metabolism imaging. J Nucl Cardiol. 2006;13:e121-51.

[53] Dilsizian V, Bacharach S, Beanlands R, et al. PET myocardial perfusion and metabolism clinical imaging. J Nucl Cardiol. 2009;16:651.

[54] Baggish AL, Boucher CA. Radiopharmaceutical agents for myocardial perfusion imaging. Circulation. 2008;118:1668-1674.

[55] Parker M, Iskander A, et al. Diagnostic accuracy of cardiac positron emission tomography versus single photon emission computed tomography for coronary artery disease, a bivariate meta-analysis. Circ Cardiovasc Imaging. 2012;5:700-707.

[56] McArdle B, Dowsley T, et al. Does Rubidium-82 PET have superior accuracy to SPECT perfusion imaging for the diagnosis of obstructive coronary artery disease? A systematic review and met-analysis. J Am Coll Cardiol. 2012;60(18):1828-1837.

[57] Jaarsma C, Leiner T, et al. Diagnostic performance of noninvasive myocardial perfusion imaging using single-photon emission computed tomography, cardiac magnetic resonance, and positron emission tomography imaging for the detection of obstructive coronary artery disease: A meta-analysis. J Am Coll Cardiol. 2012;59:1719-28.

[58] Yoshinaga K, Chow BJ, Williams K, et al. What is the prognostic value of myocardial perfusion imaging using rubidium-82 positron emission tomography? J Am Coll Cardiol. 2006;48:1029-39.

[59] Dorbala S, Hachamovitch R, Curillova Z, et al. Incremental prognostic value of gated Rb-82 positron emission tomography myocardial perfusion imaging over clinical variables and rest LVEF. JACC Cardiovasc Imaging. 2009;2:846-54.

[60] Hachamovitch R, Hayes SW, Friedman JD, et al. Comparison of the short-term survival benefit associated with revascularization compared with medical therapies in patients with no prior coronary artery disease undergoing stress myocardial perfusion single photon emission computed tomography. Circulation. 2003;107:2900-2907.

[61] Naya M, Murthy V, et al. Prognostic interplay of coronary artery calcification and underlying vascular dysfunction in patients with suspected coronary artery disease. J Am Coll Cardiol. 2013;61:2098-106.

[62] Franke A, Hoffman R, Kuhl H. Non-contrast second harmonic imaging improves interobserver agreement and accuracy of dobutamine stress echocardiography in patients with impaired image quality. Heart. 2000;83:133-40.

[63] Sozi F, Poldermans D, Bax J. Second harmonic imaging improves sensitivity of dobutamine stress echocardiography for the diagnosis of coronary artery disease. Am Heart J. 2001;142:153-9.

[64] Kasprzak JD, Paelinck B, Ten Cate FJ, et al. Comparison of native and contrast-enhanced harmonic echocardiography for visualization of left ventricular endocardial border. Am J Cardiol. 1999;83:211-217.

[65] Pellikka P, Nagueh S, Elhendy A, et al. American Society of Echocardiography Recommendations for Performance, Interpretation, and Application of Stress Echocardiography. J Am Soc Echocardiogr. 2007;20(9):1021-41.

[66] Sicari R, Nihoyannopoulos P, Evangeslista A, et al. Stress echocardiography expert consensus statement-executive summary: European Association of Echocardiography (EAE) (a registered branch of the ESC). Eur Heart Journal. 2009;30(3):278-89.

[67] Fox K, Garcia MA, Ardissino D, et al. Task Force on the Management of Stable Angina Pectoris of the European Society of Cardiology; ESC Committee for Practice Guidelines (CPG): Guidelines on the management of stable angina pectoris: Execu-

tive summary: The Task Force on the Management of Stable Angina Pectoris of the European Society of Cardiology. Eur Heart J. 2006;27:1341-81.

[68] Bjork Ingul C, Rozis E, Slordahl SA, et.al. Incremental value of strain rate imaging to wall motion analysis for prediction of outcome in patients undergoing dobutamine stress echocardiography. Circulation. 2007;115:1252-9.

[69] Ingul CB, Stoylen A, Slodahl SA, et al. Automated analysis of myocardial deformation at dobutamine stress echocardiography: An angiographic validation. J Am Coll Cardiol. 2007;49:1651-9.

[70] Nagy AI, Sahlen A, Manouras A, et al. Combination of constrast-enhanced wall motion analysis and myocardial deformation imaging using dobutamine stress echocardiography. Eur Heart J. 2015;16:88-95.

[71] Beleslin BD, Osojic M, Djordjevic-Dikie A, et al. Integrated evaluation of relation between coronary lesion features and stress echocardiography results: The importance of coronary lesion morphology. J Am Coll Cardiol. 1999;33:717-26.

[72] Marwick TH. Stress echocardiography. Heart. 2003;89:113-8.

[73] Picano E, Bedetti G, Varga A, et al. The comparable diagnostic accuracies of dobutamine stress and dipyridamole-stress echocardiographies: a meta-analysis. Coron Artery Dis. 2000;11:151e9.

[74] Ho FM, Huang PJ, Liau CS, et al. Dobutamine stress echocardiography compared with dipyridamole thallium-201 single-photon emission computed tomography in detecting coronary artery disease. Eur Heart J. 1995;16:570e5.

[75] Mahajan N, Polavaram N, Vankalaya et al. Diagnostic accuracy of myocardial perfusion imaging and stress echocardiography for the diagnosis of left main and triple vessel coronary artery disease: A comparative meta-analysis. Heart. 2010;96:956-966.

[76] Innocenti F, Lazzeretti D, Conti A, et al. Stress echocardiography in the ED: Diagnostic performance in high-risk subgroups. Am J Emerg Med. 2013;31:1309-1314.

[77] Metz LD, Beattie M, Hom R, et al. The prognostic value of normal exercise myocardial perfusion imaging and exercise echocardiography: A meta- analysis. J Am Coll Cardiol. 2007;49(2):227-37.

[78] Arruda-Olson AM, Juracan EM, Mahoney DW, et al. Prognostic value of exercise echocardiography in 5, 798 patients: Is there a gender difference: J Am Coll Cardiol. 2002;39(4):625-31.

[79] Schroder K, Wieckhorst A, Voller H. Comparison of the prognostic value of dipyridamole and dobutamine stress echocardiography in patients with known or suspected coronary artery disease. Am J Cardiol. 1997;79:1516-8.

[80] Pingitore A, Picano E, Varga A, et al. Prognostic value of pharmacological stress echocardiography in patients with known or suspected coronary artery disease: A

prospective, large-scale, multicenter, head-to-head comparison between dipyrida-mole and dobutamine test. Echo-Per- santine International Cooperative (EPIC) and Echo- Dobutamine International Cooperative (EDIC) Study Groups. J Am Coll Cardiol. 1999;34:1769-7.

[81] McCully Rb, Roger VL, Mahoney DW, et al. Outcome after abnormal exercise echo-cardiography for patients with good exercise capacity: Prognostic importance of the extent and severity of exercise related left ventricular dysfunction. J Am Coll Cardiol. 2002;39(8):1345-52.

[82] Flohr TG, Stierstorfer K, Ulzheimer S, et al. Image reconstruction and image quality evaluation for a 64-slice CT scanner with z-flying focal spot. Med Phys. 2005 Aug; 32(8):2536-47.

[83] Achenbach S, Raggi P. Imaging of coronary atherosclerosis by computed tomogra-phy. Eur H Journal. 2010;31:1442-48.

[84] Flohr TG, Mc Collough CH, Bruder H, et al. First performance evaluation of a dual-source CT (DSCT) system. Eur Radiol. 2006;16:256-268.

[85] Tsukagoshi S, Ota T, Fujii M, et al. Improvement of spatial resolution in the longitu-dinal direction for isotropic imaging in helical CT. Phys Med Biol. 2007:52(3):791-801.

[86] Arbab Zadeh A, Hoe J. Multidetector CT angiography in comparison with conven-tional angiography. Methods, caveats and implications. J Am Coll Cardiol Imag. 2011:4(2):191-202.

[87] Taylor A, Cerqueira M, Hodgson J, et al. ACCF/SCCT/ACR /AHA /ASE / ASNC/ NASCI/SCAI/SCMR 2010 Appropriate Use Criteria for Cardiac Computed Tomogra-phy. A Report of the American College of Cardiology Foundation Appropriate Use Criteria Task Force, the Society of Cardiovascular Computed Tomography, the American College of Radiology, the American Heart Association, the American Soci-ety of Echocardiography, the American Society of Nuclear Cardiology, the North American Society for Cardiovascular Imaging, the Society for Cardiovascular An-giography and Interventions, and the Society for Cardiovascular Magnetic Reso-nance. J Am Coll Cardiol. 2010;56(22):1864-1894.

[88] Budoff M, Dowe D, Jollis J, et al. Diagnostic performance of 64-multidetector row coronary computed tomographic angiography for evaluation of coronary artery stenosis in individuals without known coronary artery disease-results from the pro-spective multicenter accuracy (Assessment by Coronary Computed Tomographic Angiography of Individuals Undergoing Invasive Coronary Angiography) trial. J Am Coll Cardiol. 2008;52:1724-32.

[89] Meijboom WB, Meighem CA, Mollete NR, et al. 64-slice computed tomography coro-nary angiography in patients with high, intermediate, or low pretest probability of significant coronary artery disease. J Am Coll Cardiol. 2007;50:1469-75.

[90] Litt HI, Gatsonis C, Snyder B, et al. CT angiography for safe discharge of patients with possible acute coronary syndromes. N Engl J Med. 2012;366:1393-403.

[91] Hoffmann U, Truong QA, Schoenfeld DA, et al. Coronary CT angiography versus standard evaluation in acute chest pain. N Engl J Med. 2012;367:299-308.

[92] Goldstein JA, Chinnaiyan KM, Abidov A, et al. The CT-STAT (coronary computed tomographic angiography for systematic triage of acute chest pain patients to treatment) trial. J Am Coll Cardiol. 2011;58:1414-22.

[93] Chow BJ, Small G, Yam Y, et al. Incremental prognostic value of cardiac computed tomography in coronary artery disease using CONFIRM: COroNary computed tomography angiography evaluation for clinical outcomes: an InteRnational Multicenter registry. Circ Cardiovasc Imaging. 2011;4:463-72.

[94] Habib PJ, Green J, Butterfield RCA, et al. Association of cardiac events with coronary artery disease detected by 64-slice or greater coronary CT angiography: A systematic review and meta-analysis. Int J Cardiol. 2013; 169:112-120.

[95] Ostrom MP, Gopal A, Ahmadi N, et al. Mortality incidence and the severity of coronary atherosclerosis assessed by computed tomography angiography. J Am Coll Cardiol. 2008;52:1335-43.

[96] Detrano R, Guerci AD, Carr JJ, et al. Coronary calcium as a predictor of coronary events in four racial or ethnic groups. N Engl J Med. 2008;358:1336-1345.

[97] P. Greenland, J. S. Alpert, G. A. Beller, et al. ACCF/AHA guideline for assessment of cardiovascular risk in asymptomatic adults: A report of the American College of Cardiology Foundation/American Heart Association task force on practice guidelines. Circulation. 2010;122:584-636.

[98] Shehata ML, Basha TA, Hayeri MR, et al. MR myocardial perfusion imaging: Insights on techniques, analysis, interpretation, and findings. RadioGraphics. 2014;34:1636-57.

[99] Kim HW, Klem I, Kim R. Detection of myocardial ischemia by stress perfusion cardiovascular magnetic resonance. Cardiol Clin. 2007:25:57-70.

[100] Nagel E, Klein C, Paetsch I, et al. Magnetic resonance perfusion measurements for the noninvasive detection of CAD. Circulation. 2003;108:432-437.

[101] Cury RC, Cattani CA, Gabure LA, et al. Diagnostic performance of stress perfusion and delayed enhancement MR imaging in patients with coronary artery disease. Radiology. 2006;240:39-45.

[102] Kramer C, Barkhausen J, Flamm S, et al. Standardized cardiovascular magnetic resonance imaging (CMR) protocols, society for cardiovascular magnetic resonance: Board of trustees task force on standardized protocols. J Cardiovasc Magn Resonance. 2008;10:35. doi:10.1186/1532-429X-10-35.

[103] Hamon M, Fau G, Nee G, et al. Meta-analysis of the diagnostic performance of stress perfusion cardiovascular magnetic resonance for detection of coronary artery disease. J Cardiovasc Magn Reson. 2010;12:29.

[104] Manka R, Jahnke C, Gebker R, et al. Head-to-head comparison of first-pass MR perfusion imaging during adenosine and high-dose dobutamine/atropine stress. Int J Cardiovasc Imaging, 2011;27:995-1002.

[105] Schwitter J, Wacker C, van Rossum A, et al. MR-IMPACT: Comparison of perfusion-cardiac magnetic resonance with single-photon emission computed tomography for the detection of coronary artery disease in a multicenter, multivendor, randomized trial. Eur Heart J. 2008;29:480-489.

[106] Chen M, Bandettini W, Shanbhag S, et al. Concordance and diagnostic accuracy of vasodilator stress cardiac MRI and 320-detector row coronary CTA. Int J Cardiovasc Imaging. 2014;30:109-119.

[107] Ingkanisorn W, Kwong R, Bohme N, et al. Prognosis of negative adenosine stress magnetic resonance in patients presenting to an emergency department with chest pain. J Am Coll Cardiol. 2006;47:1427-32.

[108] Lipinski M, McVey C, Berger J, et al. Prognostic value of stress cardiac magnetic resonance imaging in patients with known or suspected coronary artery disease. A Systematic review and meta-analysis. J Am Coll Cardiol. 2013;62:826-38.

[109] Kelle S, Nagel E, Voss A, et al. A bi-center cardiovascular magnetic resonance prognosis study focusing on dobutamine wall motion and late gadolinium enhancement in 3, 138 consecutive patients. J Am Coll Cardiol. 2013;61:2310-12.

[110] Douglas P, Hoffmann U, Patel M, et al. Outcomes of anatomical versus functional testing for coronary artery disease. N Engl J Med. 2015;10.1056/NEJMoa1415516.

[111] Takx R, Blomberg B, Aidi H, et al. Diagnostic accuracy of stres myocardial perfusion imaging to invasive coronary angiography with fractional flow reserve meta-analysis. Circ Cardiovasc Imaging. 2015;8:e002666. doi:10:1161/CIRCIMAGING. 114.002666.

6

Coronary Artery Bypass and Stroke: Incidence, Etiology, Pathogenesis, and Surgical Strategies to Prevent Neurological Complications

Marco Gennari, Gianluca Polvani,
Tommaso Generali, Sabrina Manganiello,
Gabriella Ricciardi and Marco Agrifoglio

Abstract

Current data suggest that cardiac bypass surgery is the single largest cause of iatrogenic stroke. Among the strategies to decrease or eliminate aortic manipulation, there is the use of off-pump coronary artery bypass grafting (CABG) through an aortic "no touch" technique, which reduces significantly the stroke rate. However, this off-pump aortic "no touch" technique is not always applicable, and, when saphenous vein and/or free arterial aortocoronary grafts are used, there is still risk of neurological injury due to tangential aortic clamp applied during the proximal anastomosis sewing. We aim to analyze the current incidence, etiology, and physiopathology of the neurological complications after coronary artery bypass surgery. We describe the methods and techniques that provide reduction in the occurrence of neurological complications. CABG with multiple clamp technique failed to find a better outcome in terms of neuropsychological deficit in the OPCABG group. By the way, patients undergoing CABG with single clamping seems to have better outcomes, suggesting that the cross-clamping technique used and minimal aortic manipulation could have had a role in reducing neurocognitive impairment. Moreover, surprisingly, CPB seemed to be a neuroprotective factor, and this aspect could be linked to the mild hypothermia used during on-pump surgery.

Keywords: coronary artery bypass, stroke, cardiac surgery, aortic cross clamp, neurologic impairment

1. Introduction

In 1978 the World Health Organization defined a stroke as a focal or global neurologic deficit due to cerebrovascular cause that persists beyond 24 hours or is interrupted by death within 24 hours [1].

Strokes are classified by etiology into **ischemic strokes** (85%) and **hemorrhagic strokes** (15%). Ischemic strokes result from a critical reduction in blood flow and are categorized as embolic, thrombotic, hemodynamic, or hypotensive [2].

Cerebrovascular accidents (CVAs) remain one of the most common complications after surgical myocardial revascularization despite the increased quality of treatment. Cerebral injuries are associated with substantial increases in mortality, morbidity, length of hospitalization, and an impaired quality of life [3].

Ischemic stroke occurs in 1.5–5.2% of patients. Percentage varies across studies and depends on study design, patient risk profile, operative techniques, and the length of study follow-up. Although advances in surgical and medical management have occurred across the last 10 years, the risk of stroke after coronary artery bypass grafting (CABG) has not significantly declined likely because of the progressive aging of the CABG population [4].

The etiology of postoperative stroke is multifactorial. Previous studies showed that the risk factors for postoperative stroke following CABG include age, low left ventricular ejection fraction, unstable angina, atherosclerosis of the ascending aorta, chronic renal failure, chronic obstructive pulmonary disease, calcified aorta, a history of previous stroke, carotid stenosis, duration of cardiopulmonary bypass, peripheral vascular disease, smoke, and diabetes mellitus. The age seems the most important risk factor for postoperative stroke, followed by palpable calcification in the ascending aorta and arch [5, 6].

1.1. Epidemiology

The prevalence of stroke after surgery varies according to the different types of surgery and patient comorbidities. A postoperative stroke is reported to occur in 0.08–0.7% of patients after general surgery, in 0.8–3% after peripheral vascular surgery, in 4.8% after head and neck surgery, in 2–3% after carotid endarterectomy, in 8.7% after aortic repair, and in 5.7% after cardiac surgery. Furthermore, patients with advanced age, previous stroke or transient ischemic attack (TIA), or postoperative atrial fibrillation are at increased risk for postoperative strokes [7, 8].

Most postoperative strokes do not occur immediately after surgery; there is usually a symptom-free interval before ischemia becomes apparent. In a recent retrospective study, only 8% of strokes appeared in the postanesthesia care unit. Approximately 45% of occurrences are identified within the first day after surgery [9].

The incidence of early stroke within 30 days of the myocardial surgery revascularization is reported to be 2–4%. Other studies indicated that the rate of postoperative stroke in octogenarians ranged from 2 to 9% [10].

Recent studies using sensitive brain magnetic resonance imaging (MRI) with diffusion-weighted imaging report that 45% of patients who have undergone cardiac surgery have new ischemic brain lesions that are often clinically undetected. For this reason, the prevalence of stroke can be higher than documented [11, 12].

2. Incidence and etiology of neurological events after cardiac surgery

2.1. Cerebral embolism

It is possible to divide emboli into two categories: microemboli and macroemboli according to size (200 µm or greater). This distinction reflects different clinical manifestations: a single macroembolus can result in hemiplegia; instead, a microembolus is unlikely to have a noticeable effect except when these emboli are numerous. Macroemboli are unlikely to arise from the extracorporeal circuit but rather from surgical manipulation of the heart and the aorta. There are other categories: gaseous, biologic, inorganic, etc [13].

Gaseous emboli are usually derived from air or anesthetic gas (such as nitrous oxide). These emboli are introduced into the left side of the heart (during aorta or mitral valve replacement) or into the aorta (from the bypass circuit). The superiority of membrane oxygenators compared with bubble oxygenators in reducing cardiopulmonary bypass (CPB)-generated embolism has been demonstrated by ultrasound and retinal angiography [14].

Inorganic embolism which can arise from embolization of fragments of polyvinyl chloride tubing exposed to roller pump has been described.

Biologic aggregates include thrombus, platelets, and fat. Thrombus can arise from the left appendage, the left ventricular aneurysm, or from the CPB circuit. Heparin may contribute to create fat embolism by stimulating endothelial lipoprotein lipase. It seems that the principal sources of cholesterol embolism are large vessels of atherosclerotic plaques.

2.2. Cerebral hypoperfusion

Although a postoperative stroke is most often embolic in origin, an association between intraoperative hypotension and the occurrence of a postoperative stroke is often assumed.

Some authors identified the watershed infarcts; these are areas of the brain that are between non-anastomosing arterial vessels and arteries. They are termed watershed or border-zone areas. They are critically dependent on adequate perfusion pressure in the border-zone vessels. A reduction in perfusion below a critical value will result in ischemia because of inadequate collateral circulation. Infarction of watershed areas has been regarded as the hallmark of hemodynamic strokes. There are two major watershed regions. The cortical watershed areas are between the cortical branches of the anterior, middle, and posterior cerebral arteries. The internal or subcortical watershed is located in the white matter along and slightly above the lateral ventricles between the deep (lenticulostriate) and the cortical branches of the middle cerebral artery and the anterior cerebral arteries. There is much controversy about the relative contribution of low-flow pathophysiology. For example, it is hard to determine whether a local low-flow state due to hypoperfusion results in platelet microemboli or whether platelet microemboli result in local hypoperfusion. Irrespective of the sequence, there is a synergistic interaction [15, 16].

Intraoperative hypotension is a common event during surgery. Bijker et al. reviewed four major anesthesia journals for their definitions of hypotension. Almost 50 different definitions were found utilizing systolic pressure and/or mean pressure either as an absolute or as a percentage of the baseline value. Diastolic pressure was never used. The most frequent definitions were as follows [17, 18]:

1. A 20% decrease in systolic pressure from the baseline value.

2. A combination of systolic pressures below 100 mmHg or greater than 30% decrease from the baseline value.

3. A systolic pressure below 80 mmHg. A definition of "baseline" was provided in only 50% of the manuscripts but was most frequently the blood pressure immediately before induction of anesthesia.

The majority of the articles stated how frequently blood pressure was measured, but only 10% of the articles specified a minimum duration for which reduced blood pressure would constitute hypotension.

Furthermore, it is possible to found a congenital variation of the circle of Willis. A persistent complete fetal-type posterior circulation results in the complete separation of the posterior and anterior circulations and occurs in 1–4% of the population. Development of collaterals usually occurs slowly, although hypoplastic vessels may have the capacity to be more acutely dilated. The contribution of the abnormalities to perioperative stroke is unknown, although, as shown in a recent case report, they may be an important factor for some patients [19, 20].

2.3. Atherosclerosis of the aorta

Aortic atherosclerosis is characterized by the formation of intimal plaques with the usual morphologic features of atherosclerosis, including cellular proliferation, lipid accumulation, inflammation, necrosis, fibrosis, and calcifications. Ulceration of these plaques can result in embolization of plaque elements or thrombus formation, which can lead to neurologic deficit, stroke, and death. Cardiac surgery usually involves manipulation of the ascending aorta by arterial cannulation and cross clamping. All of which can increase the risk of embolization of atherosclerotic material to the brain. The prevalence of atherosclerotic disease in the ascending aorta varies across studies, depending on the patient population, the criteria used to define the disease, and the diagnostic tool implemented to detect the disease. This type of disease has significantly increased in recent years, likely due to better diagnostic methods and an increasing population of elderly. Peripheral vascular disease, age, hypertension, and diabetes have been reported to be independent predictors of atherosclerotic disease of the ascending aorta [21].

The magnitude of this problem was well illustrated in a large prospective study by Roach et al. involving 24 centers. They reported a 3.1% incidence of type 1 neurologic injury (focal injury or stupor or coma at discharge) after CABG. Affected patients had a higher in-hospital mortality rate than patients without neurologic complications (21% vs. 2%), as well as a longer hospital stay (25 days vs. 10 days). Predictors of type I outcomes were palpable proximal aortic atherosclerosis, a history of neurologic disease, and older age. A high correlation between atherosclerosis of the ascending aorta and atheroembolism during CABG surgery has been established by several studies. Observational studies have shown, for example, that atherosclerosis of the ascending aorta detected at the time of surgery is an independent risk factor for stroke. A previous study documented that the presence of atherosclerosis alone in this region in patient undergoing cardiac surgery increased the risk of early postoperative stroke from 1.8 to 8.7%. It is widely postulated that the proximate cause of atheroembolism is disruption of the atheroma during surgical manipulations such as for aortic cannulation, aortic cross clamping, or proximal coronary artery anastomosis. These interventions are associated with increases in Doppler-detected cerebral embolic signals, but the composition of these emboli cannot be determined. Disruption of atherosclerotic lesions was verified in a study of 472 patients who underwent epiaortic ultrasound before and after CPB, with new mobile lesions of the ascending aorta identified in 10 (3.4%) of patients after surgery at sites of aortic clamping or cannulation and stroke occurring in 3 of these 10 patients. A smaller study by Ribakove et al. revealed a similar rate of stroke (3 out of 10) in patients with identified mobile lesions (31). Swaminathan et al. demonstrated the potential of atheroma disruption due to the "sandblasting" effect of CPB at the site of the aortic cannula [22, 23].

Injury involving atherosclerotic lesions not only can result in emboli during surgery but may also expose lipid-laden, prothrombotic material that could promote thrombus formation postoperatively after heparin neutralization. Finally, atherosclerosis of the ascending aorta identifies patients likely to have severe atherosclerosis of cerebral arteries who are prone to cerebral injury from hypoperfusion. For this reason, avoidance of significant hypotension during and after surgery may be prudent to avoid neurologic injury [24, 25].

2.4. Atrial fibrillation

Atrial fibrillation (AF) is the most common sustained arrhythmia encountered in clinical practice. Its prevalence increases with age, affecting approximately 1% of the total population and 8% of individuals over 80 years old. The incidence of postoperative AF following coronary artery bypass grafting (CABG) surgery is high and ranges between 20 and 40% of patients. It increases the length of hospital stay and hospital costs and is associated with increased morbidity and mortality including postoperative stroke, as well as in-hospital and 6-month mortality. Postoperative AF typically develops within the first week post surgery, at a median time of 2 days after the operation. It generally resolves within 24–48 hours, and most patients are discharged in sinus rhythm. Several factors have been found to predict the risk of postoperative AF following CABG, including enlarged left atrial size and prolonged hospitalization post surgery [26].

In medical patients with chronic or recurrent AF, the cause and effect relationship between the arrhythmia and the cerebrovascular event has been unquestionably proven [27].

Lahtinen and colleagues from Finland analyzed data of 52 stroke patients after CABG operation and found that in 19 patients (36%) the first AF episode preceded the development of stroke by a mean of 21.3 hours (average, 2.5 AF episodes before stroke). The stroke was attributed to calcification in the ascending aorta in 13 patients (25%), and 16 patients (31%) had greater than 70% internal carotid artery stenosis [28].

The pathophysiology of postoperative AF is not completely understood. Apart from obvious comorbid conditions such as valvular heart disease, atrial enlargement, congestive heart failure, and history of preoperative atrial arrhythmias, several other risk factors predispose cardiac surgical patients for postoperative AF. Advanced age is the strongest, followed by systemic hypertension, left ventricular hypertrophy, peripheral vascular disease, and chronic lung disease. Longer cardiopulmonary bypass time and aortic cross-clamping time have been shown to be associated with increased incidence of postoperative AF. Postoperative pericardial fluid collection and pericarditis have also been associated with atrial arrhythmias [29].

2.5. Genetic predisposition

It has been suggested that genetic predisposition might explain the marked variability in individual susceptibility for cerebral injury from cardiac surgery despite similar risk. Tardiff was the first to show a relationship between the risk of postoperative neurocognitive dysfunction and the presence of the apolipoprotein E ε4 allele. The apolipoprotein E (APOE) ε4 genotype is a plausible candidate gene since it has been shown to increase risk for Alzheimer's disease and cognitive decline after cerebral injury. Other investigators have examined for a relationship between polymorphisms of genes involved in pathways regulating coagulation, cell adhesion, and inflammation with perioperative cerebral injury [30].

The C-reactive protein minor allele 1059G/C SNP and the P-selectin allele SELP 1087G/A allele were further found to be associated with decline in cognition 6 weeks after CABG surgery.

Grocott et al. documented that the presence of at least one minor allele at each of the two loci (CRP, 3_UTR 1846C/T; IL-6, 74G/C) is a risk factor for stroke, increasing risk more than threefold (60). The observation that the interaction of these two inflammatory SNPs contributes to perioperative stroke suggests that inflammatory pathways may be important mechanistic factors in either initiating or otherwise modulating stroke after cardiac surgery. This interpretation is consistent with the current knowledge regarding CPB initiating and IL-6 mediating a robust inflammatory response. This finding is also consistent with the view that inflammation plays an important role in the etiology of stroke in the general population [31].

2.6. Carotid stenosis

Carotid artery atherosclerosis often accompanies significant coronary atherosclerotic lesions. Hypoperfusion arising from a severely stenotic carotid artery or embolization from an ulcerated plaque, calcific debris from a diseased valve, and introduction of air during the procedure are important mechanisms. The risk of stroke in patients with carotid artery disease after CABG has been estimated 1.8% in patients with stenosis <50%, 3.2% in patients with stenosis between 50 and 99%, and 10% in patients with contralateral occlusion. It is thought that carotid intra-plaque hemorrhage can result in plaque destabilization and intimal ulceration, creating a nidus for thromboembolism. Intra-plaque hemorrhage detected by magnetic resonance imaging is associated with increase of ipsilateral stroke in symptomatic and asymptomatic nonsurgical patients. Impaired cerebral hemodynamic functional distal to carotid artery stenosis is another determinant of postoperative stroke. Maximally dilated vessels distal to carotid artery stenosis can no longer vasodilate in response to hemodynamic compromise. Therefore, perioperative reduction in blood pressure or cardiac output in this group of patients is hypnotized to lead to cerebral ischemia [32, 33].

3. Pathogenesis of neurological complications in conventional coronary artery bypass grafting (CABG)

3.1. Risk factors of stroke after myocardial revascularization

The risk factors of postoperative stroke can be divided into preoperative, intraoperative, and postoperative factors [34].

Preoperative factors include advanced age, atherosclerosis in the ascending aorta, unstable angina, hypertension, history of stroke, and redo surgery. Emergency surgery is performed for critical left main coronary artery disease (more or equal to 70% luminal narrowing with or without angina), or unstable cardiac conditions are also significant predictors of stroke after CABG procedure.

Intraoperative factors include the endurance of extracorporeal circulation and aorta clamping or operation type. Some reports demonstrate that the number of revascularized vessels (more or equal to three) is associated with a higher incidence of stroke after CABG procedure.

Finally, **postoperative factors** include atrial fibrillation, microembolism detachment, and hypotension.

The single most important risk factor for post-myocardial revascularization stroke is atrial fibrillation, newly onset or chronic. This arrhythmia occurs in up to 20% of patients following a STEMI and is associated with a significant increase in risk for an in-hospital stroke.

It is also well known that a high correlation exists between atherosclerosis of the ascending aorta and atheroembolism during CABG surgery, as several studies show.

In a prospective multicenter study including more than 2000 patients, atherosclerosis of the ascending aorta was the strongest independent predictor of stroke associated with CABG. In the study by Bergman et al., extensive atherosclerotic disease of the ascending aorta was associated with a 31% risk of postoperative stroke. The risk depends on the presence, location, and extent of disease, whenever the aorta is surgically manipulated.

Age > 75, black race, peripheral vascular disease, diabetes, renal impairment, hypertension, any frailty, and no aspirin therapy on discharge are also strong independent predictors of ischemic stroke [8]. In particular, age shows a strong correlation with stroke: for each 1 year increase in age, the odds of stroke increases by 12% [35].

In addition, the incidence of postoperative stroke in patients with a history of stroke is significantly higher than in patient with no previous history of stroke. Maybe, these data are due to associated older age and more complicated comorbidities of these patients.

3.2. Pathogenesis of stroke after myocardial revascularization

The two mechanisms responsible for stroke after CABG procedure are ischemia and hemorrhage. Some studies suggest that pan-vascular inflammation may also play a role, especially in the setting of acute coronary syndromes.

Ischemia can be due to embolic events (from cardiac chambers, aorta, or other peripheral arteries), thromboembolism of intra- or extracranial vessels, or systemic hypoperfusion. Hypoperfusion stroke arises from hemodynamic compromise distal to the carotid/cranial artery stenosis and has been associated with the patients' capacity for cerebral autoregulation [36].

Hemorrhage is instead associated with hypertension or reperfusion of infarcted area. The interaction between embolism and hypoperfusion is generally considered to be a major cause of postoperative stroke. Hypoperfusion may contribute to embolism retention. Several studies have found multiple emboli in the cortical watershed of patients who died after cardiac surgery. A recent study from Cao and co-workers suggests that unstable angina, LVEF <50%, and hypotension are risk factors of postoperative recurrent stroke. All of these factors decrease brain perfusion, leading to stroke.

Embolic ischemic stroke is generally caused by an embolus from the left atrium, as in atrial fibrillation, or from the left ventricle, as in recent AMI. Embolization of atheromatous debris from the aorta, instead, is likely to occur at the time of cannulation of the vessel to establish cardiopulmonary bypass, when the aortic clamp is applied or released or when proximal graft anastomoses are performed using side-biting clamp. Cerebral emboli often coexist with intraoperative hypoperfusion, which impairs the clearance of microemboli and may be responsible of bilateral watershed infarcts after CABG. Cerebral hypoperfusion may be exacerbated by the coexistence of carotid artery stenosis, which is another important risk factor for intraoperative stroke [37].

Thrombotic thromboembolism is related to the atherosclerotic disease of the intracranial vessels or hematologic pathologies. Thromboembolic strokes are most frequently caused by thrombus formation at the site of the ulcerated atherosclerotic plaque on the carotid/cranial arteries, although the aortic arch can also be a site of thrombus formation.

Neurological events after CABG are classified as:

- **Type 1**: in case of focal stroke, transient ischemic attack, or fatal brain damage.

- **Type 2**: in case of diffuse brain injury with disorientation and intellectual deterioration, which are normally reversible.

The stroke that occurs within the first 24 hours after the CABG is a potentially devastating complication. It is associated with the increased hospital mortality.

3.3. Risk stratification

Identification of vulnerable patients at increased risk of stroke before CABG is of paramount importance for the surgical decision-making approach and informed consent. As previously said, age, diabetes, hypertension, peripheral vascular disease, renal failure, left ventricular dysfunction, and nonelective surgery have consistently been reported as risk factors of perioperative stroke in patients undergoing CABG surgery. All these risk factors can be assessed before surgery. The combination of these variables has generated several risk stratification tools that can be implemented before surgery, to determine the individual probability of stroke in patients undergoing CABG [38].

In the Charlesworth score, generated from 33,000 consecutive patients undergoing isolated CABG, seven variables are integrated, including age, diabetes, left ventricular ejection fraction <40%, female gender, priority of surgery, renal dysfunction ,and peripheral vascular disease. In the simpler model generated by McKhann et al., only three variables are considered: age, hypertension, and history of stroke. More recently, Hornero et al. generated and validated a new risk model (Pack2 score), including priority of surgery, peripheral vascular disease, preoperative cardiac failure/left ventricular ejection fraction <40%, and chronic kidney failure. Interestingly, in patients with Pack2 score ≥ 2, off-pump CABG significantly reduced the risk of stroke compared with on-pump CABG, whereas no difference was apparent between the two strategies of revascularization in patients with Pack2 score < 2. Further studies should externally validate this score and assess whether it is useful in clinical practice to select the optimal strategy of revascularization between on-pump and off-pump CABG in high-risk patients.

However, these risk stratification tools share a major limitation in disregarding two important risk factors—atherosclerotic disease of the ascending aorta and pre-existing cerebrovascular disease. These factors should always be analyzed to make the optimal strategy of coronary revascularization within Heart Team environment.

Unfortunately, severe atherosclerosis of the ascending aorta is often an unexpected intraoperative finding during CABG, especially if preoperative risk stratification has not been accurate. It still represents a challenge for the surgeon, and sometimes the operative strategy must be changed at the time of surgery. The methods to diagnose severe atherosclerosis in the ascending aorta before surgery include computed tomography scanning, transesophageal echocardiography, or magnetic resonance imaging. Intraoperative ultrasonographic scanning of the aorta can also be used to find atherosclerotic changes in the entire ascending aorta. It is a rapid, safe, and sensitive method, and in some studies, it has been found to be more accurate than both transesophageal echocardiography and computed tomography in detecting atheromatous debris in the ascending aorta.

Assessment of the neurological risk profile of patients before CABG is another essential step to plan the surgery and predict the patients' risk for postoperative stroke. The neurological profile of the patient should be carefully characterized, seeking for a history of stroke, the presence of initial neurocognitive disorders, or the presence of pre-existing cerebrovascular disease. Recent studies have also suggested that detection of cerebral ischemia by magnetic resonance imaging before CABG is strongly associated with the risk of postoperative stroke. Searching for carotid artery disease with echo Doppler before CABG is also a safer and cheaper method of screening, especially in high-risk patients.

4. Off-pump coronary artery bypass (OPCAB) and "no touch technique" as strategies to reduce the neurological risk

CPB is still the most diffused technique used to perform CABG. Even if debate on the superiority of on-pump CABG over off-pump CABG (OPCABG) is still open, evidences of prospective studies like ROOBY trial showed better results in terms of cumulative 1-year events for myocardial infarction and revascularization procedures and better rate of venous graft patency at 1 year, along with better Fitz-Gibbon grade for on-pump CABG [39].

While other studies such as the SMART trial highlighted no significant differences between the two techniques in terms of mortality, myocardial infarction, stroke, and recurrent angina or readmission for cardiac or noncardiac events, on-pump CABG is still the gold standard procedure, and CPB is the most widely applied technique.

However, the use of CPB has been advocated to be related with a certain risk of neurocognitive sequelae linked with inflammatory response and microembolism [40].

On the other hand, cannulation itself, cross clamping, and, more widely, aortic manipulation have showed to be linked with neurocognitive impairment.

This point was also taken into consideration in ROOBY trial, where patient evaluation with neuropsychological testing was performed in every case in order to investigate memory, attention, and visuospatial skills. All the tests failed to find any clinically significant difference between the two groups, but a better scoring in the clock-drawing test was reported for the off-pump group.

This aspect was also investigated in other studies with no clear results. Remarkably, Hammon et al. prospectively analyzed 237 high-risk patients undergoing OPCABG vs. CABG with single clamp technique [41].

CABG with multiple clamp technique failed to find a better outcome in terms of neuropsychological deficit in the OPCABG group. By the way, patients undergoing CABG with single clamping had better outcome, suggesting that the cross clamping technique used and minimal aortic manipulation could have had a role in reducing neurocognitive impairment. Moreover, surprisingly, CPB seemed to be a neuroprotective factor, and this aspect could be linked to the mild hypothermia used during on-pump surgery [42].

In our study, the aim was to evaluate the acute rate of neurovascular outcome in two relatively homogeneous groups of patients, treated by the same senior surgeon in the same time frame. Neurological evaluation included clinical exam and CT scan. Five patients were found to have experienced ischemic stroke (2%) with no significant clinical sequelae, probably because of the limited interested cerebral area. However, no difference in the stroke rate between the SAC and DAC groups could be found. This is in contrast with other studies. Tsang et al. in 2003 randomized 268 patients either to single or multiple clamps with a higher rate of cerebrovascular accident in the multiple clamp group.

This fact should be taken into account if considering their results. In our study, patients were selected to be at low risk of cerebrovascular accident in order to have less confounding factors [43].

Gerriets et al. have also advocated the use of intra-aortic filter but failed to show a clinical significant benefit in their randomized trial.

Other parameters such as biochemical markers have been evaluated. Dar et al. showed that in a series of 50 patients randomized to single or multiple clamping CABG, S-100 protein levels were significantly higher in the second group; the troponin T levels were also evaluated with no significance. However, no clinically significant differences were found between the two groups.

In our cohort, none of the techniques used showed to be superior in terms of stroke incidence over the other. As each technique has its own surgical advantages and disadvantages (for instance, more space to perform proximal anastomosis in SAC and direct evaluation of graft's length in DAC), the surgeon should choose the technique with which he is more confident in order to have the best surgical result, as good outcome with very low complications rate can be achieved with both techniques. However, in selected patients, according to the literature, it can be rational to reduce aortic manipulation in the presence of aortic atheromas and to use mild hypothermia in order to have better cerebral protection, and SAC strategy could be preferred over DAC. OPCABG and the use of double mammary graft or Y configuration could be advocated in the case of porcelain aorta in order to avoid aortic manipulation [44].

An interesting aspect, as reported by Hammon et al., is that neuropsychological deficits, even if absent and even not radiologically detectable early after operation, can appear over a period of 6 months, suggesting that a closer neurological follow-up should be taken into consideration especially in high-risk patients to better estimate the real neurological outcome [45].

Regarding the so-called no touch technique, i.e., performing CABG without touching the aorta by anastomosing the grafts to the in situ left and/or right mammary arteries, the main concern is the technical feasibility and the need for adequate mammary arteries caliber and coronary arteries run-off, in order to adequately distribute the blood flow to the coronary bed [46].

5. Conclusion

In conclusion, incidence of stroke seems to be independent from cross-clamping technique, and, more generally, we could infer that the global rate of stroke after CABG is probably more influenced by the presence of subjacent risk factors as aortic atheromas, carotid stenosis, and peripheral vascular disease.

Author details

Marco Gennari[1]*, Gianluca Polvani[1,2], Tommaso Generali[3], Sabrina Manganiello[1], Gabriella Ricciardi[1] and Marco Agrifoglio[1,2]

*Address all correspondence to: marcogennari.md@gmail.com

1 Centro Cardiologico Monzino, IRCCS, Milan, Italy

2 Department of Cardiovascular Sciences and Community Health, University of Milan, Italy

3 San Donato Hospital, IRCCS, Italy

References

[1] Roach GW, Kanchuger M, Mangano CM, et al. Adverse cerebral outcomes after coronary bypass surgery: Multicenter study of Perioperative Ischemia Research Group and the Ischemia Research and Education Foundation investigators. The New England Journal of Medicine. 1996;**335**:1857-1863

[2] McKhann GM, Grega MA, Borowicz LM Jr, et al. Stroke and encephalopathy after cardiac surgery: An update. Stroke. 2006;**37**:562-571

[3] John R et al. Multicenter review of preoperative risk factors for stroke after coronary artery bypass grafting. The Annals of Thoracic Surgery. 2000;**69**:30-36

[4] D'Ancona G, Saez de Ibarra JI, Baillot R, Mathieu P, Doyle D, Metras J, et al. Determinants of stroke after coronary artery bypass grafting. European Journal of Cardio-Thoracic Surgery. 2003;**24**:552-556

[5] Filsoufi F, Rahmanian PB, Castillo JG, Bronster D, Adams DH. Incidence, topography, predictors and long term survival after stroke in patients undergoing coronary artery bypass grafting. The Annals of Thoracic Surgery. 2008;**85**:862-870

[6] Mashour GA, Shanks AM, Kheterpal S. Perioperative stroke and associated mortality after noncardiac, nonneurologic surgery. Anesthesiology. 2011;**114**:1289-1296

[7] Bateman BT, Schumacher HC, Wang S, Shaefi S, Berman MF. Perioperative acute ischemic stroke in noncardiac and nonvascular surgery: Incidence, risk factors, and outcomes. Anesthesiology. 2009;**110**:231-238

[8] Selim M. Perioperative stroke. The New England Journal of Medicine. 2007;**356**:706-713

[9] Kam PC, Calcroft RM. Peri-operative stroke in general surgical patients. Anaesthesia. 1997;**52**:879-883

[10] Hogue CW Jr, Palin CA, Aerosmith JE. Cardiopulmonary bypass management and neurologic outcomes: An evidence-based appraisal of current practices. Anesthesia and Analgesia. 2006;**103**:21

[11] Leary MC, Caplan L. Technology insight: Brain MRI and cardiac surgery-detection of postoperative brain ischemia. Nature Clinical Practice. Cardiovascular Medicine. 2007;**4**:379

[12] Padayachee TS, Parsons S, Thebold R, Linley J, Goslin RG, Deverall PB. The detection of microemboli in the middle cerebral artery during cardiopulmonary bypass: A transcranial Doppler ultrasound investigation using membrane and bubble oxygenators. The Annals of Thoracic Surgery. 1987;**44**:298-302

[13] Blauth C, Smith PL, Arnold JV, Jagoe JR, Wootton R, Taylor KM. Influence of oxygenator type on the incidence and extent of microembolic retinal ischemia during cardiopulmonary bypass. Assessment by digital image analysis. The Journal of Thoracic and Cardiovascular Surgery. 1990;**99**:61-69

[14] Blauth CJ, Cosgrove DM, Webb BW, et al. Atheroembolism from the ascending aorta. An emerging problem in cardiac surgery. The Journal of Thoracic and Cardiovascular Surgery. 1992;**103**:1104-1112

[15] Drummond JC, Lee RR, Howell JP Jr. Focal cerebral ischemia after surgery in the "beach chair" position: The role of a congenital variation of circle of Willis anatomy. Anesthesia and Analgesia. 2012;**114**:1301-1303

[16] Bijker JB, van Klei WA, Kappen TH, van Wolfswinkel L, Moons KG, Kalkman CJ. Incidence of intraoperative hypotension as a function of the chosen definition: Literature definitions applied to a retrospective cohort using automated data collection. Anesthesiology. 2007;**107**:213-220

[17] Davila-Roman VG, Barzilai B, Wareing TH, et al. Intraoperative ultrasonographic evaluation of the ascending aorta in 100 consecutive patients undergoing cardiac surgery. Circulation. 1991,**84**.III47-III53

[18] Katz ES, Tunick PA, Rusinek H, et al. Protruding aortic atheromas predict stroke in elderly patients undergoing cardiopulmonary bypass: Experience with intraoperative transesophageal echocardiography. Journal of the American College of Cardiology. 1992;**20**:70-77

[19] Bergman P, van der Linden J. Atherosclerosis of the ascending aorta as a major determinant of the outcome of cardiac surgery. Nature Clinical Practice. Cardiovascular Medicine. 2005;**2**:246-251

[20] Blauth CI. Macroemboli and microemboli during cardiopulmonary bypass. The Annals of Thoracic Surgery. 1995;**59**:1300-1303

[21] Dávila-Román VG, Murphy SF, Nickerson NJ, et al. Atherosclerosis of the ascending aorta is an independent predictor of long-term neurologic events and mortality. Journal of the American College of Cardiology. 1999;**33**:1308-1316

[22] Hogue CW, Murphy SF, Schechtman KB, et al. Risk factors for early or delayed stroke after cardiac surgery. Circulation. 1999;**100**:642

[23] Wareing TH, Davilla-Roman VG, Barzilia B. Management of the severely atherosclerotic ascending aorta during cardiac operations. The Journal of Thoracic and Cardiovascular Surgery. 1992;**103**:453

[24] Barbut D, Hinton RB, Szatrowski TP, et al. Cerebral emboli detected during bypass surgery are associated with clamp removal. Stroke. 1994;**25**:2398

[25] Stump DA, Rogers AT, Hammon JW, et al. Cerebral emboli and cognitive outcome after cardiac surgery. Journal of Cardiothoracic and Vascular Anesthesia. 1996;**10**:113

[26] Go AS, Hylek EM, Phillips KA, et al. Prevalence of diagnosed atrial fibrillation in adults: National implications for rhythm management and stroke prevention: The AnTicoagulation and Risk Factors in Atrial Fibrillation (ATRIA) Study. Journal of the American Medical Association. 2001;**285**:2370-2375

[27] Almassi GH, Schowalter T, Nicolosi AC, et al. Atrial fibrillation after cardiac surgery: A major morbid event? Annals of Surgery. 1997;**226**:501-511

[28] Mathew JP, Fontes ML, Tudor IC, et al. A multicenter risk index for atrial fibrillation after cardiac surgery. Journal of the American Medical Association. 2004;**291**:1720-1729

[29] Ahlsson AJ, Bodin L, Lundblad OH, et al. Postoperative atrial fibrillation is not correlated to C-reactive protein. The Annals of Thoracic Surgery. 2007;**83**:1332-1337

[30] Frye RL, Kronmal R, Schaff HV, Myers WO, Gersh BJ. Stroke in coronary artery bypass graft surgery: An analysis of the CASS experience. The participants in the Coronary Artery Surgery Study. International Journal of Cardiology. 1992;**36**:213-221

[31] Gardner TJ, Horneffer PJ, Manolio TA, et al. Stroke following coronary artery bypass grafting: A ten-year study. The Annals of Thoracic Surgery. 1985;**40**:574-581

[32] Angelini GD, Penny WJ, el Chamary F, et al. The incidence and significance of early pericardial effusion after open heart surgery. European Journal of Cardio-Thoracic Surgery. 1987;**1**:165-168

[33] Henderson AS, Easteal S, Jorm AF, et al. Apolipoprotein E allele epsilon 4, dementia, and cognitive decline in a population sample. Lancet. 1995;**346**:1387

[34] Charlesworth DC, Likosky DS, Marrin CAS, Maloney CT, Quinton HB, Morton JR, Leavitt BJ, Clough RA, O'Connor GT. Development and validation of a prediction model for strokes after coronary artery bypass grafting. The Annals of Thoracic Surgery. 2003;**76**:463-443

[35] Redmond M, Greene PS, Goldsborough MA, Cameron DE, Stuart RS, Sussman MS, Watkins L Jr, Laschinger JC, McKhan GM, Johnston MV, Baumgartner WA. Neurological injury in cardiac surgical patients with a history of stroke. The Annals of Thoracic Surgery. 1996;**61**:42-47

[36] Stamou SC, Hill PC, Dangas G, Pfister AJ, Boyce SW, Dullum MK, Bafi AS, Corso PJ. Stroke after coronary bypass: Incidence, predictors, and clinical outcome. Stroke. 2001;**32**:1508-1513

[37] Dutta M, Hanna E, Das P, Steinhubi SR. Incidence and prevention of ischemic stroke following myocardial infarction: Review of current literature. Cerebrovascular Disease. 2006;**22**:331-339

[38] Van der Linden J, Hadjinikolaou L, Bergman P, Lindblom D. Postoperative stroke in cardiac surgery is related to the location and extent of atherosclerotic disease in the ascending aorta. Journal of the American College of Cardiology. 2001;**38**:131-135

[39] Roach GW, Kanchuger M, Mangano CM, et al. Adverse cerebral outcomes after coronary bypass surgery. Multicenter Study of Perioperative Ischemia Research Group and the Ischemia Research and Education Foundation Investigators. New England Journal of Medicine. 1996;**335**:1857-1863

[40] Bergman P, van der Linden J. Atherosclerosis of the ascending aorta as a major determinant of the outcome of cardiac surgery. Nature Clinical Practice. Cardiovascular Medicine. 2005;**2**:246-251

[41] Lichtman JH, Krumolz HM, Wang Y, Radford M, Brass LM. Risk and predictors of stroke after myocardial infarction among the elderly. Results from co-operative cardiovascular project. Circulation. 2002;**105**:1082-1087

[42] AlWaqfi N, Ibraheem K, BaniHani M. Stroke after coronary artery surgery: Incidence and risk factors analysis. The Internet Journal of Cardiovascular Research. 2008;**7**(1)

[43] Cao et al. Risk factors for recurrent stroke after coronary artery bypass grafting. Journal of Cardiothoracic Surgery. 2011;**6**:157

[44] Grau AJ, Boddy AW, Dukovic DA, et al. Leukocyte count as an independent predictor of recurrent ischemic events. Stroke. 2004;**35**:1147-1152

[45] Schoof J, Lubahn W, Baeumer M, Kross R, Wallesch CW, Kozian A, Huth C, Goertler M. Impaired cerebral autoregulation distal to carotid stenosis occlusion is associated with increased risk of stroke at cardiac surgery with cardiopulmonary bypass. Journal of Thoracic and Cardiovascular Surgery. 2007;**134**:690-696

[46] Likosky DS, Marrin CAS, Caplan MR, Baribeu YR, Morton JR, Weintraumb MR, et al. Determination of etiologic mechanisms of stroke secondary to coronary artery bypass graft surgery. Stroke. 2003;**34**:28303-28304

7

Role and Rationale for Hybrid Coronary Artery Revascularization

Kendal M. Endicott and Gregory D. Trachiotis

Abstract

The optimal revascularization strategy for patients with multi-vessel coronary artery disease remains controversial. The advent of percutaneous coronary intervention (PCI) has challenged the superiority of coronary artery bypass graft (CABG) surgery for multi-vessel disease. In the late 1990s, an integrated approach, now referred to as "hybrid coronary revascularization" (HCR), was pioneered combining CABG and PCI to offer appropriate patients a less invasive option for revascularization while still capitalizing on the superior patency rates of the left internal mammary artery (LIMA) to the left anterior descending (LAD) artery bypass . The operative techniques continue to evolve as well as the timing strategies for intervention and use of anti-platelet therapy. While more research is needed, current data supports hybrid coronary revascularization as a promising technique to optimize outcomes in patients with multi-vessel coronary artery disease.

Keywords: Hybrid Coronary Revascularization, Coronary Artery Disease, Coronary Artery Bypass Grafting, Percutaneous Coronary Intervention, Robotics

1. Introduction

The optimal revascularization strategy for patients with multi-vessel coronary artery disease remains controversial. The advent of percutaneous coronary intervention (PCI) has challenged the superiority of coronary artery bypass graft (CABG) surgery for multi-vessel disease as PCI offers a less invasive option with faster recovery time and lower risk. Despite a survival benefit in high-risk groups and superior long-term freedom from revascularization, trends continue to move toward increasing percutaneous approaches. In the late 1990s, an integrated approach, now referred to as "hybrid coronary revascularization" (HCR), was pioneered combining CABG and PCI to offer appropriate patients a less invasive option for revascularization while still capitalizing on the superior patency rates of the left internal mammary artery (LIMA) to left anterior descending (LAD) artery bypass. The technology has evolved tremendously since the introduction of HCR with some LIMA-LAD grafts now performed completely robotically. As HCR evolves, questions regarding indications, optimal surgical technique, timing, and outcomes as well as cost-benefit analysis continue to permeate current practice and will define the future of HCR in the algorithm of coronary revascularization.

2. Rationale

CABG has long been the established standard of care to treat left main or three vessel coronary artery disease [1]. The therapeutic benefit of this approach lies in the LIMA-LAD revascularization. Patency rates of this anastomosis lie between 95%–98% at 10 years [2]. Radial arterial conduits have been explored as another option for total arterial revascularization; however, results do not compare with the long-term patency of LIMA utilization [3]. Saphenous vein grafts (SVG) also do not provide the same longevity of the LIMA-LAD revascularization. Failure of SVG is multifactorial including technical failure within 30 days, neo-intimal hyperplasia at 1–24 months, and atherosclerotic degeneration beyond 2 years. Patient risk factors such as hyperlipidemia and ongoing tobacco are also associated with accelerated graft failure. Failure rates are estimated as high as 10%–15% at 1 year after CABG with almost 50% total graft occlusion at 10 years [4]. Despite this high failure rate, SVG remain the most commonly used conduit for CABG surgery.

PCI has challenged the superiority of CABG surgery for multi-vessel disease. The use of drug-eluting stents (DES) in particular has provided a less invasive option for revascularization with faster return to normal activities and lower risk of complications. Restenosis rates and stent thrombosis of DES in non-LAD lesions are markedly lower than non-LAD SVG with rates less than 10% and 1%, respectively [5]. In addition, stenting of SVG after thrombosis introduces technical changes with higher peri-procedural rates of complications and in-hospital mortality than stenting of native arteries [4, 6]. Despite data that suggests improved outcomes with many patients including diabetics and those with left main and complex multi-vessel coronary artery disease (CAD) [2], trends continue toward increased PCI over CABG.

The strategy of HCR attempts to capitalize on the superior LIMA-LAD patency rates as well as the minimally invasive PCI approach thus eliminating the need for additional venous or arterial conduits. Patients with multi-vessel disease with significant proximal LAD disease with other lesions suitable for PCI in the left main, left circumflex, or right coronary artery territories are appropriate candidates for HCR [7]. In addition, patients with lack of suitable conduits, prior sternotomy, severe ascending aortic disease, or coronary arteries not amenable for bypass may be suitable HCR candidates. Patients generally not deemed HCR candidates and thus deferred to conventional CABG include those with chronic total occlusions, highly calcified segments, and diffusely diseased and bifurcation coronary lesions [7]. Table 1 summarizes the clinical and angiographic findings that should be taken into consideration when discussing the option for HCR. Discussions regarding treatment options are best facilitated by a multi-disciplinary approach including both an interventional cardiologist and cardiac surgeon.

	PCI	CABG	HCR
Angiographic Characteristics			
Unprotected Left Main Disease	no	yes	yes
Intra-myocardial LAD	yes	no	no
Complex LAD lesion	no	yes	yes
Complex non-LAD lesions	no	yes	no
Comorbidities			
Advanced Age	yes	no	yes
LVEF <30%	no	yes	yes
Diabetes mellitus	no	yes	yes
Renal insufficiency	no	yes	yes
Severe chronic lung disease	yes	no	no
Prior left thoracotomy	yes	yes	no
Prior sternotomy	yes	no	yes
Limited vascular access	no	yes	no
Lack of available conduits	yes	no	yes
Severe aortic calcification	yes	no	yes
Contraindication for dual anti-platelet therapy	no	yes	no

Table 1. Recommendations for Candidates for Hybrid Coronary Revascularization Versus Conventional Coronary Revascularization [2, 21]

3. Strategies and surgical approach

3.1. Surgical approaches

Minimally invasive cardiac surgery seeks to eliminate two invasive components of conventional CABG: cardiopulmonary bypass (CBP) and sternotomy. The development of stabilizer technology in the early 1990s made available off-pump CABG with the potential advantages of less blood loss, lower incidence of neurologic complications, and less pulmonary complications [8]. In conjunction with sternal sparing incisions as well as robotic techniques, a minimally invasive off-pump option for LIMA-LAD revascularization offers the key to optimizing the HCR option. The techniques described below and in Table 2 discuss the current options for minimally invasive surgical approaches to LIMA-LAD revascularization highlighting key features of the various techniques.

	Thoracic Access	LIMA Harvest	Anastomosis	Single Lung ventilation	CPB	Advantages/Disadvantages
OPCAB (Off-pump CABG)	Midline Sternotomy	Direct Vision	Direct vision with stabilizers	Not Required	No	Avoids risks associated with CBP
MIDCAB (Minimally invasive direct coronary artery bypass grafting)	Left-sided thoracotomy or lower partial sternotomy	Direct Vision	Direct Vision	Improves exposure but not required	Not required but can be performed by femoral cannulation	Avoids aortic cross-clamping and manipulation
Endo-ACAB (Endoscopic atraumatic coronary artery bypass graft surgery)	Limited rib sparing left-sided thoracotomy	Robotic or Thoracoscopic	Hand-Sutured	Required when robot is used	Not required	Decreased morbidity from thoracotomy incision yet allows for hand-sewn anastomosis
TECAB (Totally endoscopic coronary artery bypass graft surgery)	Thoracoscopic	Robotic	Robotic intracorporeal anastomosis	Required	Not required	Minimally invasive, however very technically challenging

Table 2. Surgical Techniques Used for LAD Revascularization During Hybrid Coronary Revascularization

MIDCAB: Minimally invasive direct coronary artery bypass(MIDCAB) grafting refers to an off-pump minimally invasive LIMA-LAD revascularization performed through a small left-sided thoracotomy in the fourth or fifth interspace. Costal cartilage removal or rib disarticulation is sometimes necessary for visualizing. Cardiac stabilization and LAD harvest is performed directly through the wound and does not require endoscopic or robotic skills to master the LAD harvest. Surgeon comfort with off-pump techniques is critical as well as experience with sternal sparing incisions. Single-lung ventilation is optimal for exposure; however chest cavity insufflation is not necessary. A slightly larger thoracotomy incision can allow exposure for harvest of bilateral internal mammary arteries.

Large series published since 1994 have validated short-term LAD-LIMA patency rates of this technique at 95%–97% [8]. The advantage of this technique lies in the avoidance of CBP and aortic manipulation as an off-pump strategy; however, no data exists to suggest differences in post-operative pain or pulmonary complications from conventional CABG [8]. MIDCAB may have decreased bleeding and infection rates compared to traditional sternotomy, however the need for a thoracotomy incision for the technique has prompted further exploration into various thoracoscopic and robotic techniques to capitalize on the advantages of minimally invasive strategies as discussed in the following.

Endo-ACAB: Endoscopic atraumatic coronary artery bypass (Endo-ACAB) refers to the thoracosocpic or robotic identification of the LAD with LIMA mobilization without violating the integrity of the chest wall (Figure 1). A directed, non-rib spreading or limited rib spreading thoracotomy is then employed for a hand-sewn LIMA-LAD anastomosis on the beating heart. Robotic LIMA mobilization requires single-lung ventilation and insufflation to create space in the anterior mediastinum to facilitate LIMA harvest. After the LIMA is taken down, a peri-cardial incision is made for identification of the LAD. A small (4–5cm) anterior thoracotomy without disarticulation of costal cartilage is then made to introduce an endoscopic stabilizer via an arm port, which allows for LAD stabilization and hand-sewn anastomosis.

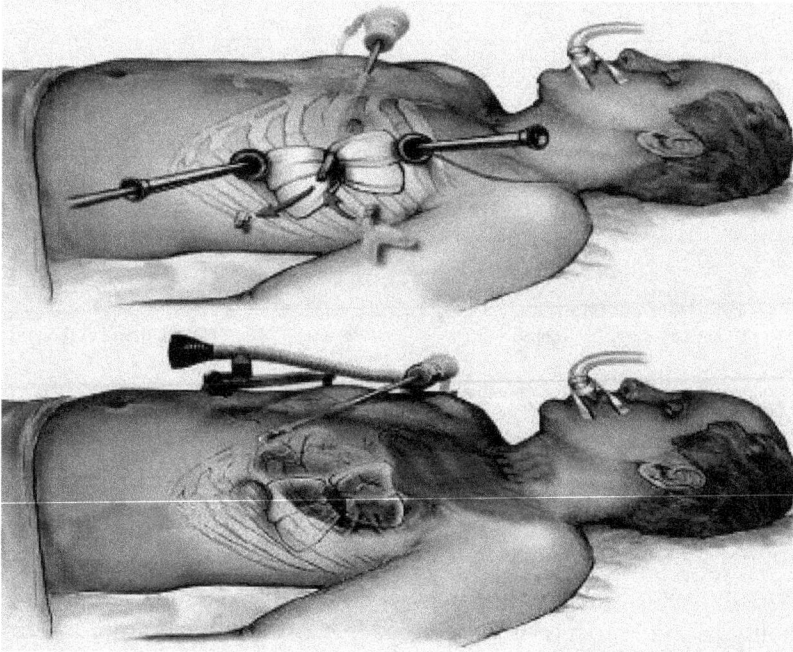

Figure 1. EndoCab technique as described above.

Multiple case series have reported excellent LIMA-LAD patency rates with thoracoscopic Endo-ACAB approaches. In new smaller series with robotic Endo-ACAB approaches, routine post-operative angiography has demonstrated no decline in LIMA-LAD patency rates. In Kiaii's series of 58 patients who underwent one-stage robotic Endo-ACAB HCR, the average length of stay in the ICU and hospital were 1 and 4 days, respectively, leading the authors to suggest benefit to patients in terms of post-operative surgical morbidity and recovery time using more minimally invasive technology [9].

TECAB: Totally endoscopic coronary artery bypass grafting (TECAB) utilizes a robotically sewn, intracorporeal anastomosis, which negates the need for even a small thoracotomy. This technique was first explored on an arrested heart during CBP; however, the associated complications of CPB have led most robotic surgeons to employ an off-pump TECAB. The operation itself is technically challenging without widespread adoption of this technique owning to the need for robotic technology and surgeon expertise.

One of the largest series published in 2012 reported on 226 patients with 5-year outcomes [10]. Perioperative results were consistent with the standards of open CABG. The authors report a dramatically decreased time to recovery owning to the lack of need for sternal precautions. In the 10 cases requiring conversion to thoracotomy, these patients averaged 2- day longer hospital stays with increased ventilator time and return to normal activities [10]. Overall results in other case series support the safety and feasibility of this technique; however, Harskamp reports that only approximately one-third of HCRs from 2011–2013 reported in the Society of Thoracic Adult Cardiac Database utilize robotic technology [11]. Expansion of the TECAB approach is currently limited by the cost and learning curve associated with the implementation of robotic technology.

Graft Assessment: Off-pump (OP) and minimally invasive techniques for LAD-LIMA grafting have appropriately been scrutinized with regard to patency rate outcomes compared to the classical on-pump CABG via a midline sternotomy. The recent Randomized On/Off Bypass (ROOBY) trial as well as other smaller trails have demonstrated that the patency rates of LIMA-LAD grafts between off-pump coronary artery bypass (OPCAB) and conventional CABG were similar (95.3 and 96.2, respectively) [12]. As the HCR approach relies upon the durability and integrity of this anastomosis, the ability of the surgeon to assess the LIMA-LAD graft intra-operatively becomes increasingly important. In fact, the European Society of Cardiology (ESC) and the European Association for Cardio-Thoracic Surgery (EACTS) recommends graft evaluation before leaving the operating room [13].

Graft assessment includes the traditional methods such as inspection, palpation, electrocardiography (ECG), and echocardiography (ECHO). Other methods include conventional coronary angiography, which is the gold standard, transit-time flow measurement (TTFM), and intra-operative fluorescence imaging (IFI). As the causes of early graft failure are often technical, this technology seeks to eliminate these errors by objectively evaluating graft function. Certainly, a clear advantage of single stage HCR with CABG followed by PCI lies in the opportunity for angiographic graft assessment with readily available operative access for reintervention; however, when angiographic assessment is not available, the most commonly utilized technique among cardiovascular surgeons over the last decade has become TTFM. Retrospective studies have demonstrated the ability of TTFM to detect grafts with impaired flow thus predicting graft failure within 6 months after CABG [14]; however, little is known about how TTFM relates to long-term graft patency and patient survival.

TTFM relies on the principles of transit-time ultrasound technology. The surgeon can obtain both quantitative data of average blood flow volume and several calculated derivatives of the flow of blood in the graft displayed in waveform. TTFM cannot, however, differentiate physiologic conditions accounting for low blood flow versus technical quality of a surgical anastomosis. While clear cut-off values for graft revision have not been set, a mean flow <15ml min $^{-1}$ for grafts to the left coronary system and less than 20ml min $^{-1}$ for grafts to the right coronary system were predictive of failure. A pulsatility index (PI) greater than 0.5 is predictive of graft failure. Another important value is the diastolic flow percentage (DF%) or diastolic flow divided by total flow through the graft. This value should be greater than 50% for all grafts and territories and ideally greater than 65%. When the PI and DF% both demonstrate adequate measurements, the graft can be objectively presumed adequate [15]. Figure 2 demonstrates the intra-operative TTFM tracings utilizing the MediStim ASA technology, which is one of the more commonly utilized flowmeters.

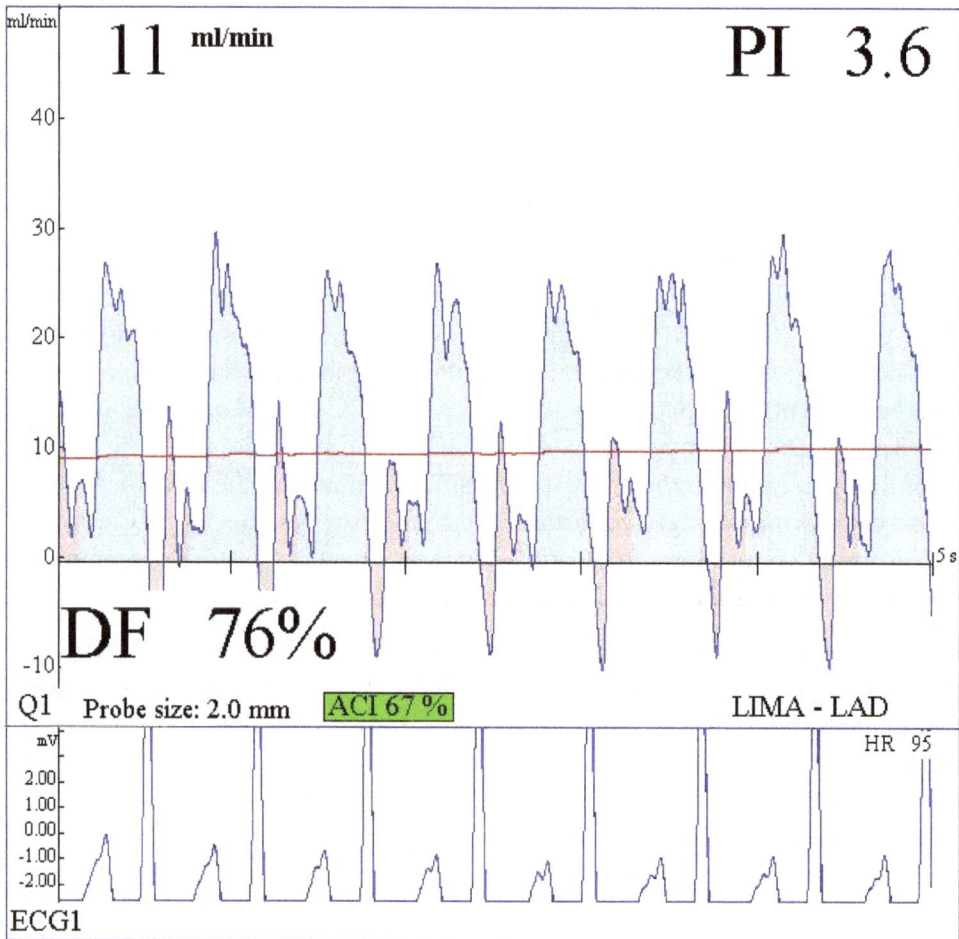

Figure 2. Transit Time Flow Assessment.

3.2. Timing strategies

HCR began in the 1990s as a staged procedure with LIMA-LAD revascularization performed first followed by PCI. The use of DESs and anti-platelet therapy as well as the use of hybrid operating room suites has introduced questions as to the most optimal timing for open and

PCI revascularization. Currently, three options for timing strategies exist: PCI followed by CABG, CABG followed by PCI, and one-stage hybrid HCR. Each option introduces different benefits and challenges, and at this time no clear consensus exists on the optimal strategy for timing of revascularization (Table 3). Patient characteristics, operator skill, and availability of facilities should be considered when choosing the most appropriate approach.

One-Stage HCR	Two-Stage HCR	
Simultaneous CABG and PCI	CABG then PCI	PCI then CABG
Advantages:	**Advantages:**	**Advantages:**
Ability to study LIMA-LAD graft	Ability to study LIMA-LAD graft	Pre-operative angiographic imaging of LIMA size
Protected LAD to allow PCI to high-risk non-LAD lesions	Protected LAD to allow PCI to high-risk non-LAD lesions	Lower risk of ischemia during CABG given non-LAD territory revascularization
Single anesthetic exposure	Reduced risk of post-surgical bleedingas no need for anti-platelet therapy post CABG	Useful in acute coronary syndromeswith non-LAD culprits
Can convert to conventional CABG if PCI fails	After LIMA-LAD revascularization, asymptomatic patients may require no further intervention	If stents unsuccessful, conventional CABG has to be subsequently performed
Single procedure reduces cost and hospital length of stay		
Disadvantages:	**Disadvantages:**	**Disadvantages:**
Requires hybrid suite	Risk of ischemia during CABG in non-LAD lesions	No ability to angiographically evaluate LIMA-LAD anastomosis
Increased risk of post-operative bleeding due to need for anti-platelet after surgery	Unsuccessful PCI may lead to need for surgical reintervention	Increased peri-operative bleeding due to need for anti-platelet therapy
Risk of stent thrombosis due to post-operative inflammatory state		Potential for LAD territory ischemia between stages
CKD patients exposed to dual nephrotoxic insults with surgery and PCI contrast use		Higher risk of stent thrombosis due to inflammatory response of CABG and potential need to hold anti-platelet therapy
High degrees of coordination needed between teams		

Table 3. Advantages and Disadvantages of One and Two-Staged HCR Procedures

One-Stage HCR: Simultaneous CABG and PCI: The advent of hybrid operating room suites has introduced the option for simultaneous CABG and PCI. This approach allows for complete revascularization before leaving the operating room. Routine imaging of the LIMA-LAD anastomosis is also available before chest closure. More aggressive percutaneous approaches can be taken to otherwise challenging lesions given the safety net of open revascularization options. The patient benefits from a single anesthetic exposure and decreased hospitalization time. One ongoing concern however is the post-operative risk of bleeding given the need for dual anti-platelet therapy after DES placement in conjunction with incomplete heparin reversal. Concerns also exist regarding the relationship of the inflammatory response in the post-operative setting and risk for acute stent thrombosis.

Two-Stage: PCI Followed by CABG: This option confers several advantages. In revascularizing the non-LAD lesion first and thus providing collateralization, the potential risks of ischemia during LAD occlusion are minimized. PCI firstly also provides the interventional cardiologist a safety net should revascularization be unsuccessful percutaneously. The most important benefit of this approach occurs in the setting of acute coronary syndrome with a non-LAD culprit. The acutely affected lesion may be stented followed by LAD revascularization at a later time. This strategy does however introduce the difficulty of the need for anti-platelet therapy with DES. Even brief discontinuation of anti-platelet therapy can risk stent thrombosis; however this must be weighed with intra-operative bleeding risk. Investigation is underway regarding the use of newer anti-platelet agents and potential decreased bleeding risk. It again should be noted that the pro-inflammatory trauma from surgery could also put new stents at risk for thrombosis.

Two-Stage: CABG Followed by PCI: This strategy has become the most widely adopted one for HCR. With PCI post-CABG, the concern for surgical bleeding while on anti-platelet therapy is negated. Like hybrid HCR, LIMA-LAD graft patency can be confirmed during PCI angiography. Pre-PCI protection of the LAD also provides the interventional cardiologist the option to approach lesions that would perhaps have otherwise been at higher risk. This includes both left main lesions and diagonal bifurcation lesions [8]. For the minimally invasive surgeon, the unrevascularized collateral lesions could manifest as intra-operative ischemia. Careful attention must be paid to hemodynamics during insufflation, and the use of peripheral CPB should be considered if needed. In the scenario of a PCI complication or failure, this approach could necessitate a return to the operating room with emergent CABG. The optimal time frame for PCI following CABG remains unclear. Some teams opt for PCI during the index hospitalization and thus avoid patient discharge with an incomplete revascularization, however other teams propose a more extended period of waiting from 1 to several weeks. Economic factors also become an increasing concern given questions of reimbursement.

Overall, no clear optimal timing strategy has been clearly defined. While some studies demonstrate increased post-operative bleeding risks on dual-anti-platelet therapy, others suggest that the minimally invasive surgical approaches negate this risk traditionally associated with sternotomy. Harskamp's analysis of recent STS data suggests that the need for post-operative transfusion was actually lower in the one-stage procedure group with comparable reoperation for bleeding [11]. This analysis also reports that patients undergoing one-stage procedures were more likely to have peripheral vascular disease and stroke history compared to other groups [11]. Further studies are needed to outline the specific clinical scenarios and patient characteristics, which should dictate the timing of CABG and PCI. Certainly, cost analysis and patient preferences will also factor into future decision-making regarding timing strategies.

Anti-platelet management: As discussed, the use of anti-platelet therapy is a complicated balance of post-surgical bleeding versus risk of acute stent thrombosis. Currently, no guidelines exist to define the optimal strategy. This question of anti-platelet therapy poses two questions regarding the order of staging as well as timing of initiation of therapy. Different authors have reported their experience with varying strategies and outcomes. In cases of two staged procedures with CABG first, most authors performed CABG on aspirin alone followed by a second anti-platelet agent greater than 4 h post-operatively after ensuring that there were no bleeding complications [16]. In the two stage procedures, which performed PCI first, anti-platelet therapy was begun before PCI and continued uninterrupted during CABG. In one-stage procedures, the most common strategies administered anti-platelet therapy after undergoing the LIMA-LAD graft, just before its completion, or immediately after PCI. Others administered anti-platelet therapy at the induction of anesthesia or in the pre-operative area owning to the fact that maximal platelet inhibition occurs 4–24 h after administration [16]. None of these strategies differed in reported rate of acute stent thrombosis [5]. In some studies, the rate of blood transfusion was actually lower in the HCR group as was the need for reoperation for bleeding [11]. Newer anti-platelet agents that are more potent and have a faster onset of action and reversal have also been employed; however, there is currently no data to support the use of these new agents in HCR.

4. Outcomes

Multiple case series from single institution experiences have been published on HCR since the first report in 1996. This includes a population of over 3,000 patients [16]. Data from these series suggest that in experienced hands, the safety profile of HCR is excellent. Multiple studies comparing outcomes after HCR versus CABG and multi-vessel disease have also been published (Table 4). Among cohort studies, the single-stage HCR was most commonly employed. Across these studies, age averaged around 60 years with a male predominance. Left ventricular ejection fraction (LVEF) was preserved or mildly reduced in the majority of patients. With the exception of data from Leacche et al., overall in-hospital mortality, stroke and reoperation for bleeding rates were comparable and low [0% to 2.6%). The outlier reported by Leacche et al. was among the high SYNTAX-HCR group with a reported in-hospital mortality of 23% leading the authors to suggest that HCR should be approached with caution in patients with high (≥33] SYNTAX scores [17]. These reports collectively suggest that HCR may be a comparable option to CABG in patients with non-LAD lesions accessible by PCI.

Author, Year Type of Study	N	Surgical Technique	Timing of PCI	Age, years	Male, %	LVEF %	SYNTAX Score	In-Hospital Mortality	Follow-Up Period	Survival
Shen et al., 2013 Retrospective, matched cohort study (propensity matched) Recruitment: 2007-2010 (23)	141 HCR 141 CABG 141 PCI	Lower partial mini-sternotomy CABG (on and off pump)	One Stage	62±9.9 62.4±7.8 61.7±10.3	88.7 90.1 87.2	62.7±7.1 62.6±8.0 62.1±9.3	27.6±7.9 28.2±9.4 26.0±8.2	N/A	30 days	99.3% 97.2% 96.5%
Leacche et al., 2013 Retrospective cohort study (group stratification) Recruitment: 2005-2009 (17)	80 HCR SYNTAX≤32 (67) SYNTAX>32 (13) 301 CABG SYNTAX≤32 (226) SYNTAX>32 (75)	OP 22% OP 31% OP 15% OP 16%	One Stage	62 (32-85) 74 (32-84) 63 (32-89) 62 (32-83)	79 62 75 83	50 (20-70) 50 (20-65) 55 (10-80) 50 (10-70)	N/A	****	30 days	N/A
Bachinsky et al., 2012 Prospective cohort study, no matching Recruitment: 2009-2011 (24)	25 HCR 27 CABG	OP MIDCab (Robotic) 100% OP CABG (thoracotomy)	One Stage	63.2±10.5 66.78±10.7	80 59	55.3±10.4 51.48±12.0	33.52±8 34.89±8.2	0% 4%	30 days	100% 96%
Halkos et al., 2011 Retrospective matched cohort study (propensity matching) Recruitment: 2003-2010 (25)	147 HCR 588 CABG	OP EndoACAB OP CABG	Surgery and PCI within 2-3 day (137); One stage (10)	64.3±12.8 64.3±12.5	38.1 28.6	54.7±8.7 54.6±8.7	N/A	0.7% 0.9%	3.2 years	5-year survival: 86.8% 84.3%
Vassiliades et al., 2009 Retrospective cohort study (no matching, propensity score adjustment) Recruitment: 2003-2007 (26)	91 HCR 4175 CABG	OP EndoACAB OP CABG	85 CABG first 6 PCI first	64.7±13.7 62.8±11.7	40.7 37.3	51.5±9.4 50.9±12.7	N/A	0% 1.8%	3 years	94.0% 89.2%
Zhao et al., 2009 Retrospective cohort study (no matching) Recruitment: 2005-2007 (27)	112 HCR 20 CABG	Reversed-J inferior sternotomy OP CABG	One Stage	63 (32-85) 63 (32-89)	71 76	50 (15-70) 54 (10-72)	N/A	2.6% 1.5%	N/A	N/A
Reicher et al., 2008 Prospective, matched cohort study (propensity matching) 2005-2006 (28)	12 HCR 26 CABG	OP MidCab OP CABG (sternotomy)	CABG first	62±10 64±10	80 83	31 (EF <40%) 27 (EF <40%)	N/A	0% 0%	30 days	100% 100%
Kon et al., 2008 Matched prospective cohort study, unclear matching method Recruitment: 2005-2006 (29)	15 HCR 30 CABG	OP MidCab OP CABG (sternotomy)	One Stage	61±10 65±10	73 63	47±14 45±14	N/A	0% 0%	12 mo.	100% 100%

**** see text

Table 4. Studies Comparing Outcomes After HCR Versus CABG or PCI in the Drug Eluting Stent Era [5, 22]

Harskamp et al. published a meta-analysis in 2014 reporting clinical outcomes after HCR in 1,190 patients in single-center registries [18]. This study incorporated six observational studies (one case control and five propensity adjusted) that included adjustments for differences in baseline characteristics. Comparisons of individual components showed no differences in all-cause mortality, MI, or stroke at one year follow-up (odds ratio: 0.49; 95% confidence interval: 0.2 -1.24; p=0.13), however the HCR group demonstrated a higher repeat revascularization rate compared with CABG. These findings were irrespective of the order in which LIMA-LAD graft and PCI were performed.

The only current randomized control trial comparing HCR and CABG was published in 2014 [19]. Two-hundred consecutive patients from a single institution with angiographically confirmed multi-vessel disease involving the proximal LAD and a significant (>70%) lesion in at least one major non-LAD epicardial vessel amenable to both PCI and CABG were randomized in a 1:1 fashion. The primary endpoint was the evaluation of the safety of HCR. The HCR group (n=98) utilized MIDCAB and cobalt chromium DES with a two-stage HCR with PCI performed within 36 h of initial MIDCAB, versus the conventional CABG group (n=102) in which 85.0% of the procedures were performed off-pump. Pre-operative characteristics were similar. Regarding HCR procedures, 6.1% patients were converted to CABG with no adverse early or late outcomes, and HCR was feasible in 93.9% of patients. At 1 year, the two groups had similar all-cause mortality (CABG 2.9% versus HCR 2%; p=NS) and MACE-free survival rates (CABG 92.2% versus HCR 89.8%; p log-rank =0.54). Larger studies are needed to power conclusions regarding long-term mortality data; however, this study suggests that HCR is feasible and safe.

Harskamp et al. recently published a study of practice patterns and clinical outcomes after HCR, in the United States, using the Society of Thoracic Surgeons Adult Cardiac Surgery Database from July 2011 to March 2013 [11]. This analysis demonstrated that HCR represented 0.48% (n=950; staged=809, concurrent=141) of the total CABG volume (n=198,622) over the studied time. HCR was performed in approximately one-third of participating centers (n=361). Interestingly, patients who underwent HCR had high-risk profiles but less extensive coronary disease. There was no statistically significant association between operative approach and operative mortality when comparing the HCR and conventional CABG treatment groups [11].

5. Conclusions

Hybrid coronary revascularization has emerged as a promising technique that combines the superior patency of the LIMA-LAD graft with the superior patency of DES to SVG grafts for non-LAD vessels. As with any new technique, ongoing research will benefit from standardized definitions as well as sub-classification for HCR procedures [20]. Current evidence also lacks direction as to which patient population benefits most from HCR. Current data supports HCR as a feasible alternative to CABG, however, the future of these techniques will rely on improved patient satisfaction, recovery, and financial feasibility. Current reported quality of life assessments 1 year post-operatively are remarkably better in patients undergoing HCR versus OPCAB [5]. Likely reasons include decreased post-operative pain and decreased length of intensive care and hospital stay with quicker return to work and normal activities. Cost analysis have been reported both equal and in favor of HCR; however, these analysis did not examine the hidden cost of construction of a cardiac hybrid operating room as well as training of personal [5]. Further studies are needed to firmly establish improved outcomes and financial benefits of HCR before this novel technique establishes itself as a widespread option in the algorithm of coronary revascularization.

Author details

Kendal M. Endicott[2] and Gregory D. Trachiotis[1,2*]

*Address all correspondence to: gregory.trachiotis@va.gov

1 Division of Cardiothoracic Surgery, Veterans Affairs Medical Center, Washington, DC, USA

2 Division of Cardiothoracic Surgery, The George Washington University, Washington, DC, USA

References

[1] Serruys PW, Morice MC, et al. Percutaneous Coronary Intervention versus Coronary-Artery Bypass Grafting for Severe Coronary Artery Disease. *N Engl J Med*. 2009;360:961-972.

[2] Popma JJ, Nathan S, et al. Hybrid Myocardial Revascularization: An Integrated Approach to Coronary Revascularization. *Catheterization and Cardiovascular Interventions*. 2010;75:S28-S34.

[3] Tatoulis J, Buxton BF, et al. Patencies of 2,127 Arterial to Coronary Conduits Over 15 Years. *Ann Thorac Surg*. 20004;77:93-101.

[4] Harskamp RE, Lopes RD, et al. Saphenous Vein Graft Failure after Coronary Artery Bypass Surgery: Pathophysiology, Management, and Future Directions. *Ann Surg*. 2013;257:824-833.

[5] Harskamp RE, Zheng Z, et al. Status Quo of Hybrid Coronary Revascularization for Multi-Vessel Coronary Artery Disease. *Ann Thorac Surg*. 2013;96:2268-2277.

[6] Brilakis ES, Rao SV, et al. Percutaneous Coronary Intervention in Native Arteries versus Bypass Grafts in Prior Coronary Artery Bypass Grafting Patients. *J Am Coll Cardiol Intv*. 2011;4:844-50.

[7] Green KD, Lynch DR, et al. Combining PCI and CABG: the Role of Hybrid Revascularization. *Curr Cardiol Rep*. 2013;15,351:1-8.

[8] Narasimhan S, Srinivas V, et al. Hybrid Coronary Revascularization. *Cardiology in Review*. 2011;19:101-107.

[9] Kiaii B, McClure S, et al. Simultaneous Integrated Coronary Artery Revascularization with Long-Term Angiographic Follow-Up. *J Thorac Cardiovasc Surg*. 2008;136:702-708.

[10] Bonatti JO, Zimrin D, et al. Hybrid Coronary Revascularization using Robotic Totally Endoscopic Surgery: Perioperative Outcoes and 5-Year Results. *Ann Thorac Surg*. 2012;94:1920-1926.

[11] Harskamp RE, Brennan, JM, et al. Practice Patters and Clinical Outcomes after Hybrid Coronary Revascularization in the United States: An Analysis from the Society of Thoracic Surgeons Adult Cardiac Database. *Circulation*. 2014;130:872-879.

[12] Shroyer AL, Grover FL et al.; The ROOBY Study Group. On-Pump versus Off-Pump Coronary-Artery Bypass Surgery. *N Engl J Med*. 2009;361:1827-1837.

[13] The Task Force on Myocardial Revascularization of the European Society of Cardiology (ESC) and the European Association for Cardio-Thoracic Surgery (EACTS): Guidelines on Myocardial Revascularization. *European Heart Journal*. 2010;31:2501-2505.

[14] Jokinen JJ, Werkkala K. Clinical Value of Intra-operative Transit-time Flow Measurement for Coronary Artery Bypass Grafting: a Prospective Angiography-Controlled Study. *Eur J Cardiothorac Surg*. 2011;39:918-923.

[15] Trachiotis GD. Value of Diastolic Flow with Transit-time Flow Meters in Coronary Artery Bypass Surgery. *Eur J Cardiothorac Surg*. 2011;39:424-437.

[16] Panoulas V, Colombo A. Hybrid Coronary Revascularization: Promising, But yet to Take Off. *J Am Coll Cardiol*. 2015;65:85-97.

[17] Leacche M, Byrne JG, et al. Comparison of 30-day Outcomes of Coronary Artery Bypass Grafting Surgery versus Hybrid Coronary Revascularization Stratified by SYNTAX and euroSCORE. *J Thorac Cardiovasc Surg*. 2013;145:1004-1012.

[18] Harskamp RE, Bagai A, et al. Clinical Outcomes after Hybrid Coronary Revascularization versus Coronary Artery Bypass Surgery: a Meta-analysis of 1,190 Patients. *Am Heart J*. 2014;166, 4:585-592.

[19] Gasior M, Zembala MO, et al. Hybrid Revascularization for Multivessel Coronary Artery Disease. *J Am Coll Cardiol Intv*. 2014;7:1277-1283.

[20] Harskamp RE, Bonatti, JO, et al. Standardizing Definitions for Hybrid Coronary Revascularization. *J Thorac Cardiovasc Surg*. 2014;147:556-560.

[21] Fihn SD, Gardin JM, et al. 2012 ACCF/AHA/ACP/AATS/PCNA/SCAI/STS Guideline for the diagnosis and management of patients with stable ischemic heart disease: a

report of the American College of Cardiology Foundation/American Heart Association Task Force on Practice Guidelines, and the American College of Physicians, American Association for Thoracic Surgery, Preventive Cardiovascular Nurses Association, Society for Cardiovascular Angiography and Interventions, and Society of Thoracic Surgeons. *Circulation*. 2012;126:e354-e471.

[22] Gosain P, Yamani N, et al. Hybrid Coronary Revascularization: A Systematic Review. *Cardiology in Review*. 2015;23:87-93.

[23] Shen L, Hu S, et al. One-Stop Hybrid Coronary Revascularization versus Coronary Artery Bypass Grafting and Percutaneous Coronary Intervention for the Treatment of Multivessel Coronary Artery Disease. *J Am Coll Cardiol*. 2013;61:2525-2533.

[24] Bachinsky WB. Abdelsalam M, et al. Comparative Study of Same Sitting Hybrid Coronary Artery Revascularization versus Off-Pump Coronary Artery Bypass in Multivessel Coronary Artery Disease. *J Interven Cardiol*. 2012;25:160-468.

[25] Halkos ME, Vassiliades TA, et al. Hybrid Coronary Revascularization versus Off-Pump Coronary Artery Bypass Grafting for the Treatment of Multivessel Coronary Artery Disease. *Ann Thorac Surg*. 2011;92:1695-1702.

[26] Vassiliades TA, Kilgo PD, et al. Clinical Outcomes after Hybrid Coronary Revascularization versus Off-Pump Coronary Artery Bypass. *Innovations*. 2009;4:299-306.

[27] Zhao DX, Leacche M, et al. Routine Intraoperative Completion Angiography after Coronary Artery Bypass Grafting and 1-Stop Hybrid Revascularization: Results from a Fully Integrated Hybrid Catheterization Laboratory/Operating Room. *J Am Coll Cardiol*. 2009;53:232-241.

[28] Reicher B, Poston RS, et al. Simultaneous "Hybrid" Percutaneous oronary Intervention and Minimally Invasive Surgical Bypass Grafting: Feasibility, Safety, and Clinical Outcomes. *Am Heart J*. 2008;155:661-667.

[29] Kon ZN, Brown EN, et al. Simultaneous hybrid coronary revascularization reduces postoperative morbidity compared with results from conventional off-pump coronary artery bypass. J Thorac Cardiovasc Surg. 2008;125:367-75.

8

Arrhythmias Post Coronary Artery Bypass Surgery

Bandar Al-Ghamdi

Abstract

Arrhythmias are common after cardiac surgery such as coronary artery bypass grafting surgery. Although most of these arrhythmias are transient and have a benign course, it may represent a significant source of morbidity and mortality. Postoperative arrhythmias (POAs) include atrial tachyarrhythmias, ventricular arrhythmias, and bradyarrhythmias. The incidence of POAs has not changed despite improvements in anesthetic and surgical techniques. The tachyarrhythmias in the postoperative period include atrial fibrillation, atrial flutter, supraventricular tachycardia, and ventricular tachycardia. The clinical significance of each arrhythmia depends on several factors that include cardiac function, patient's comorbidities, arrhythmia duration, and ventricular response rate. Tachycardia with uncontrolled ventricular rates can cause diastolic and later on systolic dysfunction, reduce cardiac output, and result in hypotension or myocardial ischemia. In the other hand, bradyarrhythmias may have a remarkable influence on patients with systolic or diastolic ventricular dysfunction. Arrhythmia management starts preoperatively with optimizing the patient's condition and controlling patient's risk factors, intra-operatively with careful attention to hemodynamic changes during surgery and uses appropriate anesthesia, and postoperatively with correction of temporary and correctable predisposing factors, as well as specific therapy for the arrhythmia itself. The POAs treatment urgency and management options are determined by the clinical presentation of the arrhythmia.

Keywords: coronary artery bypass surgery, arrhythmias, atrial fibrillation, ventricular arrhythmias, bradyarrhythmias

1. Introduction

Arrhythmias are common after cardiac surgery such as coronary artery bypass grafting (CABG) surgery and represent a significant source of morbidity and mortality. Although most of these arrhythmias are transient and have a benign course, it may prolong intensive care and hospital stay, and in rare instances, it may lead to mortality. Postoperative arrhythmias (POAs) include atrial tachyarrhythmias (ATs) and to a lesser extent ventricular arrhythmias (VAs) and bradyarrhythmias [1]. The incidence of POAs has not changed despite improvements in anesthetic and surgical techniques, and evidence suggests that its incidence may be increasing [2].

The clinical significance of each arrhythmia depends on several factors that include underlying cardiac function, patient's comorbidities, arrhythmia duration, and ventricular response rate. So, POAs could be tolerated in some patients and a source of morbidity and mortality in others, depending on the interaction between these factors [1, 3]. Rapid ventricular rates with tachycardia can cause diastolic and later on systolic dysfunction, reduce cardiac output, and result in hypotension or myocardial ischemia [4, 5]. Bradydysrhythmias, particularly with the loss of atrial function, may have a remarkable influence on patients with systolic or diastolic ventricular dysfunction [6].

Arrhythmia management starts preoperatively with optimization of the patient's condition and controlling patient's risk factors. Intraoperatively, it includes careful attention to hemodynamic changes during surgery and uses appropriate anesthesia. Postoperatively, it includes correction of temporary and correctable predisposing factors, as well as specific therapy for the arrhythmia itself [7]. The POAs treatment urgency and management options are determined by the clinical presentation of the arrhythmia [7]. Self-terminating arrhythmias without overt cardiac disease often need no therapy. However, arrhythmias with hemodynamic instability, especially in patients with critical stress conditions like systemic infections or persistent pericardial effusion need urgent intervention to restore a stable clinical status [7].

The aim of this chapter is to review post-CABG arrhythmias pathophysiology and management.

2. Pathophysiology

The primary function of CABG is to reestablish perfusion to ischemic myocardium with utilizing autologous arteries and veins. This may be achieved by using different surgical techniques. The POAs pathophysiology, incidence, and clinical course may vary depending on the surgical techniques used. Initially, cardiac surgeries were performed on a beating heart, but with the development of cardiopulmonary bypass (CPB) machine and cardioplegia, most CABG surgeries were performed on a pump. However, interest in off-pump coronary artery bypass (OPCAB) surgery had revived in the 1990s [8]. Reported potential benefits of OPCAB include lower end-organ damage with less cerebrovascular accidents (CVA), fewer cognitive deficits, renal failure, less psychomotor defects, reduced systemic inflammation, and lower transfusion rates [9]. However, variable outcomes have been reported in studies comparing these strategies [9]. Minimally invasive surgery without use of CPB and through smaller incisions- and robotic-assisted approaches have also been developed [9]. This method is most often used for left internal mammary artery (LIMA) to left anterior descending artery (LAD) grafts. Additional benefits may also include reduced operative time, reduced recovery time, decreased the need for blood transfusion, less time under anesthesia, reduced duration of ICU stay, less pain, and an estimated 40% savings over conventional CABG [10].

The development of POAs is related to factors that influence the atrial and ventricular myocardium. These primarily include: a previous *anatomic substrate*, caused by degenerative changes typical of age and underlying disease, and *electrical substrate* derived from the perioperative processes that alter the membrane potentials, increase the dispersion of the refractory periods, and decrease the conduction velocity [11]. Inflammation and hyperadrenergic state appear to play a fundamental role in the development of postoperative tachyarrhythmias, favoring automatism [11]. Hypokalemia and hypomagnesemia characteristic of this period alter phase III of the membrane action potential, increasing the automatism, and slowing the conduction speed [11]. Atrial and ventricular ischemia due to hypoxemia is another contributing factor [11].

Several perioperative risk factors have been implicated in atrial and ventricular susceptibility to POAs, but their relative role is still uncertain. Risk factors for POAs may be classified into patient- and surgery-related factors [7].

2.1. Patient-related risk factors

Various patient-related risk factors have been described to cause POAs. These include:

2.1.1. Age

Increasing age is associated with age-related structural and electrophysiological changes that may lead to postoperative atrial tachyarrhythmias in the elderly. Old age has been demonstrated to be correlated with the development of POAs [2, 3, 12–14].

2.1.2. Underlying structural heart disease

Patients with underlying structural heart disease are at higher risk of developing POAs compared to patients with a normal heart. Structural heart disease in the atria and ventricles provides a substrate for arrhythmia via abnormal automaticity, triggered activity, or reentry. Cardiac surgery patients often have the substrate of atrial enlargement and elevation of atrial pressures may function as a substrate for atrial arrhythmias. It is well known that large atrial size and fibrosis supports propagation of atrial reentrant circuits and helps in maintaining atrial fibrillation (AF). Similarly, patients with ventricular dysfunction, ventricular dilation, or fibrosis are at higher risk of having ventricular arrhythmias [4]. Other important risk factors for POAs include previous history of arrhythmias (e.g., AF), cardiac surgery, and POAs. Also, severe right coronary artery stenosis [15], sinus nodal or atrioventricular nodal branch disease [13, 16, 17], and mitral valvular disease (particularly rheumatic mitral stenosis) have been reported as risk factors for POAs. The preoperative brain natriuretic peptide plasma concentration is another predictor of POAs [18].

2.1.3. Other comorbidities

Noncardiac comorbidities have been reported to increase the risk of POAs especially AF. These include obesity [19], previous stroke, and history of chronic obstructive pulmonary disease [20].

2.2. Surgery-related risk factors

Cardiac surgery may lead to POAs via multiple surgery-related mechanisms and risk factors that include:

2.2.1. Trauma and inflammation

Cardiac surgery provokes a vigorous inflammatory response due to a variety of metabolic, endocrine, and immune changes known as the "stress response," which has important clinical implications [21, 22] (**Figure 1**). Surgical trauma, blood loss or transfusion, hypothermia, and CPB are nonspecific activators of the inflammatory response [18, 19]. Surgical trauma may contribute to a higher degree of the inflammatory response compared to CPB [23]. These effects predispose to atrial and ventricular arrhythmias in the early postoperative period. Inflammatory mechanisms have been proposed for the development of postoperative AF (POAF) as its incidence peaks at early postoperative days. Inflammation may be related to the development of clinically aberrant or silent pericarditis. Unfortunately, clinical criteria, such as fever, pleuritic chest pain, pericardial rubs, and electrocardiogram changes correlate poorly with postoperative pericarditis and supraventricular arrhythmias [7]. However, patients with pericardial effusion in one study had a higher incidence of supraventricular arrhythmias (63% compared with 11% in patients without effusions) [24].

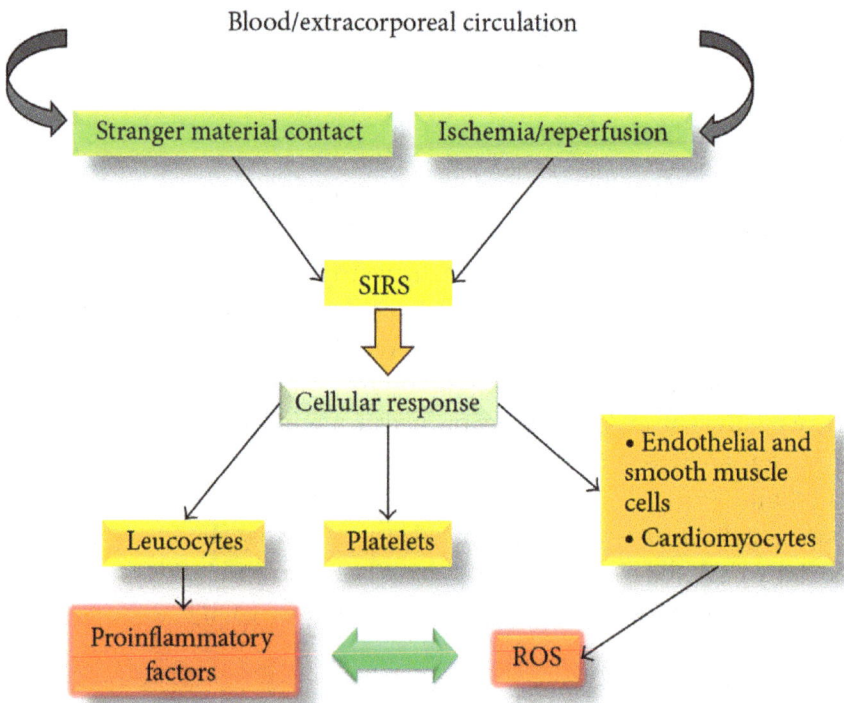

Figure 1. Pathophysiologic changes in response to cardiopulmonary bypass and the extracorporeal circulation. ROS, reactive oxygen species; SIRS, systemic inflammatory response syndrome (from Ref. [22]).

2.2.2. Hemodynamic stress

Atrial and ventricular hemodynamic changes during CABG predispose to POAs. The risk factors for POAs include atrial changes at the time of cardiac surgery, such as acute atrial trauma from cannulation, enlargement, hypertension, and ischemia [7]. Postoperative pulmonary edema and postoperative pleural effusion requiring thoracentesis have also been described as possible risk factors [25]. Hemodynamic changes might trigger focal arrhythmias [7]. It is possible that atrial stretch, hypertension, pressure and volume shifts, and heightened catecholamine states can trigger AF foci from the pulmonary veins [26].

2.2.3. Ischemic injury

The coronary blood flow is interrupted during CABG surgery and CPB, and the heart is put under circulatory arrest. This interruption of coronary blood flow causes ischemia-reperfusion injury that is exacerbated by adverse neutrophil-mediated myocardial inflammation and injury [27–29]. Atrial and ventricular ischemia or infarction triggers POAs [30]. Myocardial focal ischemia may occur due to endogenous or exogenous catecholamines, hypoxemia, hypercarbia, acid-base imbalances, drug effects, and mechanical factors. CPB, cross-clamp times, type of cardioplegia, and CABG surgical technique are also critical in determining ischemic injury. The incidence of AF has been demonstrated to be lower after OPCAB than conventional CABG. OPCAB is also associated with a lesser degree of inflammation [21].

2.2.4. Perioperative drugs

Beta-blocker withdrawal has been associated with an increased rate of postoperative supraventricular arrhythmias [31]. In contrary, some studies showed that preoperative digoxin use is a risk factor for POAs [2, 32], but not in the others [33]. Intravenous inotropic agents may be associated with POAs in some patients. The reported primary arrhythmias are sinus tachycardia (ST) and premature ventricular beats (PVCs), although other supraventricular (SVT) or ventricular arrhythmias (VT) have been reported. Clinically significant proarrhythmic effects with these agents appear to occur rarely. At conventional doses, intravenous inotropic agents are relatively safe concerning proarrhythmic effects. Inotropic agents increase sinoatrial node automaticity and decrease atrioventricular (AV) nodal conduction time [34, 35]. Dobutamine use has been reported to induce ventricular ectopic activity in 3–15% of patients [34]. Dopamine is more likely to be associated with a dose-related ST or AF [34]. Finally, short-term intravenous administration of the phosphodiesterase inhibitors amrinone and milrinone has been reported to cause PVCs and short runs of VT in up to 17% of patients [34]. Amiodarone and sotalol are useful and can be considered appropriate alternatives in high-risk patients [36]. Patients who need urgent CABG may benefit from intravenous and oral amiodarone combination in addition to beta-blockers. Although corticosteroids are associated with risk, it may be considered in selected CABG patients [36].

2.2.5. Electrolytes disorders

Hypokalemia leads to alteration of the electrophysiologic properties of cardiac myocytes with an increase in the action potential duration (increase in phase-3 depolarization), enhanced automaticity (increased slope of diastolic depolarization), and decreased conduction velocity [37]. These changes may provoke POAs [37]. Preoperative serum potassium levels of <3.5 mmol/L have a significant association with perioperative arrhythmias in patients undergoing elective CABG surgery [37].This association might be particularly evident in the atria, where changes in inward-rectifier potassium currents are supposed to act as profibrillatory mechanisms [38]. However, hypokalemia is more likely to be associated with VAs [38]. Moreover, it is worth noting that arrhythmogenesis is often multifactorial. Catecholamine release increases cellular potassium uptake and thus decreases serum potassium levels [39]. Serum potassium levels greater than 5.5 mmol/L appear to be associated with the development of POAF and atrial flutter (AFL) [37]. The role of magnesium remains controversial. The low serum magnesium levels—which is frequently seen after cardiac surgery—correlate with an increased incidence of POAs [7]. However, magnesium supplementation has produced conflicting results. Magnesium supplementation should be considered in all patients with hypomagnesemia [40–41].

2.2.6. Other factors

The human epicardial fat pads (FPs) contain parasympathetic ganglia [42]. There are two posterior FPs with the first one located in the superior vena caval-atrial junction and contains postganglionic fibers that lead to the sinoatrial (SA) node. The second FP is located at the pulmonary vein-left atrium and contains postganglionic fibers that lead to the atrioventricular (AV) node [43–45]. The anterior epicardial FP located in the aortopulmonary window that is routinely dissected and removed in CABG because it is located where the aortic cross-clamp is typically placed. Preservation of the human anterior epicardial FP during CABG decreases the incidence of POAF in one study [46], but not in another more recent study [47].

3. Postoperative atrial tachyarrhythmias (POATs)

3.1. Postoperative atrial fibrillation (POAF)

3.1.1. Epidemiology

AF is the most common complication seen after CABG surgery. The incidence of POAF is approximately 30% after isolated CABG, 40% after valve replacements or repair, and about 50% after combined CABG and valve surgeries [2, 48–51]. The incidence of POAF increases with older age [2, 52, 53].

3.1.2. Diagnosis

The diagnosis of POAF is confirmed based on the telemetry and 12-lead electrocardiogram (ECG) recordings with an abrupt change in heart rate and rhythm, and loss of P waves [16, 54]. Atrial electrograms obtained from temporary atrial epicardial pacing wires that are often routinely placed at the time of cardiac surgery can be helpful in confirming the diagnosis of AF, AFL, and other forms of supraventricular tachycardia (SVTs) [54].

3.1.3. Clinical course

POAF usually occurs within 2–4 days after cardiac surgery, with a peak incidence on the second postoperative day [12, 55]. In POAF patients without a prior history of atrial arrhythmias, AF is usually self-limited. About 15–30% of POAF convert to sinus rhythm within 2 h and up to 80% within 24 h [56, 57]. The mean duration of AF in one report was 11–12 h [57], and >90% of the patients were in sinus rhythm 6–8 weeks after surgery [57, 58]. In another study, only 2 out of 112 patients who had paroxysmal AF after CABG were still in AF at 6 weeks [59].

3.1.4. Prognosis

Although POAF is often self-limiting, its clinical effects depend on ventricular rate, ventricular function, arrhythmia duration, symptoms, hemodynamic stability, and risk of thromboembolism. [60]. POAF is associated with increased postoperative thromboembolic risk and stroke [25, 60–62]. In a series of 4507 patients, the incidence of stroke was significantly higher in those who devel oped POAF (3.3 versus 1.4%) [2]. Patient's underlying comorbidities, such as older age, previous cerebrovascular disease (CVA), the presence of a carotid bruit, peripheral vascular disease (PVD), and CPB time, have an important role in the development of in-hospital stroke [63–65]. In a review of 2972 patients undergoing CABG and/or valve surgery, POAF was associated with late onset stroke only if accompanied by a low cardiac output syndrome (3.9 versus 1.9%) [66]. Besides, POAF development is associated with a prolonged length of hospitalization [2, 25, 54]. The POAF is associated with an additional 2–4 days hospital stay after CABG surgery with an additional cost [54]. However, this effect seems to be less prominent with current cardiac surgical care [67]. Additionally, POAF may result in hemodynamic compromise [68], ventricular dysrhythmias [2], and iatrogenic complications associated with therapeutic interventions [53]. POAF may result in increased in-hospital and long-term mortality in a subset of patients [3, 60]. In a retrospective study of 6475 patients undergoing CABG at a single institution: 994 patients (15%) developed POAF. Higher in-hospital (7.4 versus 3.4%) and 4-year mortality (26 versus 13%) was noted in POAF patients but also with more comorbidities (i.e., older age, hypertension, and left ventricular hypertrophy) [60].

3.1.5. POAF management

The management of POAF should include the strategy for prevention and treatment of POAF when it develops. PAOF management starts with the optimization of medical comorbidities, if possible (e.g., hypoxia), and the correction of underlying electrolyte disturbances (e.g., potassium and magnesium abnormalities) [53]. POAF is treated similarly to AF in nonsurgical patients by rhythm control via pharmacological or electrical approach or heart rate control, and appropriate antithrombotic therapy.

3.1.5.1. Rhythm control versus heart rate control

In the atrial fibrillation follow-up investigation of rhythm management (AFFIRM) trial, the rate control versus rhythm control in nonsurgical patients with AF was studied and found that the use of rhythm control had no survival advantage, and it was associated with more frequent hospitalizations and adverse drug effects [69]. However, some studies involving patients with AF after cardiac surgery have suggested that rhythm control may offer advantages over rate control. This is still controversial and the evidence is inconclusive [11, 70–72].

Treatment strategies of POAF aim to reduce symptoms, limit adverse hemodynamic effects, decrease the length of hospital stay, prevent readmissions, and improve survival [73]. The rhythm control strategy has the advantage of a rapid conversion to sinus rhythm, which restores atrial activity, functional capacity, and might reduce thromboembolic. The rate control strategy has the advantage of avoiding the potential adverse effects of antiarrhythmic drugs and complications associated with cardioversion [73]. In a recent trial, there was no difference in hospital admissions during a 60-day follow-up, with randomizing POAF patients to either rhythm control therapy with amiodarone or rate control [73]. As a result, the main aim of rhythm control therapy in POAF patients should be to improve AF-related symptoms. In asymptomatic patients and those with acceptable symptoms, rate control or deferred cardioversion preceded by anticoagulation is a reasonable approach [73].

In the following paragraph, rate control and rhythm control options will be discussed briefly.

(A) Rate control strategy: the rate control may be achieved by using beta-blockers, nondihydropyridine calcium channel blockers, digoxin, or a combination of these medications. Beta-blocker agents are the drug of choice, particularly for ischemic heart disease patients, because of the increased adrenergic stress in the postoperative period [53, 73, 74]. However, beta-blockers might be poorly tolerated or relatively contraindicated in patients with known bronchial asthma or bronchospastic lung diseases, active congestive heart failure, or AV conduction block [53]. The nondihydropyridine calcium channel blocker agents represent an alternative AV nodal blocking agent. Digoxin is less effective when the adrenergic tone is as high as in the postoperative period, but it may be used in patients with congestive heart failure. Amiodarone is another agent that can be used as it has been reported to be effective in controlling heart rate. Also, intravenous amiodarone administration has been associated with improved hemodynamic status [75, 76]. For further information about drugs used in AF rate control see **Table 1**.

(B) Rhythm control: the rhythm control could be archived by using a direct current cardioversion (electrical cardioversion) or antiarrhythmic drugs (pharmacological cardioversion). Electrical cardioversion is indicated on an urgent basis in hemodynamically unstable patients, acute heart failure, or myocardial ischemia. Also, it may be used electively to restore sinus rhythm when a pharmacologic attempt has failed to resume a sinus rhythm [53]. Rhythm control with antiarrhythmic medications is preferred in symptomatic patients despite rate control trial, or when the control of ventricular response is hard to achieve. Amiodarone [77–79] or vernakalant [79, 80] have been efficient in converting POAF to sinus rhythm. Other antiarrhythmic medications that may be used include procainamide [80], ibutilide [81], and sotalol [82]. With ibutilide use, electrolyte imbalance should be corrected to avoid polymorphic ventricular tachycardia [82]. For further information about drugs used in AF rhythm control see **Table 2**.

3.1.5.2. Anticoagulation

POAF is associated with poor short- and long-term outcomes, including high rates of early and late stroke, and late mortality as mentioned earlier. However, the indication and timing of anticoagulation in POAF patients should take into consideration the risk of postoperative bleeding.

Drug	Route of admintration and doses	Side effects sects	Remarks
Beta-blockers			
Atenolol	Oral 25–100 mg QD	Bradycardia, hypotension, fatigue, depression, negative inotropy, bronchospasm, AVB	Decrease dose if CrCl <35
Bisoprolol	Oral 2.5–10 mg QD	As above	Good choice for HF patients
Carvedilol	Oral 3.125–25 mg BID	As above	Good choice for HF patients
Esmolol	I.V. 500 mcg/kg bolus over 1 min, then 50–300 mcg/kg/min	As above	Only IV Higher rate of hypotension
Metoprolol tartrate	IV 2.5–5.0 mg bolus over 2 min; up to 3 doses Oral 25–100 mg BID	As above	
Metoprolol XL (succinate)	Oral 50 100 mg QD	As above	Good choice for HF patients
Nadolol	Oral 10 (usual initial adult dose 40 mg)–240 mg QD	As above	Dosage adjustments based on CrCl
Propranolol	IV 1 mg over 1 min, up to 3 doses at 2-min intervals Oral 10–40 mg up to 160–320 mg/day divided in BID to QID doses 80–160 to 320 mg QD (ER)	As above	
Calcium channel blockers			
Diltiazem	IV 0.25 mg/kg bolus over 5 min followed by 0.05–0.15 mg/kg/h continuous infusion Oral 30 mg TID/QID up to 480 mg/day 120–360 to 480 mg Q D (ER)	Bradycardia, hypotension, ankle swelling, exacerbation of HF, AVB	Do not use in HF Drug interaction via CYP3A4 including digoxin and warfarin
Verapamil	IV 5–10 mg (0.075–0.15 mg/kg) over bolus at least 2 min; may give an additional 10 mg (0.15 mg/kg) after 30 min if no response, then 0.005 mg/kg/min infusion Oral 80–120 mg TID up to 480 mg/day 180–480 mg QD or 240 BID (ER)	Bradycardia, AVB, hypotension, constipation, exacerbation of HF	As diltiazem
Others			
Digoxin	IV 0.25 mg IV with repeat dosing to a maximum of 1.5 mg over 24 h Oral 0.125–0.25 mg QD	Bradycardia, AVB, nausea, vomiting, visual disturbance	Narrow therapeutic window Adjust for renal failure Drug interactions via p-glycoprotein
Amiodarone	IV 150 mg over 10 min, followed by 1 mg/min continuous IV infusion for 6 h, then 0.5 mg/min continuous infusion for 18 h Oral 400–800 mg/day PO in divided doses for 2–4 weeks to a total load of up to 10 g, then 100–200 mg QD	Bradycardia, hypotension, AV block, QTc prolongation, phlebitis on chronic use: Ocular, pulmonary, hepatic, hematological, neurological complications	Monitor thyroid, liver and lung functions

AVB, atrioventricular block; CrCl, creatinine clearance; BID, twice daily; h, hour; ER, extended release; HF, heart failure; IV, intravenous; mg milligram; min, minute; QD, once daily; QID, 4 times a day; QTc, correct QT interval; TID, 3 times a day.

Table 1. Medications commonly used for atrial fibrillation **rate control** with its dosage and common possible side effects.

Drug	Usual doses	Side effects sects	Additional information
Vaughan Williams class IA			
Disopyramide	Oral IR 100–200 mg q 6 h ER 200–400 mg q 12 h	HF Prolonged QT interval Prostatism Glaucoma	Metabolized by CYP3A4: caution with inhibitors (e.g., verapamil, diltiazem, ketoconazole, macrolide antibiotics, protease inhibitors, grapefruit juice) and inducers (e.g., phenytoin, phenobarbital, rifampin) Avoid other QT interval prolonging drugs
Procainamide	IV 15–17 mg/kg infused at a rate of 20–30 mg/min or alternatively100 mg IV every 5 min, max. 1 g MD 1–4 mg/min	HF Prolonged QT interval May cause hypotension, myopathies, blood dyscrasias, and SLE-like syndrome	Drug of choice for WPW with AF Avoid other QT interval prolonging drugs Adjust for renal failure
Quinidine	Oral IR 200–300 mg q 6–8 h up to 600 mg q 6 h ER 324 mg–648 mg q 8–12 h	Prolonged QT interval Diarrhea Bradycardia, AV block, bundle-branch block, digitalis toxicity	Inhibits CYP2D6: ⇧ concentrations of metoprolol, tricyclic antidepressants, antipsychotics; ⇩ efficacy of codeine Inhibits P-glycoprotein:⇧ digoxin concentration
Vaughan Williams class IC			
Flecainide	IV 1.5–3 mg/kg over 10-20 min Oral LD 200 (wt < 70 kg)–300 mg (wt > 70 kg), MD 50–200 mg BID max. 400 mg/day	Sinus or AV node dysfunction HF CAD Atrial flutter Brugada syndrome Renal or liver disease May cause blurred vision	Metabolized by CYP2D6 (inhibitors include quinidine, fluoxetine, tricyclics; also genetically absent in 7–10% of population) and renal excretion (dual impairment can ⇧⇧ plasma concentration) Decrease dose if CrCl < 35
Propafenone	IV 1.5–2 mg/kg over 10–20 min Oral IR: 150–300 mg q 8 h ER: 225–425 mg q 12 h (Oral LD 450 mg (wt < 70 kg)–600 mg (wt > 70 kg), MD 450–900 mg/d divided into q 8 h (IR), or 12 h (ER))	Sinus or AV node dysfunction or Infranodal conduction disease HF CAD Atrial flutter Brugada syndrome Liver disease Asthma may cause dysgeusia	Metabolized by CYP2D6 (inhibitors include quinidine, fluoxetine, tricyclics; also genetically absent in 7–10% of population)—poor metabolizers have ⇧beta blockade Inhibits P-glycoprotein: ⇧digoxin concentration Inhibits CYP2C9: ⇧warfarin concentration (⇧INR 25%) Decrease dose in hepatic failure
Vaughan Williams class III			
Amiodarone	IV LD 150 mg over 10 min; followed by 1 mg/min for 6 h; then 0.5 mg/min for 18 h or change to oral dosing; after 24 h, consider decreasing dose to 0.25 mg/min Oral 400–600 mg daily in divided doses for 2–4 wk; maintenance typically 100–200 mg QD	Sinus or AV node dysfunction Infranodal conduction disease Lung disease Prolonged QT interval	Inhibits most CYPs to cause drug interaction: ⇧concentrations of warfarin (⇧INR between 0–200%), statins, many other drugs Inhibits P-glycoprotein: ⇧digoxin concentration

Drug	Usual doses	Side effects sects	Additional information
Dronedarone	Oral 400 mg BID	Bradycardia HF Liver disease Thyriod disease pulmonary fibrosis Prolonged QT interval	Metabolized by CYP3A: caution with inhibitors (e.g., verapamil, diltiazem, ketoconazole, macrolide antibiotics, protease inhibitors, grapefruit juice) and inducers (e.g., phenytoin, phenobarbital, rifampin) Inhibits CYP3A, CYP2D6, P-glycoprotein: ⇧concentrations of some statins, digoxin, beta blockers, sirolimus, tacrolimus Avoid in long-standing persistent or permanent AF and HF
Dofetilide	Oral 125–500 mcg BID if CrCl >60, 250 mcg if CrCl 40–60, 125 mcg if CrCl 20–40 Decrease MD if QTc increased by >15% of >500 ms 2–3 h after dose or consider discontinuing it	Prolonged QT interval and torsades de pointes Renal disease Hypokalemia hypomagnesacmia AV block, bradycardia, sick sinus syndrome	Adjust dose for renal function, body size, and age (avoid if CrCl < 20) Drug interactions via CYP3A4: CI to use with verapamil, cimetidine, ketoconazole, trimethoprim, prochlorperazine, HCTZ, and megestrol Discontinue amiodarone at least 3 m before initiation Avoid other QT interval prolonging drugs
Ibutilide	IV 1 mg over 10 min; may repeat 1 mg once if necessary (if weight <60 kg, use 0.01 mg/kg)	Prolonged QT interval and torsade de pointes hypotension CAD HF	Mointor K and mg level
Sotalol	Oral 40–160 mg q12 h IV 75–150 mg QD or BID over 5 h (only if patient cannot take oral)	Prolonged QT interval Sinus or AV nodal dysfunction HF	Renal excretion: CI if Cr Cl <40 decrease dose if CrCl 40–60 Risk of torsade de pointes (do not initiate sotalol therapy if the baseline QTc is longer than 450 ms. If the QT interval prolongs to 500 ms or greater, the dose must be reduced, the duration of the infusion prolonged or the drug discontinued) Avoid other QT interval prolonging drugs correct hypokalemia/hypomagnesemia

ACC AF [74]; JACC [53]. AF, atrial fibrillation; AV, atrioventricular; BID, twice daily; CAD, coronary artery disease; CI, contraindicated; CrCl, creatinine clearance; ER, extended release; h, hour; HCTZ, hydrochlorothiazide; HF, heart failure; IL, immediate release; IV, intravenous; LD, loading dose; INR, international normalized ratio; MD, maintenance dose; min, minute; max, maximum; SLE, systemic lupus erythematosus; Q, every; QD, once daily; wt, weight. http://www.pdr.net/

Table 2. Medications commonly used for atrial fibrillation Rythm Control with its dosage and major pharmacokinetic and drug interactions.

Oral anticoagulation at discharge has been associated with a reduced long-term mortality in patients with POAF [83] but without evidence from controlled trials [75]. POAF that persists for longer than 48 h should be anticoagulated with warfarin or nonvitamin K antagonist oral anticoagulants (NOACs). The NOACs are available for the treatment of nonvalvular AF. NOACs have been found to be as efficacious or even superior to warfarin in the prevention of stroke in nonvalvular AF patients with high risk of thromboembolism, with similar to lower rates of major bleeding, and also lower rates of intracranial hemorrhage [84].

3.1.6. Prevention of POAF

Beta-blockers are effective in reducing POAF and SVTs. Propranolol uses reduced POAF incidence from 31.7% in the control group to 16.3% in the treatment group [85]. In the majority of beta-blocker studies, it is administered postoperatively [86]. Amiodarone reduced the incidence of POAF and hospital stay compared to beta-blocker therapy in several meta-analyses [86–89]. Prophylactic administration of sotalol may be considered for patients at risk of developing AF after cardiac surgery [76, 90, 91]. Also, administration of colchicine postoperatively may reduce POAF [75, 92]. Statin use preoperatively did not prevent POAF in a prospective controlled trial [93], despite that initial reports from meta-analyses were encouraging [94–96].

Other therapies for the prevention of POAF have been studied in small trials, but have not demonstrated clear beneficial effects [76]. These include angiotensin converting enzyme inhibitors (ACEIs) [97], magnesium [85, 98, 99], n-3 polyunsaturated fatty acids [100–108], corticosteroids [109–111], and posterior pericardiectomy [112]. Conflicting results have also been reported for acetylcysteine [113], and sodium nitroprusside [114].

Nonpharmacologic therapy with atrial pacing has been tested in various studies [7]. One meta-analysis showed a significant reduction in POAF with atrial pacing (OR 0.57, 95% CI 0.38–0.84) [67], and most [115–117] but not all [118, 119] published studies showed benefit with this therapy. Besides, there are conflicting findings as to the relative value of the different types of atrial pacing [115, 116].

3.2. Postoperative atrial flutter (POAFL)

Unlike POAF, POAFL after CABG is not well studied. In a single-center study with 80 consecutive patients who underwent CABG with no previous history of AFL, 16 patients (20%) had documented POAFL. Ten of these patients showed temporary AFLs that were curable without radiofrequency catheter ablation (RFCA), and 37.5% of the patients with POAFL (i.e., 7.5% of the patients after CABG) showed sustained or repeated AFL with subjective symptoms [120]. In another study that looked at ATs late after open heart surgery, it was found that cavotricuspid isthmus (CTI)-dependent AFL was the most common. Atypical AFL becomes progressively more widespread with more extensive atriotomy [121]. AFL and ATs that developed late after cardiac surgery are believed to be due to scars created by incisions applied to the right and/or left atrium either for establishing extracorporeal circulation or access to intracardiac structures (coronary sinus, interatrial or interventricular septum, atrioventricular valves, etc.) [122]. The scars created by these incisions play a significant role in the development of ATs, months or years after surgery [123, 124].

AFL in the early postoperative period is managed as POAF with rate control or rhythm control and anticoagulation based on arrhythmia duration and patient risk factors. On long-term catheter ablation of AFL is an effective, safe, and potentially curative procedure.

3.3. Supraventricular tachycardia (SVT)

3.3.1. Epidemiology

Sinus tachycardia (ST) represents an appropriate autonomic response to a physiological stress. The upper limit of normal rate for sinus tachycardia is calculated from the formula

(220 bpm minus age) [125]. Inappropriate ST may be seen in some patients, especially with young age, but it is rare and should be considered a diagnosis of exclusion [125]. The term 'SVT' refers to paroxysmal tachyarrhythmias that require atrial or AV nodal tissue, or both, for their initiation and maintenance [126]. It is typical of a sudden or paroxysmal onset and includes AV nodal reentrant tachycardias (AVNRT), AV reentrant tachycardias (AVRT), and atrial tachycardias. The overall incidence of perioperative arrhythmias in noncardiac surgery varies from 16 to 62% with intermittent ECG monitoring and up to 89% with continuous Holter monitoring [127]. It is more likely to be supraventricular than ventricular in origin [127]. In small study, the incidence of persistent SVT in noncardiac surgery patients was 2% during surgery and 6% in the postoperative period [128].

3.3.2. Diagnosis

12-lead ECG and rhythm strips during tachycardia are diagnostic and may give an impression about the most likely diagnosis. Although ST is usually easy to diagnose on 12-lead ECG, the presence of first-degree AV block, which is not uncommon after cardiac surgery, may give ECG appearance that mimics SVT due to P wave merge with T wave (P wave hidden within T wave). ECG features of ATs including SVTs are shown in **Table 3**.

3.3.3. Clinical course

ATs occur most frequently 2–3 days postsurgery and are likely related to sympathetic stimulation associated with an inflammatory response [129]. Patients with known SVT may have an exacerbation of their tachycardia in the perioperative period. However, SVT may be diagnosed for the first time in the perioperative period [2, 7, 130, 131]. SVT is often associated with a high sympathetic tone, but other precipitants may contribute to its occurrence. The clinical symptoms, time of onset, and natural course of ATs are identical in patients with cardiac, thoracic, or other surgery.

3.3.4. Prognosis

The prognosis of perioperative SVTs is good, but it may be associated with increased hospital stay [128].

3.3.5. Management

The SVT management, in general, depends on the hemodynamic status of the patient. If the patient with SVT is hemodynamically unstable, synchronized cardioversion is recommended for acute termination of the tachycardia when vagal maneuvers or adenosine is ineffective or not feasible [132]. Before initiating specific drug therapy for acute SVT in hemodynamically stable patients, it is important to assess and correct possible precipitating factors such as respiratory failure or electrolyte imbalance. SVT may respond to vagal maneuver if the patient can do it. Adenosine might be used if there is no contraindication. SVT also responds to rate control drugs such as beta-blockers (e.g., esmolol, metoprolol, bisoprolol) or nondihydropyridine calcium channel antagonists (e.g., diltiazem, verapamil). Intravenous (IV) digoxin, IV amiodarone, adenosine, IV or oral beta-blockers, diltiazem, and verapamil are potentially harmful in acute treatment in patients with pre-excited AF (AF in patients with Wolff-Parkinson-White (WPW) syndrome) [133]. Of note, atrial tachycardia unifocal or multifocal usually respond to rate control drugs but are not amenable to direct current cardioversion. Cardiac electrophysiology study with catheter ablation is an effective long-term management for recurrent SVT.

4. Postoperative ventricular tachyarrhythmias (POVTAs)

The postoperative ventricular tachyarrhythmias (POVTAs) range from isolated PVC to VT or ventricular fibrillation (VF).

4.1. Premature ventricular complexes (PVCs)

4.1.1. Epidemiology

Isolated PVCs including nonsustained ventricular tachycardia (NSVT) are seen in about 50% of patients during and after cardiac surgery [134]. PVCs can be related to electrolyte or other metabolic imbalances [7].

4.1.2. Diagnosis

PVCs may be seen on continuous telemetric monitoring and 12-lead ECG, however, careful evaluation of the ECG tracing is needed to be distinguished from atrial ectopy with aberrant ventricular conduction [7].

4.1.3. Clinical course

Patients with postoperative PVCs may be asymptomatic or may have palpitations with a skipped beat, or dizziness. It is rarely associated with hemodynamic instability.

4.1.4. Prognosis

Patients with isolated and noncomplicated PVCs postoperatively do not exhibit increased risk of malignant VAs [135, 136]. On the contrary, frequent PVCs (>30 per hour) may reduce ventricular function and therefore have an adverse impact on the short-term outcome. There was no significant difference in mortality in patients with versus patients without frequent postoperative PVCs and NSVT (8 versus 5%), at an average follow-up of 3 years, in a study including 185 postoperative patients [137]. However, in another study of 126 patients with postoperative PVCs, it was shown that patients with left ventricular ejection fraction (LVEF) of <40% had a 75% mortality rate and 33% incidence of sudden death at an average follow-up of 15 months, whereas none of the patients with preserved left ventricular function had sudden death [135]. Thus, PVCs are not related to mortality with good LV function, and long-term outcome after cardiac surgery seems to be closely related to the left ventricular function.

4.1.5. Management

Correction of any reversible cause of ventricular arrhythmias should be performed. Hemo dynamically stable and asymptomatic PVCs do not usually need treatment with antiarrhythmic therapy on short or long-term. Lidocaine has been used with a successful result in reducing hemodynamically significant or symptomatic PVCs, but without improving mortality. Empirical use of class I antiarrhythmic drugs for suppression of frequent and/or complex PVCs had no beneficial effects on mortality rate and may be harmful as shown in several studies in another setting [138, 139]. Additionally, overdrive pacing, using either atrial or atrioventricular sequential pacing, has been used without significant results [138, 139]. Patients with asymptomatic NSVT after cardiac surgery and preserved LVEF generally have a favorable long-term prognosis and do not require invasive workup with an electrophysiology study. The use of implantable cardioverter defibrillators (ICDs) has shown no benefits in improving prognosis in this population [140].

4.2. Ventricular tachyarrhythmias

4.2.1. Epidemiology

Sustained VT and VF rarely occur after cardiac surgery with an incidence of 0.4–1.7% in most of the studies [138, 141], but an incidence of 3.1% has been reported [142]. Furthermore, it is life threatening and affects outcome [134, 143].

4.2.2. Pathophysiology and risk factors

Pathophysiology of POAs, in general, was disused in item 2. Coronary artery disease (CAD) leads to a broad spectrum of changes and may trigger arrhythmia mechanisms via enhanced automaticity, triggered activity, and reentry. While myocardial infarction (MI) related scar constitutes the clinical model of reentry [144], focal activation due to abnormal automaticity is the primary mechanism involved in the VT during acute ischemia [145]. Early and delayed after depolarization result from focal discharge by calcium overload and triggered activity is another likely mechanism of VT initiation in ischemia, but this needs to be proven experimentally thus far [146, 147]. Acute ischemia activates the adenosine triphosphate-sensitive potassium (K-ATP) channels, causing an increase in extracellular potassium along with acidosis and hypoxia in the cardiac muscle. As a result of the minor increases in extracellular potassium depolarize the myocardiocyte's resting membrane potential, which can increase tissue excitability in early phases of ischemia [145]. The mechanism underlying the VT associated with healed or healing MI is reentry in more than 95% of cases [144].

Complex ventricular arrhythmias (VAs) are associated with multiple risk factors [7]. Based on clinical studies, the conditions associated with VAs after cardiac surgery may include: increased age, female gender, presence of unstable angina, congestive cardiac failure, hemodynamic instability, preoperative use of inotropes, preoperative use of IABP, emergency surgery, electrolyte disturbances, hypoxia, hypovolemia, myocardial ischemia/infarction, acute graft closure, reperfusion after cessation of CPB, and inotropes antiarrhythmic drugs use, on-pump surgery, and PVD [134, 135, 141, 143, 148].

	Heart rate (bpm)	Regularity	Onset	Atrial activity	Response to adenosine	Rhythm strip
AF	A: 350-500 V: 100- 220	Irregular	Sudden	No discrete P-waves	Transient slowing of ventricular rate	
AFL	A: 250-350 V: 150 (slower or faster depends on AV conduction)	Regular (irregular with variable AV conduction)	Sudden	Flutter waves "saw-tooth" pattern)	Transient slowing of ventricular rate	
ST	220-age	Regular	Gradual	Normal P-waves	Transient slowing	
AT	150-250	Regular	Sudden	Abnormal P-waves morphology	-Transient slowing of ventricular rate -May terminate tachycardia in 70% of the cases	
AVNRT	150-250	Regular	Sudden	No obvious P-waves as P- wave is in or just after QRS (Pseudo r' in V1 or S wave in inferior leads)	Termination of tachycardia	

	Heart rate (bpm)	Regularity	Onset	Atrial activity	Response to adenosine	Rhythm strip
AVRT (WPW)	150-250	Regular	Sudden	**ORT:** P-waves may be buried in QRS complex, or retrograde P wave may be seen at the end of the QRS complex or in the early part of the ST segment	Termination of tachycardia	
				ART: P wave normal with short PR and delta wave (wide QRS complexes due to abnormal ventricular depolarization via accessory pathway)	Termination of tachycardia	
				AF: no P-wave, irregular rhythm, and wide QRS complex	Should not be used	

Table 3. Differential diagnosis of atrial tachyarrhythmias.

4.2.3. Diagnosis

In addition to a clinical history and a physical exam, the general evaluation of a patient with CAD and suspected or documented VAs includes performing a 12-lead ECG and an echocardiogram. Telemetry monitoring with careful evaluation of VAs initiation and termination is very helpful. Based on ECG criteria, wide complex tachycardias (WCT) may be either ventricular or SVT with aberrancy. However, in patients with structural heart disease like prior infarction, the diagnosis is mostly VT. If feasible, a 12-lead ECG and atrial electrograms through temporary epicardial wires placed at the time of cardiac surgery should be obtained. The presence of AV dissociation strongly suggests VT [138]. Although the ECG diagnosis of a WCT is challenging, it is important to remember that VT is the cause in at least 80% of cases [149].

4.2.4. Clinical course

Clinical presentation of patients post cardiac surgery with VTs is variable. The hemodynamic state of these patients depends mainly on the rate of the tachyarrhythmia and the left ventricular function. Therefore, some patients may be asymptomatic. Other patients with VT may complain of palpitations, dyspnea, or chest discomfort as their main symptoms. VTs may present with syncope and sudden cardiac death as a result of hemodynamic compromise. Incessant VT, even if it is hemodynamically stable, can lead to hemodynamic deterioration and heart failure [150, 151].

4.2.5. Prognosis

The prognosis is correlated with the type of arrhythmia and the type and degree of structural heart disease [7]. As mentioned earlier, PVCs and NSVT generally have no impact on the outcome. However, patients with sustained VAs have poorer short- and long-term prognosis.

POVAs predicts higher in-hospital mortality (21.7–31.5%) compared with (1.4–2.9%) in control [134, 143, 148]. In one study, POVAs was associated with increased long-term mortality over a mean follow-up of 3.5 years. Patients with POVAs had a high risk of death in the POVAs group during the first 6 postsurgical months (6-month survival of POVAs 59.8 versus 93.8% for POVAs free group). This difference in survival persisted over time [148].

4.2.6. Management of POVAs

Asymptomatic PVCs and hemodynamically stable short runs of NSVT do not need specific intervention, and the correction of any reversible cause of VAs is generally sufficient. Postoperative sustained VAs treatment follows the ICD indications used in other clinical settings [150, 152]. However, the postoperative patients require close attention to the identification and treatment of reversible causes of arrhythmia like electrolyte or other metabolic disturbances, myocardial ischemia, or mechanical complications of surgery [7]. Sustained VAs should be promptly cardioverted either by drugs infusion or electrically based on hemodynamic stability. Hemodynamically stable sustained VTs may be initially treated with antiarrhythmic drugs infusion.

4.2.6.1. Pharmacological treatment

It includes antiarrhythmic medication use and standard medical therapy. The most commonly used antiarrhythmic agents include:

- Amiodarone: IV amiodarone is frequently used as a first-line treatment for VAs as it is better tolerated in patients with low ejection fraction than the other antiarrhythmic drugs. The recommended starting dose of Cordarone I.V. is 1000 mg over the first 24 h of therapy. It is usually delivered by bolus infusion of 150 mg over 10–15 min, followed by 1 mg/min for 6 h, then 0.5 mg/min infusion for 18 h. The alternative dose would be 300 mg over 1 h then infusion at 50 mg/h. Additional 150 mg blouses may be given but frequent boluses during the first 24 h should be limited due to the risk of hepatic toxicity [153].

- Lidocaine: it is generally a good choice if ischemia is suspected. Lidocaine is administered as a bolus of 0.75–1.5 mg/kg, followed by an IV infusion of 1–4 mg/min (the maximal dose is 3 mg/kg/h). In elderly patient and patients with congestive heart failure or hepatic dysfunction, the lidocaine dose should be reduced [153].

- Procainamide: it is often a second line drug, and it is given as loading dose of 15–18 mg/kg administered as a slow infusion over 25–30 min or 100 mg/dose. The infusion rate should not exceed 50 mg/min. The loading dose may be repeated every 5 min as needed to a total dose of 1 g. However, it should be stopped if hypotension occurs, or QRS complex widens by 50% of its original width. This is followed by a maintenance dose of 1–4 mg/min by continuous infusion. The procainamide maintenance infusion should be reduced by 1/3 in patients with moderate renal or cardiac impairment and by 2/3 in patients with severe renal or cardiac impairment [153].

Standard medical therapy includes beta-blockers, and ACEIs drugs have been demonstrated to improve long-term survival particularly in patients with left ventricular dysfunction.

4.2.6.2. Nonpharmacological management

- Overdrive pacing: in patients with slower VTs who have ventricular epicardial wires, overdrive pacing may be performed. Electrical cardioversion/defibrillation should be easily available because of the possibility of acceleration of the VT or degeneration to VF [154].

- Electrical cardioversion/defibrillation: in patients with cardiac arrest, basic life support (BLS) and advanced cardiovascular life support (ACLS) should be followed. Electrical defibrillation should be performed for VF, pulseless VT, and hemodynamically unstable VT. Electrical cardioversion may be used for stable sustained VT as the first choice or for those who do not respond to antiarrhythmic medications. The recommended energy with current biphasic defibrillators ranges from 150 to 200 Joules. Sedation with short-acting agents should precede cardioversion in awake patients [154].

- Emergency mechanical support: in postoperative patients who are not responding to standard resuscitation maneuvers, initiation of emergency CPB in the intensive care unit may be considered. In one study, CPB use in a postoperative cardiac arrest was associated with a 56% long-term survival rate with a 22% incidence of soft tissue infections and no mediastinitis [154].

- Implantable cardioverter-defibrillator (ICD) therapy:

In the absence of a reversible cause of sustained VT or cardiac arrest after CABG, long-term management may include electrophysiology study and eventually an ICD implantation. Patients with NSVT, prior MI, and left ventricular dysfunction (LVEF <40%) may be considered for electrophysiology testing and implantation of an ICD if a sustained ventricular arrhythmia is induced [152, 155]. Multicenter automatic defibrillator implantation trial (MADIT) study [152] excluded subjects within 2 months after CABG and 3 months after percutaneous transluminal coronary angioplasty (PTCA), and MADIT-II study [156] excluded subjects within 3 months after revascularization. Conversely, early revascularization was permitted in MUSTT (Multicenter Unsustained Tachycardia Trial) study [155], which enrolled subjects at least 4 days after revascularization, and sudden cardiac death in heart failure trial (SCD-HeFT) study [157] made no specific exclusion on the timing of revascularization. However, in SCD-HeFT, the median time from CABG to enrollment was 3.1 years, and from PCI to enrollment was 2.3 years. Therefore, ICD implantation within 90 days of coronary revascularization for patients who otherwise meet ICD implant criteria for primary prevention of sudden cardiac death (SCD) is not addressed in the published device-based therapy guidelines. Revascularization has significant time-dependent benefits. In fact, MADIT-II study showed that the efficacy of ICD therapy in patients with ischemic left ventricular dysfunction is time dependent, with a significant life-saving benefit in patients receiving device implantation more than 6 months after coronary revascularization (CR). The lack of ICD benefit early after CR may be related to a relatively small risk of SCD during this period [158]. Although, sudden cardiac arrest (SCA) has a higher incidence in patients with reduced LVEF in the months after acute MI and/or following revascularization [159, 160]. The two randomized controlled trials, defibrillator in acute myocardial infarction (DINAMIT) and immediate risk stratification improves survival (IRIS), showed that early ICD implantation does not reduce mortality [161, 162]. In both of those trials, there was a reduction in arrhythmic death, which was counteracted by a concomitant increase in death due to other causes [163]. Similarly, the coronary artery bypass graft (CABG)-patch trial [164] examined ICD implantation at the time of elective CABG surgery showed a small decrease in arrhythmic death, but no benefit for overall mortality in patients with preoperative LVEF ≤35%. However, one should keep in mind that the epicardial ICDs tested in this trial differed significantly from the current transvenous endocardial ICD systems. A retrospective study evaluating ICD implantation within 3 months of cardiac surgery suggested the benefit of ICD implantation for secondary prevention. In this study, 164 patients were with ICD implantation within 3 months of cardiac surgery; 93 of these patients had an ICD for sustained pre or postoperative VT or VF requiring resuscitation. During the mean follow-up of 49 months; the primary endpoint was total mortality (TM) and/or appropriate ICD therapy (ICD-T), and secondary endpoints are the TM and ICD-T, and individual end points of TM and ICD-T were observed in 52 (56%), 35 (38%), and 28 (30%) patients, respectively, with 55% of TM, and 23% of ICD-T occurring within 2 years of implant [165].

Overall, ICD for *primary prevention* of SCD *can be useful* in patients who are within 90 days of revascularization and who are not within 40 days of an acute MI if:

- they are previously qualified for primary prevention of SCD or

- revascularization is unlikely to result in an improvement in LVEF to level >35% [166].

ICD for *secondary prevention* (i.e., in patients resuscitated from cardiac arrest due to VT/VF) *is recommended* for patients within 90 days of revascularization who have:

- previously satisfied criteria for ICD implantation if they have abnormal left ventricular function or

- SCD is unlikely related to myocardial ischemia/injury and have normal left ventricular function [166].

ICD implantation *can be useful* in patients who are within 90 days of revascularization if SCD was not related to acute myocardial ischemia/injury and who were subsequently found to have coronary artery disease that is revascularized with normal left ventricular function, or SCD was not related to acute myocardial ischemia/injury and who were subsequently found to have coronary artery disease that is revascularized with normal left ventricular function [166]. ICD is *not recommended* in patients within 90 days of revascularization who were resuscitated from cardiac arrest due to VT that was related to acute MI/injury, with normal left ventricular function, and who undergo complete coronary revascularization [166]. ICD with appropriately selected pacing capabilities *is recommended* in patients within 90 days of revascularization who require nonelective permanent pacing, who would also meet primary prevention criteria for implantation of an ICD, and in whom recovery of left ventricular function is uncertain or not expected [166].

An alternative approach for primary prevention of SCD in patients with ischemic cardiomyopathy and low LVEF undergoing revascularization would be the use the wearable cardioverter-defibrillator vest during the 3 months waiting period after revascularization until LVEF is reassessed and design made about permanent ICD implantation [163].

- Ventricular tachycardia ablation:

There are no studies of VT ablation in POVAs situation. In patients with extensive structural abnormalities, especially those with prior MI, multiple morphologies of VT might develop. Therefore, VT ablation does not eliminate the need for ICD and/or antiarrhythmic therapy. VT episodes might occur in up 0–60% of patients who have received an ICD for secondary prevention and in 2.5–12% of patients with ICD implanted for primary prevention [167]. Because antiarrhythmic drugs do not eliminate the risk of VAs, VT catheter ablation may be needed to reduce the frequency of VT episodes, especially patients with incessant VT or frequent ICD therapy [149]. Ablation is usually indicated in cases of recurrent, monomorphic VT arising from a specific substrate that can be targeted by mapping techniques.

5. Postoperative bradyarrhythmias (POBAs)

5.1. Epidemiology

Bradyarrhythmias (BAs) are common after cardiac surgery, but it mostly consists of transient episodes of low ventricular heart rate. The conduction defects post cardiac surgery include sinus node dysfunction, partial and complete bundle branch blocks, and various degrees of atrioventricular (AV) block. The right bundle branch block (RBBB) was the most frequently noted abnormality [168]. Bradyarrhythmias may decrease cardiac output in patients with relatively fixed stroke volumes. The risk of developing conduction disturbances after CABG or valvular surgery leading to permanent pacemaker (PPM) implantation is about 0.4–1.1% of patients after isolated CABG and 3–6% after heart valve operations [169–171]. It seems that in the current surgical era that the incidence of postoperative PPM implantation has decreased due to improvements in surgical techniques, technological innovations and enhanced understanding of the mechanisms of injury [172]. However, some studies have shown an increased incidence of PPM implantation after cardiac surgery after the year 2000 [173].

5.2. Pathophysiology and risk factors

Conduction disorders after cardiac surgery are explained by one of the following two mechanisms: (1) direct trauma to the conduction system in operative procedures in proximity to the sinoatrial or AV nodes or the His bundle; or (2) ischemic injury to the conduction system due to extensive coronary artery disease might compromise myocardial protection during intraoperative cardioplegic arrest [174].

The risk factors for POBAs may be classified as preoperative, operative, and postoperative factors. Preoperative risk factors include age >75 years, the use of rate lowering cardiac medications (e.g., beta-blockers, calcium channel blockers, digoxin, and antiarrhythmic drugs), the presence of conduction system disease preoperatively, right bundle branch block (RBBB) or left bundle branch block (LBBB), first-degree AV block or left anterior fascicular block (LAFB) [169–171, 175–178].

Operative risk factors include myocardial ischemia, inadequate cardiac protection during surgery, and direct surgical injury to conduction system, prolonged CPB time and cross-clamp time, and reoperation [171, 172, 174, 179, 180].

Postoperative risk factors include postoperative conduction disturbances and high-grade AV block [174, 175, 181].

5.3. Clinical course and management

Temporary electrical pacing may be required in symptomatic bradycardias. It is common practice nowadays to place temporary epicardial atrial and ventricular pacing wires placed at the time of surgery to facilitate temporary pacing when needed. In some cases, as mentioned above, the conduction defect does not revert, and permanent pacing may be necessary. Chronotropic medications, such as theophylline or aminophylline, have been used for sinus bradycardia after transplantation to improve SSS [182] or high-grade AVB [183] and may decrease the need for permanent pacing but its long-term effect is not encouraging.

The challenge with POBAs is often to determine when to implant the PPM as the sinus node function or AV conduction may recover in some patients. Recovery of conduction system is common with long-term follow-up. Only 30–40% of patients with a permanent pacemaker due to sinus node disease remain pacemaker dependent. However, the rate of recovery is less in patients with postoperative AVB, as 65–100% of patients with complete heart block, remain pacemaker dependent. Currently, the usual practice is to implant a PPM if postoperative symptomatic complete AVB or severe sinus node dysfunction persists longer than 5–7 days [184]. PPM implantation may be considered earlier if the underlying intrinsic rhythm is absent or temporary pacing leads fail.

6. Conclusion

Arrhythmias are common after CABG. Although tachyarrhythmias are frequent, they are usually transient and have a benign course. POAF represents the most frequently observed ATs. VAs are less common but have an adverse impact on the short and long-term outcome. POTAs management includes optimization of the patient's condition, controlling patient's risk factors, and careful attention to hemodynamic changes during surgery with using appropriate anesthesia. Postoperatively, it is important to correct reversible arrhythmia predisposing factors, followed by specific therapy based on the arrhythmia type and its hemodynamic effect.

On the other hand, bradyarrhythmias are also frequently observed after cardiac surgery. However, most of the conduction disturbances are transient and recovered spontaneously. PPM implantation may be required in patients with persistent symptomatic bradycardia due to sick sinus syndrome or second degree type 2, third degree, or high-grade AV block.

Author details

Bandar Al-Ghamdi[1,2]*

*Address all correspondence to: balghamdi@kfshrc.edu.sa

1 Heart Centre, King Faisal Specialist Hospital and Research Centre, Riyadh, Saudi Arabia

2 College of Medicine, Alfaisal University, Riyadh, Saudi Arabia

References

[1] Herzog L, Lynch C. Arrhythmias accompanying cardiac surgery. In: Lynch C, editor. Clinical Cardiac Electrophysiology. 3rd ed. Philadelphia, PA, USA: JB Lippincott; 1994. pp. 231-258.

[2] Creswell LL, Schuessler RB, Rosenbloom M, Cox JL. Hazards of postoperative atrial arrhythmias. The Annals of Thoracic Surgery. 1993;**56**:539-549. DOI: https://doi.org/10.1016/0003-4975(93)90894-N

[3] Mathew JP, Fontes ML, Tudor IC, Ramsay J, Duke P, Mazer CD, Barash PG, Hsu PH, Mangano DT, Investigators of the Ischemia Research and Education Foundation, Multicenter Study of Perioperative Ischemia Research Group. A multicenter risk index for atrial fibrillation after cardiac surgery. JAMA. 2004;**291**:1720-1729. DOI: 10.1001/ jama.291.14.1720

[4] Steinbach K, Merl O, Frohner K, Hief C, Nurnberg M, Kalten-brunner W, Podczeck A, Wessely E. Hemodynamics during ventricular tachyarrhythmias. American Heart Journal. 1994;**127**:1102-1106. DOI: http://dx.doi.org/10.1016/0002-8703(94)90095-7

[5] Fenelon G, Wigjns W, Andries E, Brugada P. Tachycardiomyopathy: Mechanisms and clinical implications. PACE. 1996;**19**:95-106. DOI: 10.1111/j.1540-8159.1996.tb04796.x

[6] Baig MW, Perrins EJ. The hemodynamics of cardiac pacing. Progress in Cardiovascular Diseases. 1991;**33**:283-298. DOI: https://doi.org/10.1016/0033-0620(91)90021-D

[7] Peretto G, Durante A, Limite LR, Cianflone D. Postoperative arrhythmias after cardiac surgery: Incidence, risk factors, and therapeutic management. Cardiology Research and Practice. 2014;**2014**:615987. DOI: 10.1155/2014/615987

[8] Diodato M, Chedrawy EG. Coronary artery bypass graft surgery: The past, present, and future of myocardial revascularisation. Surgery Research and Practice. 2014;**2014**:726158. DOI: 10.1155/2014/726158

[9] Møller CH, Penninga L, Wetterslev J, Steinbruchel DA, Gluud C. Off-pump versus on-pump coronary artery bypass grafting for ischaemic heart disease. Cochrane Database of Systematic Reviews. 2012 March 14;**3**:CD007224. DOI: 10.1002/14651858.CD007224.pub2

[10] Mack M, Acuff T, Yong P, Jett GK, Carter D. Minimally invasive thoracoscopically assisted coronary artery bypass surgery. European Journal of Cardio-Thoracic Surgery. 1997;**12**:20-24. DOI: https://doi.org/10.1016/S1010-7940(97)00141-3

[11] Enríquez F, Jiménez A. Post-operative tachyarrhythmias in adult cardiac surgery: Prophylaxis. Cirugia Cardiovascular. 2010;**17**:259-274. DOI: Https://doi.org/10.1016/S1134-0096(10)70100-5 (in Spanish: Taquiarritmias postoperatorias en la cirugía cardíaca del adulto. Profilaxis)

[12] Zaman AG, Archbold RA, Helft G, Atrial Paul EA, Curzen NP, Mills PG. Atrial fibrillation after coronary artery bypass surgery: A model for preoperative risk stratification. Circulation. 2000;**101**:1403-1408. DOI: https://doi.org/10.1161/01.CIR.101.12.1403

[13] Leitch JW, Thomson D, Baird DK, Harris PJ. The importance of age as a predictor of atrial fibrillation and flutter after coronary artery bypass grafting. The Journal of Thoracic and Cardiovascular Surgery. 1990;**100**:338-342 PMID: 2391970

[14] Premaratne S, Premaratne ID, Fernando ND, Williams L, Hasaniya NW. Atrial fibrillation and flutter following coronary artery bypass graft surgery: A retrospective study and review. JRSM Cardiovascular Disease. 2016;**5**:2048004016634149. DOI: 10. 1177/2048004016634149

[15] Mendes LA, Connelly GP, McKenney PA, Podrid PJ, Cupples LA, Shemin RJ, Ryan TJ, Davidoff R. Right coronary artery stenosis: An independent predictor of atrial fibrillation after coronary artery bypass surgery. Journal of the American College of Cardiology. 1995;**25**:198-202. DOI: https://doi.org/10.1016/0735-1097(94)00329-O

[16] Helgadottir S, Sigurdsson MI, Ingvarsdottir IL, Arnar DO, Gudbjartsson T. Atrial fibrillation following cardiac surgery: Risk analysis and long-term survival. Journal of Cardiothoracic Surgery. 2012;**7**:87. DOI: 10.1186/1749-8090-7-87

[17] Kolvekar S, D'Souza A, Akhtar P, Reek C, Garratt C, Spyt T. Role of atrial ischaemia in development of atrial fibrillation following coronary artery bypass surgery. European Journal of Cardio-Thoracic Surgery. 1997;**11**:70-75. DOI: 10.1016/S1010-7940(96)01095-0

[18] Wazni OM, Martin DO, Marrouche NF, Latif AA, Ziada K, Shaaraoui M, Almahameed S, Schweikert RA, Saliba WI, Gillinov AM, Tang WH, Mills RM, Francis GS, Young JB, Natale A. Plasma B-type natriuretic peptide levels predict postoperative atrial fibrillation in patients undergoing cardiac surgery. Circulation. 2004;**110**:124-127. DOI: https://doi.org/10.1161/01.CIR.0000134481.24511.BC

[19] Zacharias A, Schwann TA, Riordan CJ, Durham SJ, Shah AS, Habib RH. Obesity and risk of new-onset atrial fibrillation after cardiac surgery. Circulation. 2005;**112**:3247-3255 https://doi.org/10.1161/CIRCULATIONAHA.105.553743

[20] Maesen B, Nijs J, Maessen J, Allessie M, Schotten U. Post-operative atrial fibrillation: A maze of mechanisms. Europace. 2012;**14**:159-174. DOI: https://doi.org/10.1093/europace/eur208

[21] Warltier DC, Laffey JG, Boylan JF, Cheng DCH. The systemic inflammatory response to cardiac surgery: Implications for the anesthesiologist. Anesthesiology. 2002;**97**:215-252 PMID: 12131125

[22] Bulow NMH, Colpo E, Duarte MF, Correa EFM, Schlosser RS, Lauda A, Kade IJ, Rocha JBT. Inflammatory response in patients under coronary artery bypass grafting surgery and clinical implications: A review of the relevance of Dexmedetomidine use. ISRN Anesthesiology. 2014;**2014**:1-28 http://dx.doi.org/10.1155/2014/905238

[23] Prondzinsky R, Knüpfer A, Loppnow H, Redling F, Lehmann DW, Stabenow I, Witthaut R, Unverzagt S, Radke J, Zerkowski HR, Werdan K. Surgical trauma affects the proinflammatory status after cardiac surgery to a higher degree than cardiopulmonary bypass. The Journal of Thoracic and Cardiovascular Surgery. 2005;**129**:760-766. DOI: https://doi.org/10.1016/j.jtcvs.2004.07.052

[24] Angelini GD, Penny WJ, el-Ghamary F, West RR, Butchart EG. The incidence and significance of early pericardial effusion after open heart surgery. European Journal of Cardio-Thoracic Surgery. 1987;**1**:165-168. DOI: https://doi.org/10.1016/1010-7940(87)90034-0

[25] Stamou SC, Dangas G, Hill PC, Pfister AJ, Dullum MK, Boyce SW, Bafi AS, Garcia JM, Corso PJ. Atrial fibrillation after beating heart surgery. The American Journal of Cardiology. 2000;**86**:64-67. DOI: https://doi.org/10.1016/S0002-9149(00)00829-8

[26] Haïssaguerre M, Jaïs P, Shah DC, Takahashi A, Hocini M, Quiniou G, Garrigue S, Le Mouroux A, Le Métayer P, Clémenty J. Spontaneous initiation of atrial fibrillation by ectopic beats originating in the pulmonary veins. The New England Journal of Medicine. 1998;**339**:659-666. DOI: 10.1056/NEJM199809033391003

[27] Vinten-Johansen J. Involvement of neutrophils in the pathogenesis of lethal myocardial reperfusion injury. Cardiovascular Research. 2004;**61**:481-497. DOI: 10.1016/j. cardiores.2003.10.011

[28] Butler J, Parker D, Pillai R, Westaby S, Shale DJ, Rocker GM. Effects of cardiopulmonary bypass on systemic release of neutrophil elastase and tumour necrosis factor. The Journal of Thoracic and Cardiovascular Surgery. 1993;**105**:25-30 PMID:8419705

[29] Wakayama F, Fukuda I, Suzuki Y, Kondo N. Neutrophil elastase inhibitor, sivelestat, attenuates acute lung injury after cardiopulmonary bypass in the rabbit endotoxemia model. The Annals of Thoracic Surgery. 2007;**83**:153-160. DOI: 10.1016/j.athoracsur.2006.08.023

[30] Atlee JL. Perioperative cardiac dysrhythmias: Diagnosis and management. Anesthesiology. 1997;**86**:1397-1424

[31] Salazar C, Frishman W, Friedman S, Patel J, Lin YT, Oka Y, Frater RW, Becker RM. β-blockade therapy for supraventricular tachyarrhythmias after coronary surgery: A propranolol withdrawal syndrome? Angiology. 1979;**30**:816-819. DOI: 10.1177/000331977903001204

[32] Deliargyris EN, Raymond RJ, Guzzo JA, Dehmer GJ, Smith SC, Weiner MS, Roberts CS. Preoperative factors predisposing to early postoperative atrial fibrillation after isolated coronary artery bypass grafting. The American Journal of Cardiology. 2000;**85**:763-764. DOI: http://dx.doi.org/10.1016/S0002-9149(99)00857-7

[33] Rubin DA, Nieminski KE, Reed GE, Herman MV. Predictors, prevention, and long-term prognosis of atrial fibrillation after coronary artery bypass graft operations. The Journal of Thoracic and Cardiovascular Surgery. 1987;**94**:331-335 PMID: 3306163

[34] Tisdale JE, Patel R, Webb CR, Borzak S, Zarowitz BJ. Electrophysiologic and proarrhythmic effects of intravenous inotropic agents. Progress in Cardiovascular Diseases. 1995;**38**:167-180. DOI: http://dx.doi.org/10.1016/S0033-0620(05)80005-2

[35] Williams JB, Hernandez AF, Li S, Dokholyan RS, O'Brien SM, Smith PK, Ferguson TB, Peterson ED. Postoperative inotrope and vasopressor use following CABG: Outcome data from the CAPS-care study. Journal of Cardiac Surgery. 2011;**26**:572-578. DOI: 10.1111/j.1540-8191.2011.01301.x

[36] Haghjoo M. Pharmacological and nonpharmacological prevention of atrial fibrillation after coronary artery bypass surgery. The Journal of Tehran Heart Center. 2012;**7**:2-9 PMCID: PMC3466882

[37] Wahr JA, Parks R, Boisvert D, Comunale M, Fabian J, Ramsay J, Mangano DT. Preoperative serum potassium levels and perioperative outcomes in cardiac surgery patients. Multicenter study of perioperative ischemia research group. JAMA. 1999;**281**:2203-2210. DOI: 10.1001/jama.281.23.2203

[38] Luo X, Pan Z, Shan H, Xiao J, Sun X, Wang N, Lin H, Xiao L, Maguy A, Qi XY, Li Y, Gao X, Dong D, Zhang Y, Bai Y, Ai J, Sun L, Lu H, Luo XY, Wang Z, Lu Y, Yang B, Nattel S. MicroRNA-26 governs profibrillatory inward-rectifier potassium current changes in atrial fibrillation. The Journal of Clinical Investigation. 2013;**123**:1939-1951. DOI: 10.1172/JCI62185

[39] Pinski SL. Potassium replacement after cardiac surgery: It is not time to change practice, yet. Critical Care Medicine. 1999;**27**:2581-2582 PMID: 10579291

[40] England MR, Gordon G, Salem M, Chernow B. Magnesium administration and dysrhythmias after cardiac surgery: A placebo-controlled, double-blind, randomized trial. JAMA. 1992;**268**:2395-2402. DOI: 10.1001/jama.1992.03490170067027

[41] Aglio LS, Stanford GC, Maddi R, Boyd III JL, Nussbaum S, Chernow B. Hypomagnesemia is common following cardiac surgery. Journal of Cardiothoracic and Vascular Anesthesia. 1991;**5**:201-208. DOI: http://dx.doi.org/10.1016/1053-0770(91)90274-W

[42] Singh S, Johnson PI, Lee RE, Orfei E, Lonchyna VA, Sullivan HJ, Montoya A, Tran H, Wehrmacher WH, Wurster RD. Topography of cardiac ganglia in the adult human heart. The Journal of Thoracic and Cardiovascular Surgery. 1996;**112**:943-953. DOI: 10.1016/S0022-5223(96)70094-6

[43] Quan KJ, Lee JH, Geha AS, Biblo LA, Van Hare GF, Mackall JA, Carlson MD. Characterization of sinoatrial parasympathetic innervation in humans. Journal of Cardiovascular Electrophysiology. 1999;**10**:1060-1065. DOI: 10.1111/j.1540-8167.1999.tb00278.x

[44] Quan KJ, Lee JH, Van Hare GF, Biblo LA, Mackall JA, Carlson MD. Identification and characterization of atrioventricular parasympathetic innervation in humans. Journal of Cardiovascular Electrophysiology. 2002;**13**:735-739. DOI: 10.1046/j.1540-8167.2002.00735.x

[45] Carlson MD, Geha AS, Hsu J, Martin PJ, Levy MN, Jacobs G, Waldo AL. Selective stimulation of parasympathetic nerve fibers to the human sinoatrial node. Circulation. 1992;**85**:1311-1317. DOI: https://doi.org/10.1161/01.CIR.85.4.1311

[46] Cummings JE, Gill I, Akhrass R, Dery Biblo LA, Quan KJ. Preservation of the anterior fat pad paradoxically decreases the incidence of postoperative atrial fibrillation in humans. Journal of the American College of Cardiology. 2004;**17**(43):994-1000. DOI: 10.1016/j.jacc.2003.07.055

[47] CM W, Sander S, Coleman CI, Gallagher R, Takata H, Humphrey C, Henyan N, Gillespie EL, Kluger J. Impact of epicardial anterior fat pad retention on postcardiothoracic surgery atrial fibrillation incidence: The AFIST-III study. Journal of the American College of Cardiology. 2007;**49**:298-303. DOI: 10.1016/j.jacc.2006.10.033

[48] Mitchell LB. Incidence, timing and outcome of atrial tachyarrhythmias after cardiac surgery. In: Steinberg JS, editor. Atrial Fibrillation after Cardiac Surgery. Boston: Kluwer Academic Publishers; 2000. pp. 37-50.

[49] Maisel WH, Rawn JD, Stevenson WG. Atrial fibrillation after cardiac surgery. Annals of Internal Medicine. 2001;**135**:1061-1073. DOI: 10.7326/0003-4819-135-12-200112180-00010

[50] Blomstrom Lundqvist C. Post CABG atrial fibrillation: What are the incidence, predictors, treatment, and long-term outcome? In: Raviele A, editor. Cardiac Arrhythmias 2005. Venice, Italy: Springer; 2005. pp. 131-136.

[51] Pavri BB, O'Nunain SS, Newell JB, Ruskin JN, William G. Prevalence and prognostic significance of atrial arrhythmias after orthotopic cardiac transplantation. Journal of the American College of Cardiology. 1995;**25**:1673-1680. DOI: https://doi.org/10.1016/0735-1097(95)00047-8

[52] Mathew JP, Parks R, Savino JS, Friedman AS, Koch C, Mangano DT, Browner WS. Atrial fibrillation following coronary artery bypass graft surgery: Predictors, outcomes, and resource utilization. JAMA. 1996;**276**:300-306. DOI: 10.1001/jama.1996.03540040044031

[53] Echahidi N, Pibarot P, O'Hara G, Mathieu P. Mechanisms, prevention, and treatment of atrial fibrillation after cardiac surgery. Journal of the American College of Cardiology. 2008;**51**:793-801. DOI: 10.1016/j.jacc. 2007.10.043

[54] Shingu Y, Kubota S, Wakasa S, Ooka T, Tachibana T, Matsui Y. Postoperative atrial fibrillation: Mechanism, prevention, and future perspective. Surgery Today. 2012;**42**:819-824. DOI: 10.1007/s00595-012-0199-4

[55] Aranki SF, Shaw DP, Adams DH, Rizzo RJ, Couper GS, VanderVliet M, Collins JJ Jr, Cohn LH, Burstin HR. Current trends and impact on hospital resources. Circulation. 1996;**94**:390-397. DOI: https://doi.org/10.1161/01.CIR.94.3.390

[56] Soucier RJ, Mirza S, Abordo MG, Berns E, Dalamagas HC, Hanna A, Silverman DI. Predictors of conversion of atrial fibrillation after cardiac operation in the absence of class I or III antiarrhythmic medications. The Annals of Thoracic Surgery. 2001;**72**:694-697. DOI: http://dx.doi.org/10.1016/S0003-4975(01)02817-X

[57] Lee JK, Klein GJ, Krahn AD, Yee R, Zarnke K, Simpson C, Skanes A, Spindler B. Rate-control versus conversion strategy in postoperative atrial fibrillation: A prospective, randomized pilot study. American Heart Journal. 2000;**140**:871-877. DOI: 10.1067/mhj.2000.111104

[58] Landymore RW, Howell F. Recurrent atrial arrhythmias following treatment for postoperative atrial fibrillation after coronary bypass operations. European Journal of Cardio-Thoracic Surgery. 1991;**5**:436-439. DOI: https://doi.org/10.1016/1010-7940(91)90191-L

[59] Kowey PR, Stebbins D, Igidbashian L, Goldman SM, Sutter FP, Rials SJ, Marinchak RA. Clinical outcome of patients who develop PAF after CABG surgery. Pacing and Clinical Electrophysiology. 2001;**24**:191-193. DOI: 10.1046/j.1460-9592.2001.00191.x

[60] Villareal RP, Hariharan R, Liu BC, Kar B, Lee VV, Elayda M, Lopez JA, Rasekh A, Wilson JM, Massumi A. Postoperative atrial fibrillation and mortality after coronary artery bypass surgery. Journal of the American College of Cardiology. 2004;**43**:742-748. DOI: 10.1016/j.jacc.2003.11.023

[61] Fuller JA, Adams GG, Buxton B. Atrial fibrillation after coronary artery bypass grafting: Is it a disorder of the elderly? The Journal of Thoracic and Cardiovascular Surgery. 1989;**97**:821-825 PMID: 2566713

[62] Lahtinen J, Biancari F, Salmela E, Mosorin M, Satta J, Rainio P, Rimpiläinen J, Lepojärvi M, Juvonen T. Postoperative atrial fibrillation is a major cause of stroke after on-pump coronary artery bypass surgery. The Annals of Thoracic Surgery. 2004;**77**:1241-1244. DOI: 10.1016/j.athoracsur.2003.09.077

[63] Reed GL, III, Singer DE, Picard EH, DeSanctis RW. Stroke following coronary-artery bypass surgery. A case-control estimate of the risk from carotid bruits. The New England Journal of Medicine. 1988;**319**:1246-1250. DOI: 10.1056/NEJM198811103191903

[64] Newman MF, Wolman R, Kanchuger M, Marschall K, Mora-Mangano C, Roach G, Smith LR, Aggarwal A, Nussmeier N, Herskowitz A, Mangano DT. Multicenter pre-operative stroke risk index for patients undergoing coronary artery bypass graft surgery. Multicenter study of perioperative ischemia (McSPI) research group. Circulation. 1996;**94**(9 Suppl):II74-II80 PMID: 8901723

[65] Mickleborough LL, Walker PM, Takagi Y, Ohashi M, Ivanov J, Tamariz M. Risk factors for stroke in patients undergoing coronary artery bypass grafting. The Journal of Thoracic and Cardiovascular Surgery. 1996;**112**:1250-1259. DOI: 10.1016/S0022-5223(96)70138-1

[66] Hogue CW Jr, Murphy SF, Schechtman KB, Dávila-Román VG. Risk factors for early or delayed stroke after cardiac surgery. Circulation. 1999;**100**:642-647. DOI: https://doi.org/10.1161/01.CIR.100.6.642

[67] Kim MH, Deeb GM, Morady F, Bruckman D, Hallock LR, Smith KA, Karavite DJ, Bolling SF, Pagani FD, Wahr JA, Sonnad SS, Kazanjian PE, Watts C, Williams M, Eagle KA. Effect of postoperative atrial fibrillation on length of stay after cardiac surgery (the postoperative atrial fibrillation in cardiac surgery study [PACS2]). The American Journal of Cardiology. 2001;**87**:881-885. DOI: http://dx.doi.org/10.1016/S0002-9149(00)01530-7

[68] Lauer MS, Eagle KA, Buckley MJ, DeSanctis RW. Atrial fibrillation following coronary artery bypass surgery. Progress in Cardiovascular Diseases. 1989;**31**:367-378. DOI: http://dx.doi.org/10.1016/0033-0620(89)90031-5

[69] Wyse DG, Waldo AL, DiMarco JP, Domanski MJ, Rosenberg Y, Schron EB, Kellen JC, Greene HL, Mickel MC, Dalquist JE. Atrial fibrillation follow-up investigation of rhythm management (AFFIRM) investigators a comparison of rate control and rhythm control in patients with atrial fibrillation. The New England Journal of Medicine. 2002;**347**:1825-1833. DOI: 10.1056/NEJMoa021328.

[70] Jongnarangsin K, Oral H. Postoperative atrial fibrillation. Cardiology Clinics. 2009;**27**:69-78. DOI: 10.1016/j.ccl.2008.09.011

[71] Mayson SE, Greenspon AJ, Adams S, Decaro MV, Sheth M, Weitz HH, Whellan DJ. The changing face of postoperative atrial fibrillation prevention: A review of current medical therapy. Cardiology in Review. 2007;**15**:231-241. DOI: 10.1097/CRD.0b013e31813e62bb

[72] Al-Khatib SM, Hafley G, Harrington RA, Mack MJ, Ferguson TB, Peterson ED, Califf RM, Kouchoukos NT, Alexander JH. Patterns of management of atrial fibrillation complicating coronary artery bypass grafting: Results from the PRoject of ex-vivo vein graft ENgineering via transfection IV (PREVENT-IV) trial. American Heart Journal. 2009;**158**:792-798. DOI: 10.1016/j.ahj.2009.09.003

[73] Gillinov AM, Bagiella E, Moskowitz AJ, Raiten JM, Groh MA, Bowdish ME, Ailawadi G, Kirkwood KA, Perrault LP, Parides MK, Smith RL II, Kern JA, Dussault G, Hackmann AE, Jeffries NO, Miller MA, Taddei-Peters WC, Rose EA, Weisel RD, Williams DL,

Mangusan RF, Argenziano M, Moquete EG, O'Sullivan KL, Pellerin M, Shah KJ, Gammie JS, Mayer ML, Voisine P, Gelijns AC, O'Gara PT, Mack MJ, CTSN. Rate control versus rhythm control for atrial fibrillation after cardiac surgery. The New England Journal of Medicine. 2016;**374**:1911-1921. DOI: 10.1056/NEJMoa1602002.

[74] January CT, Wann LS, Alpert JS, Calkins H, Cigarroa JE, Cleveland JC Jr, Conti JB, Ellinor PT, Ezekowitz MD, Field ME, Murray KT, Sacco RL, Stevenson WG, Tchou PJ, Tracy CM, Yancy CW; ACC/AHA Task Force Members. 2014 AHA/ACC/HRS guideline for the management of patients with atrial fibrillation: Executive summary: A report of the American College of Cardiology/American Heart Association Task Force on Practice Guidelines and the Heart Rhythm Society. Circulation 2014;**130**:2071-2104. DOI: 10.1161/CIR.0000000000000040

[75] Kirchhof P, Benussi S, Kotecha D, Ahlsson A, Atar D, Casadei B, Castellá M, Diener HC, Heidbuchel H, Hendriks J, Hindricks G, Manolis AS, Oldgren J, Alexandru Popescu B, Schotten U, Van Putte B, Vardas P. 2016 ESC guidelines for the management of atrial fibrillation developed in collaboration with EACTS. European Heart Journal. 2016 Oct 7;**37**(38):2893-2962. DOI: 10.1093/eurheartj/ehw210

[76] Clemo HF, Wood MA, Gilligan DM, Ellenbogen KA. Intravenous amiodarone for acute heart rate control in the critically ill patient with atrial tachyarrhythmias. The American Journal of Cardiology. 1998;**81**:594-598. DOI: http://dx.doi.org/10.1016/S0002-9149(97)00962-4

[77] Daoud EG, Strickberger SA, Man KC, Goyal R, Deeb GM, Bolling SF, Pagani FD, Bitar C, Meissner MD, Morady F. Preoperative amiodarone as prophylaxis against atrial fibrillation after heart surgery. The New England Journal of Medicine. 1997;**337**:1785-1791. DOI: 10.1056/NEJM199712183372501

[78] Dunning J, Treasure T, Versteegh M, Nashef SA, EACTS Audit and Guidelines Committee. Guidelines on the prevention and management of de novo atrial fibrillation after cardiac and thoracic surgery. European Journal of Cardiothoracic Surgery. 2006;**30**:852-872. DOI: 10.1016/j.ejcts.2006.09.003

[79] Heldal M, Atar D. Pharmacological conversion of recent-onset atrial fibrillation: A systematic review. Scandinavian Cardiovascular Journal. Supplement. 2013;**47**:2-10. DOI: 10.3109/14017431.2012.740572

[80] Kowey PR, Dorian P, Mitchell LB, Pratt CM, Roy D, Schwartz PJ, Sadowski J, Sobczyk D, Bochenek A, Toft E, Atrial Arrhythmia Conversion Trial Investigators. Vernakalant hydrochloride for the rapid conversion of atrial fibrillation after cardiac surgery: A randomized, double-blind, placebo-controlled trial. Circulation. Arrhythmia and Electrophysiology. 2009;**2**:652-659. DOI: 10.1161/CIRCEP.109.870204

[81] VanderLugt JT, Mattioni T, Denker S, Torchiana D, Ahern T, Wakefield LK, Perry KT, Kowey PR. Efficacy and safety of ibutilide fumarate for the conversion of atrial arrhythmias after cardiac surgery. Circulation. 1999;**100**:369-375. DOI: https://doi.org/10.1161/01.CIR.100.4.369

[82] Gomes JA, Ip J, Santoni-Rugiu F, Mehta D, Ergin A, Lansman S, Pe E, Newhouse TT, Chao S. Oral d,l sotalol reduces the incidence of post-operative atrial fibrillation in coronary artery

bypass surgery patients: A randomized, double-blind, placebo-controlled study. Journal of the American College of Cardiology. 1999;**34**:334-339. DOI: https://doi.org/10.1016/S0735-1097(99)00213-2

[83] El-Chami MF, Kilgo P, Thourani V, Lattouf OM, Delurgio DB, Guyton RA, Leon AR, Puskas JD. New-onset atrial fibrillation predicts long-term mortality after coronary artery bypass graft. Journal of the American College of Cardiology. 2010;**55**:1370-1376. DOI: 10.1016/j.jacc.2009.10.058

[84] Anderson E, Dyke C, Levy JH. Anticoagulation strategies for the management of postoperative atrial fibrillation. Clinics in Laboratory Medicine. 2014;**34**:537-561. DOI: 10.1016/j.cll.2014.06.012

[85] Arsenault KA, Yusuf AM, Crystal E, Healey JS, Morillo CA, Nair GM, Whitlock RP. Interventions for preventing post-operative atrial fibrillation in patients undergoing heart surgery. Cochrane Database of Systematic Reviews. 2013;**1**:CD003611. DOI: 10.1002/14651858.CD003611.pub3

[86] Khan MF, Wendel CS, Movahed MR. Prevention of post-coronary artery bypass grafting (CABG) atrial fibrillation: Efficacy of prophylactic beta-blockers in the modern era: A meta-analysis of latest randomized controlled trials. Annals of Noninvasive Electrocardiology. 2013;**18**:58-68. DOI: 10.1111/anec.12004

[87] Burgess DC, Kilborn MJ, Keech AC. Interventions for prevention of post-operative atrial fibrillation and its complications after cardiac surgery: A meta-analysis. European Heart Journal. 2006;**27**:2846-2857. DOI: 10.1093/eurheartj/ehl272

[88] Chatterjee S, Sardar P, Mukherjee D, Lichstein E, Aikat S. Timing and route of amiodarone for prevention of postoperative atrial fibrillation after cardiac surgery: A network regression meta-analysis. Pacing and Clinical Electrophysiology. 2013;**36**:1017-1023. DOI: 10.1111/pace.12140

[89] Zhu J, Wang C, Gao D, Zhang C, Zhang Y, Lu Y, Gao Y. Meta-analysis of amiodarone versus beta-blocker as a prophylactic therapy against atrial fibrillation following cardiac surgery. Internal Medicine Journal. 2012;**42**:1078-1087. DOI: 10.1111/j.1445-5994.2012.02844.x

[90] Koniari I, Apostolakis E, Rogkakou C, Baikoussis NG, Dougenis D. Pharmacologic prophylaxis for atrial fibrillation following cardiac surgery: A systematic review. Journal of Cardiothoracic Surgery. 2010;**5**:121. DOI: 10.1186/1749-8090-5-121

[91] Shepherd J, Jones J, Frampton GK, Tanajewski L, Turner D, Price A. Intravenous magnesium sulphate and sotalol for prevention of atrial fibrillation after coronary artery bypass surgery: A systematic review and economic evaluation. Health Technology Assessment. 2008;**12**:iii-iv, ix-95(1-49). DOI: https://dx.doi.org/10.3310/hta12280

[92] Imazio M, Brucato A, Ferrazzi P, Rovere ME, Gandino A, Cemin R, Ferrua S, Belli R, Maestroni S, Simon C, Zingarelli E, Barosi A, Sansone F, Patrini D, Vitali E, Trinchero R, Spodick DI I, Adler Y, COPPS Investigators. Colchicine reduces postoperative atrial fibrillation: Results of the colchicine for the prevention of the Postpericardiotomy syndrome (COPPS) atrial fibrillation substudy. Circulation. 2011;**124**:2290-2295. DOI: 10.1161/CIRCULATIONAHA.111.026153

[93] Zheng Z, Jayaram R, Jiang L, Emberson J, Zhao Y, Li Q, Du J, Guarguagli S, Hill M, Chen Z, Collins R, Casadei B. Perioperative Rosuvastatin in cardiac surgery. The New England Journal of Medicine. 2016;**374**:1744-1753. DOI: 10.1056/NEJMoa1507750

[94] Liakopoulos OJ, Kuhn EW, Slottosch I, Wassmer G, Wahlers T. Preoperative statin therapy for patients undergoing cardiac surgery. Cochrane Database of Systematic Reviews. 2012;**4**:Cd008493. DOI: 10.1002/14651858.CD008493.pub2

[95] Fauchier L, Clementy N, Babuty D. Statin therapy and atrial fibrillation: Systematic review and updated meta-analysis of published randomized controlled trials. Current Opinion in Cardiology. 2013;**28**:7-18. DOI: 10.1097/HCO.0b013e32835b0956

[96] Zheng H, Xue S, ZL H, Shan JG, Yang WG. The use of statins to prevent postoperative atrial fibrillation after coronary artery bypass grafting: A meta-analysis of 12 studies. Journal of Cardiovascular Pharmacology. 2014 Sep;**64**(3):285-292. DOI: 10.1097/FJC.0000000000000102

[97] Mathew JP, Fontes ML, Tudor IC, Ramsay J, Duke P, Mazer CD, Barash PG, Hsu PH, Mangano DT, Investigators of the Ischemia Research and Education Foundation, Multicenter Study of Perioperative Ischemia Research Group. A multicenter risk index for atrial fibrillation after cardiac surgery. Journal of the American Medical Association. 2004;**14**(291):1720-1729. DOI: 10.1001/jama.291.14.1720

[98] Cook RC, Yamashita MH, Kearns M, Ramanathan K, Gin K, Humphries KH. Prophylactic magnesium does not prevent atrial fibrillation after cardiac surgery: A meta-analysis. The Annals of Thoracic Surgery. 2013;**95**:533-541. DOI: 10.1016/j.athoracsur.2012.09.008

[99] De Oliveira GS, Jr Knautz JS, Sherwani S, McCarthy RJ. Systemic magnesium to reduce postoperative arrhythmias after coronary artery bypass graft surgery: A meta-analysis of randomized controlled trials. Journal of Cardiothoracic and Vascular Anesthesia. 2012;**26**:643-650. DOI: 10.1053/j.jvca.2012.03.012

[100] Costanzo S, di Niro V, Di Castelnuovo A, Gianfagna F, Donati MB, de Gaetano G, Iacoviello L. Prevention of postoperative atrial fibrillation in open heart surgery patients by preoperative supplementation of n-3 polyunsaturated fatty acids: An updated meta-analysis. The Journal of Thoracic and Cardiovascular Surgery. 2013;**146**:906-911. DOI: 10.1016/j.jtcvs.2013.03.015

[101] Farquharson AL, Metcalf RG, Sanders P, Stuklis R, Edwards JR, Gibson RA, Cleland LG, Sullivan TR, James MJ, Young GD. Effect of dietary fish oil on atrial fibrillation after cardiac surgery. The American Journal of Cardiology. 2011;**108**:851-856. DOI: 10.1016/j.amjcard.2011.04.036

[102] Heidarsdottir R, Arnar DO, Skuladottir GV, Torfason B, Edvardsson V, Gottskalksson G, Palsson R, Indridason OS. Does treatment with n-3 polyunsaturated fatty acids prevent atrial fibrillation after open heart surgery? Europace. 2010;**12**:356-363. DOI: 10.1093/europace/eup429

[103] Mariani J, Doval HC, Nul D, Varini S, Grancelli H, Ferrante D, Tognoni G, Macchia A. N-3 polyunsaturated fatty acids to prevent atrial fibrillation: Updated systematic

review and meta-analysis of randomized controlled trials. Journal of the American Heart Association. 2013;2:e005033. DOI: 10.1161/JAHA.112.005033

[104] Rodrigo R, Korantzopoulos P, Cereceda M, Asenjo R, Zamorano J, Villalabeitia E, Baeza C, Aguayo R, Castillo R, Carrasco R, Gormaz JG. A randomized controled trial to prevent post-operative atrial fibrillation by antioxidant reinforcement. Journal of the American College of Cardiology. 2013;62:1457-1465. DOI: 10.1016/j.jacc.2013.07.014

[105] Saravanan P, Bridgewater B, West AL, O'Neill SC, Calder PC, Davidson NC. Omega-3 fatty acid supplementation does not reduce risk of atrial fibrillation after coronary artery bypass surgery: A randomized, double-blind, placebo-controlled clinical trial. Circulation. Arrhythmia and Electrophysiology. 2010;3:46-53. DOI: 10.1161/CIRCEP.109.899633

[106] Wu JH, Marchioli R, Silletta MG, Macchia A, Song X, Siscovick DS, Harris WS, Masson S, Latini R, Albert C, Brown NJ, Lamarra M, Favaloro RR, Mozaffarian D. Plasma phospho-lipid omega-3 fatty acids and incidence of postoperative atrial fibrillation in the OPERA trial. Journal of the American Heart Association. 2013;2:e000397. DOI: 10.1161/JAHA.113.000397

[107] Xin W, Wei W, Lin Z, Zhang X, Yang H, Zhang T, Li B, Mi S. Fish oil and atrial fibrilla-tion after cardiac surgery: A meta-analysis of randomized controlled trials. PloS One. 2013;8:e72913. DOI: 0.1371/journal.pone.0072913

[108] Zhang B, Zhen Y, Tao A, Bao Z, Zhang G. Polyunsaturated fatty acids for the preven-tion of atrial fibrillation after cardiac surgery: An updated meta-analysis of randomized controlled trials. Journal of Cardiology. 2014;63:53-59. DOI: 10.1016/j.jjcc.2013.06.014

[109] Ho KM, Tan JA. Benefits and risks of corticosteroid prophylaxis in adult cardiac sur-gery a dose-response meta-analysis. Circulation. 2009;119:1853-1866. DOI: 10.1161/CIRCULATIONAHA.108.848218

[110] Cappabianca G, Rotunno C, de Luca Tupputi Schinosa L, Ranieri VM, Paparella D. Protective effects of steroids in cardiac surgery: A meta-analysis of randomized dou-ble-blind trials. Journal of Cardiothoracic and Vascular Anesthesia. 2011;25:156-165. DOI: 10.1053/j.jvca.2010.03.015

[111] Viviano A, Kanagasabay R, Zakkar M. Is perioperative corticosteroid administration associated with a reduced incidence of postoperative atrial fibrillation in adult car-diac surgery? Interactive Cardiovascular and Thoracic Surgery. 2014;18:225-229. DOI: https://doi.org/10.1093/icvts/ivt486

[112] Kaleda VI, McCormack DJ, Shipolini AR. Does posterior pericardiotomy reduce the incidence of atrial fibrillation after coronary artery bypass grafting surgery? Interactive Cardiovascular and Thoracic Surgery. 2012;14:384-389. DOI: 10.1093/icvts/ivr099

[113] Ozaydin M, Peker O, Erdogan D, Kapan S, Turker Y, Varol E, Ozguner F, Dogan A, Ibrisim E. N-acetylcysteine for the prevention of postoperative atrial fibrillation: A prospective, randomized, placebo-controlled pilot study. European Heart Journal. 2008;29:625-631. DOI: 10.1093/eurheartj/ehn011

[114] Cavol Cavolli R, Kaya K, Aslan A, Emiroglu O, Erturk S, Korkmaz O, Oguz M, Tasoz R, Ozyurda U. Does sodium nitroprusside decrease the incidence of atrial fibrillation after myocardial revascularization? A pilot study. Circulation. 2008;**118**:476-481. DOI: 10.1161/CIRCULATIONAHA.107.719377

[115] Fan K, Lee KL, Chiu CS, Lee JW, He GW, Cheung D, Sun MP, Lau CP. Effects of biatrial pacing in prevention of postoperative atrial fibrillation after coronary artery bypass surgery. Circulation. 2000;**102**:755-760. DOI: https://doi.org/10.1161/01.CIR.102.7.755

[116] Daoud EG, Dabir R, Archambeau M, Morady F, Strickberger SA. Randomized, double-blind trial of simultaneous right and left atrial epicardial pacing for prevention of post-open heart surgery atrial fibrillation. Circulation. 2000;**102**:761-765. DOI: https://doi.org/10.1161/01.CIR.102.7.761

[117] Levy T, Fotopoulos G, Walker S, Rex S, Octave M, Paul V, Amrani M. Randomized controlled study investigating the effect of biatrial pacing in prevention of atrial fibrillation after coronary artery bypass grafting. Circulation. 2000;**102**:1382-1387. DOI: https://doi.org/10.1161/01.CIR.102.12.1382

[118] Gerstenfeld EP, Hill MR, French SN, Mehra R, Rofino K, Vander Salm TJ, Mittleman RS. Evaluation of right atrial and biatrial temporary pacing for the prevention of atrial fibrillation after coronary artery bypass surgery. Journal of the American College of Cardiology. 1999;**33**:1981-1988. DOI: https://doi.org/10.1161/01.CIR.102.12.1382

[119] Chung MK, Augostini RS, Asher CR, Pool DP, Grady TA, Zikri M, Buehner SM, Weinstock M, McCarthy PM. Ineffectiveness and potential proarrhythmia of atrial pacing for atrial fibrillation prevention after coronary artery bypass grafting. The Annals of Thoracic Surgery. 2000;**69**:1057-1063. DOI: http://dx.doi.org/10.1016/S0003-4975(99)01338-7

[120] Mori SS, Fujii GG, Ishida HH, Tomari SS, Matsuura AA, Yoshida KK. Atrial flutter after coronary artery bypass grafting: Proposed mechanism as illuminated by independent predictors. Annals of Thoracic and Cardiovascular Surgery. 2003;**9**:50-56 PMID: 12667130

[121] Pap R, Kohári M, Makai A, Bencsik G, Traykov VB, Gallardo R, Klausz G, Zsuzsanna K, Forster T, Sághy L. Surgical technique and the mechanism of atrial tachycardia late after open heart surgery. Journal of Interventional Cardiac Electrophysiology. 2012;**35**:127-135. DOI: 10.1007/s10840-012-9705-2

[122] Hammon JW, Hines MH. Extracorporeal circulation: Perfusion system. In Cohn LH editor. Cardiac Surgery in the Adult. 4th ed. New York: McGraw-Hill; 2008. pp. 350-370. Ch12

[123] Anné W, van Rensburg H, Adams J, Ector H, Van de Werf F, Heidbüchel H. Ablation of post-surgical intra-atrial reentrant tachycardia. Predilection target sites and mapping approach. European Heart Journal. 2002;**23**;1609-1616. PMID: 12323161

[124] Nakagawa H, Shah N, Matsudaira K, Overholt E, Chandrasekaran K, Beckman KJ, Spector P, Calame JD, Rao A, Hasdemir C, Otomo K, Wang Z, Lazzara R, Jackman WM. Characterization of reentrant circuit in macroreentrant right atrial tachycardia after surgical repair of congenital heart disease: Isolated channels between scars allow "focal" ablation. Circulation. 2001 Feb 6;**103**:699-709. DOI: https://doi.org/10.1161/01.CIR.103.5.699

[125] Stewart AM, Greaves K, Bromilow J. Supraventricular tachyarrhythmias and their management in the perioperative period. Continuing Education in Anesthesia, Critical Care and Pain. 2015;**15**:90-97. DOI: https://doi.org/10.1093/bjaceaccp/mku018

[126] Delacrétaz E. Clinical practice. Supraventricular tachycardia. The New England Journal of Medicine. 2006;**354**:1039-1051. DOI: 10.1056/NEJMcp051145

[127] Poldermans D, Bax JJ, Boersma E, De Hert S, Eeckhout E, Fowkes G, Gorenek B, Hennerici MG, Iung B, Kelm M, Kjeldsen KP, Kristensen SD, Lopez-Sendon J, Pelosi P, Philippe F, Pierard L, Ponikowski P, Schmid JP, Sellevold OF, Sicari R, Van den Berghe G, Vermassen F, Hoeks SE, Vanhorebeek I, Vahanian A, Auricchio A, Bax JJ, Ceconi C, Dean V, Filippatos G, Funck-Brentano C, Hobbs R, Kearn P, McDonag T, McGregor K, Popescu BA, Reiner Z, Sechtem U, Sirnes PA, Tendera M, Vardas P, Widimsky P, De Caterina R, Agewall S, Al Attar N, Andreotti F, Anker SD, Baron-Esquivias G, Berkenboom G, Chapoutot L, Cifkova R, Faggiano P, Gibbs S, Hansen HS, Iserin L, Israel CW, Kornowski R, Eizagaechevarria NM, Pepi M, Piepoli M, Priebe HJ, Scherer M, Stepinska J, Taggart D, Tubaro M, Task Force for Preoperative Cardiac Risk Assessment and Perioperative Cardiac Management in Non-cardiac Surgery of European Society of Cardiology (ESC), European Society of Anaesthesiology (ESA). Guidelines for pre-operative cardiac risk assessment and perioperative cardiac Management in non-Cardiac Surgery. The task force for preoperative cardiac risk assessment and perioperative cardiac management in non-cardiac surgery of the European Society of Cardiology (ESC) and endorsed by the European Society of Anaesthesiology (ESA). European Journal of Anaesthesiology. 2010;**27**:92-137. DOI: 10.1097/EJA.0b013e328334c017

[128] Polanczyk CA, Goldman L, Marcantonio ER, Orav EJ, Lee TH. Supraventricular arrhythmia in patients having noncardiac surgery: Clinical correlates and effect on length of stay. Annals of Internal Medicine. 1998;**129**:279-285. DOI: 10.7326/0003-4819-129-4-199808150-00003

[129] Amar D. Perioperative atrial tachyarrhythmias. Anesthesiology. 2002;**97**:1618-1623 PMID: 12459693

[130] Amar D, Roistacher N, Burt M, Reinsel RA, Ginsberg RJ, Wilson RS. Clinical and echocardiographic correlates of symptomatic tachydysrhythmias after noncardiac thoracic surgery. Chest. 1995;**108**:349-354. DOI: https://doi.org/10.1378/chest.108.2.349

[131] Maisel WH, Rawn JD, Stevenson WG. Atrial fibrillation after cardiac surgery. Annals of Internal Medicine. 2001;**18**(135):1061-1073. DOI: 10.7326/0003-4819-135-12-200112180-00010

[132] Roth A, Elkayam I, Shapira I, Sander J, Malov N, Kehati M, Golovner M. Effectiveness of prehospital synchronous direct-current cardioversion for supraventricular tachyarrhythmias causing unstable hemodynamic states. The American Journal of Cardiology. 2003;**91**:489-491. DOI: http://dx.doi.org/10.1016/S0002-9149(02)03257-5

[133] Page RL, Joglar JA, Caldwell MA, Calkins H, Conti JB, Deal BJ, Estes NA 3rd, Field ME, Goldberger ZD, Hammill SC, Indik JH, Lindsay BD, Olshansky B, Russo AM, Shen WK, Tracy CM, Al-Khatib SM. 2015 ACC/AHA/HRS guideline for the Management of

Adult Patients with Supraventricular Tachycardia: A report of the American College of Cardiology/American Heart Association task force on clinical practice guidelines and the Heart Rhythm Society. Journal of the American College of Cardiology. 2016;**67**(13):e27-e115. DOI: 10.1016/j.jacc.2015.08.856

[134] Ascione R, Reeves BC, Santo K, Khan N, Angelini G. Predictors of new malignant ventricular arrhythmias after coronary surgery: A case control study. Journal of the American College of Cardiology. 2004;**43**:1630-1638. DOI: 10.1016/j.jacc.2003.11.056

[135] Huikuri HV, Yli-Mäyry S, Korhonen UR, Airaksinen KE, Ikäheimo MJ, Linnaluoto MK, Takkunen JT. Prevalence and prognostic significance of complex ventricular arrhythmias after coronary arterial bypass graft surgery. International Journal of Cardiology. 1990;**27**:333-339. DOI: 10.1016/0167-5273(90)90290-L

[136] Smith RC, Leung JM, Keith FM, Merrick S, Mangano DT, Study of Perioperative Ischemia (SPI) Research Group. Ventricular dysrhythmias in patients undergoing coronary artery bypass graft surgery: Incidence, characteristics, and prognostic importance. American Heart Journal. 1992;**123**:73-81. DOI: https://doi.org/10.1016/0002-8703(92)90749-L

[137] Pinto RP, Romerill DB, Nasser WK, Schier JJ, Surawicz B. Prognosis of patients with frequent premature ventricular complexes and nonsustained ventricular tachycardia after coronary artery bypass graft surgery. Clinical Cardiology. 1996;**19**:321-324. DOI: 10.1002/clc.4960190408

[138] Topol EJ, Lerman BB, Baughman KL, Platia EV, Griffith LS. De novo refractory ventricular tachyarrhythmias after coronary revascularization. The American Journal of Cardiology. 1986;**57**:57-59. DOI: http://dx.doi.org/10.1016/0002-9149(86)90951-3

[139] King FG, Addetia AM, Peters SD, Peachey GO. Prophylactic lidocaine for postoperative coronary artery bypass patients, a double-blind, randomized trial. Canadian Journal of Anaesthesia. 1990;**37**:363-368. DOI: 10.1007/BF03005592

[140] Chung MK. Cardiac surgery: Postoperative arrhythmias. Critical Care Medicine. 2000;**28**(10):N136-N144 PMID: 11055682

[141] Sapin PM, Woelfel AK, Foster JR. Unexpected ventricular tachyarrhythmias soon after cardiac surgery. The American Journal of Cardiology. 1991;**68**(10):1099-1100. DOI: http://dx.doi.org/10.1016/0002-9149(91)90505-F

[142] Steinberg JS, Gaur A, Sciacca R, Tan E. New-onset sustained ventricular tachycardia after cardiac surgery. Circulation. 1999;**99**:903-908. DOI: https://doi.org/10.1161/01.CIR.99.7.903

[143] Yeung-Lai-Wah JA, Qi A, McNeill E, Abel JG, Tung S, Humphries KH, Kerr CR. New-onset sustained ventricular tachycardia and fibrillation early after cardiac operations. The Annals of Thoracic Surgery. 2004;**77**:2083-2088. DOI: 10.1016/j.athoracsur.2003.12.020

[144] Josephson ME. Recurrent ventricular tachycardia. In: Josephson ME, editor. Clinical Cardiac Electrophysiology: Techniques and Interpretations. 4th ed. Philadelphia: Lippincott Williams &Wilkins; 2008. pp. 446-642

[145] Carmeliet E. Cardiac ionic currents and acute ischemia: From channels to arrhythmias. Physiological Reviews. 1999;**79**:917-1017 PMID: 10390520

[146] Rubart M, Zipes DP. Mechanisms of sudden cardiac death. The Journal of Clinical Investigation. 2005;**115**:2305-2315. DOI: 10.1172/JCI26381

[147] Coronel R, Wilms-Schopman FJ, Dekker LR, Janse MJ. Heterogeneities in [K+]o and TQ potential and the inducibility of ventricular fibrillation during acute regional ischemia in the isolated perfused porcine heart. Circulation. 1995;**92**:120-129. DOI: https://doi.org/10.1161/01.CIR.92.1.120

[148] El-Chami MF, Sawaya FJ, Kilgo P, Stein W 4th, Halkos M, Thourani V, Lattouf OM, Delurgio DB, Guyton RA, Puskas JD, Leon AR.Ventricular arrhythmia after cardiac surgery: Incidence, predictors, and outcomes. Journal of the American College of Cardiology. 2012;**60**:2664-2671. DOI: 10.1016/j.jacc.2012.08.1011

[149] Miller J, Das M. Differential diagnosis for wide QRS complex tachycardia. In: Zipes D, Jalife J, editors. Cardiac Electrophysiology: From Cell to Bedside. 5th ed. Philadelphia: Elsevier International;2010. P.823-831.

[150] Zipes DP, Camm AJ, Borggrefe M, Buxton AE, Chaitman B, Fromer M, Gregoratos G, Klein G, Moss AJ, Myerburg RJ, Priori SG, Quinones MA, Roden DM, Silka MJ, Tracy C, Priori SG, Blanc JJ, Budaj A, Dean V, Deckers JW, Despres C, Dickstein K, Lekakis J, McGregor K, Metra M, Morais J, Osterspey A, Tamargo JL, Zamorano JL, Smith SC Jr, Jacobs AK, Adams CD, Antman EM, Anderson JL, Hunt SA, Halperin JL, Nishimura R, Ornato JP, Page RL, Riegel B; American College of Cardiology; American Heart Association Task Force; European Society of Cardiology Committee for Practice Guidelines; European Heart Rhythm Association; Heart Rhythm Society. ACC/AHA/ESC 2006 guidelines for management of patients with ventricular arrhythmias and the prevention of sudden cardiac death: A report of the American College of Cardiology/American Heart Association task force and the European Society of Cardiology Committee for practice guidelines (writing committee to develop guidelines for management of patients with ventricular arrhythmias and the prevention of sudden cardiac death) developed in collaboration with the European Heart Rhythm Association and the Heart Rhythm Society. Europace. 2006;**8**:746-837. DOI: 10.1093/europace/eul108

[151] Benito B, Josephson ME. Rev Esp Cardiol (Engl Ed). 2012;**65**:939-955. DOI: 10.1016/j.recesp.2012.03.027

[152] Moss AJ, Hall WJ, Cannom DS, Daubert JP, Higgins SL, Klein H, Levine JH, Saksena S, Waldo AL, Wilber D, Brown MW, Heo M. Improved survival with an implanted defibrillator in patients with coronary disease at high risk for ventricular arrhythmia. The New England Journal of Medicine. 1996 Dec;**335**(26, 26):1933-1940. DOI: 10.1056/NEJM199612263352601

[153] Fogel RI, Prystowsky EN. Management of malignant ventricular arrhythmias and cardiac arrest. Critical Care Medicine. 2000;**28**:N165-N169 PMID: 11055686

[154] Rousou JA, Engelman RM, Flack JE 3rd, Deaton DW, Owen SG. Emergency cardiopul-monary bypass in the cardiac surgical unit can be a lifesaving measure in postoperative cardiac arrest. Circulation. 1994;**90**:280-284. PMID: 7955266

[155] Buxton AE, Lee KL, Fisher JD, Josephson ME, Prystowsky EN, Hafley G. A randomized study of the prevention of sudden death in patients with coronary artery disease. The New England Journal of Medicine. 1999;**341**:1882-1890. DOI: 10.1056/NEJM199912163412503

[156] Moss AJ, Zareba W, Hall WJ, Klein H, Wilber DJ, Cannom DS, Daubert JP, Higgins SL, Brown MW, Andrews ML, for the Multicenter Automatic Defibrillator Implantation Trial II Investigators. Prophylactic implantation of a defibrillator in patients with myo-cardial infarction and reduced ejection fraction. The New England Journal of Medicine. 2002;**346**:877-883. DOI: 10.1056/NEJMoa013474

[157] Bardy GH, Lee KL, Mark DB, Poole JE, Packer DL, Boineau R, Domanski M, Troutman C, Anderson J, Johnson G, McNulty SE, Clapp-Channing N, Davidson-Ray LD, Fraulo ES, Fishbein DP, Luceri RM, Ip JH, Sudden Cardiac Death in Heart Failure Trial (SCD-HeFT) Investigators. Amiodarone or an implantable cardioverter-defibrillator for con-gestive heart failure. The New England Journal of Medicine. 2005;**352**:225-237. DOI: 10.1056/NEJMoa043399

[158] Goldenberg I, Moss AJ, McNitt S, Zareba W, Hall WJ, Andrews ML, Wilber DJ, Klein HU, Investigators MADIT-II. Time dependence of defibrillator benefit after coronary revascu-larization in the multicenter automatic defibrillator implantation trial (MADIT)-II. Journal of the American College of Cardiology. 2006;**47**:1811-1817. DOI: 10.1016/j.jacc.2005.12.048

[159] Solomon SD, Zelenkofske S, McMurray JJ, Finn PV, Velazquez E, Ertl G, Harsanyi A, Rouleau JL, Maggioni A, Kober L, White H, Van de Werf F, Pieper K, Califf RM, Pfeffer MA, Valsartan in Acute Myocardial Infarction Trial (VALIANT) Investigators. Sudden death in patients with myocardial infarction and left ventricular dysfunction, heart fail-ure, or both. The New England Journal of Medicine. 2005;**352**:2581-2588. DOI: 10.1056/NEJMoa043938

[160] Zishiri ET, Williams S, Cronin EM, Blackstone EH, Ellis SG, Roselli EE, Smedira NG, Gillinov AM, Glad JA, Tchou PJ, Szymkiewicz SJ, Chung MK. Early risk of mortality after coronary artery revascularization in patients with left ventricular dysfunction and potential role of the wearable cardioverter defibrillator. Circulation. Arrhythmia and Electrophysiology. 2013;**6**:117-128. DOI: 10.1161/CIRCEP.112.973552

[161] Hohnloser SH, Kuck KH, Dorian P, Roberts RS, Hampton JR, Hatala R, Fain E, Gent M, Connolly SJ, DINAMIT Investigators. Prophylactic use of an implantable cardioverter-defibrillator after acute myocardial infarction. The New England Journal of Medicine. 2004;**351**:2481-2488. DOI: 10.1056/NEJMoa041489

[162] Steinbeck G, Andresen D, Seidl K, Brachmann J, Hoffmann E, Wojciechowski D, Kornacewicz-Jach Z, Sredniawa B, Lupkovics G, Hofgärtner F, Lubinski A, Rosenqvist M, Habets A, Wegscheider K, Senges J, Investigators IRIS. Defibrillator implantation early after myocardial infarction. The New England Journal of Medicine. 2009;**361**:1427-1436. DOI: 10.1056/NEJMoa0901889

[163] Morin DP. The Role and Indications of ICD in Patients with Ischemic Cardiomyopathy Undergoing Revascularization [Internet]. 2016. Available from: http://www.acc.org/lat-est-in-cardiology/articles/2016/03/21/07/42/the-role-and-indications-of-icd-in-patients-with-ischemic-cardiomyopathy-undergoing-revascularization. [Accessed: June 3, 2017]

[164] Bigger JT Jr, for the Coronary Artery Bypass Graft (CABG) Patch Trial Investigators. Prophylactic use of implanted cardiac defibrillators in patients at high risk for ven-tricular arrhythmias after coronary-artery bypass graft surgery. Coronary artery bypass graft (CABG) patch trial investigators. The New England Journal of Medicine. 1997;337:1569-1575. DOI: 10.1056/NEJM199711273372201

[165] Nageh MF, Kim JJ, Chen LH, Yao JF. Implantable defibrillators for secondary prevention of sudden cardiac death in cardiac surgery patients with perioperative ventricular arrhythmias. Journal of the American Heart Association. 2014;3:e000686. DOI: 10.1161/JAHA.113.000686

[166] Kusumoto FM, Calkins H, Boehmer J, Buxton AE, Chung MK, Gold MR, Hohnloser SH, Indik J, Lee R, Mehra MR, Menon V, Page RL, Shen WK, Slotwiner DJ, Stevenson LW, Varosy PD, Welikovitch L, Heart Rhythm Society, American College of Cardiology, American Heart Association. HRS/ACC/AHA expert consensus statement on the use of implantable Cardioverter-defibrillator therapy in patients who are not included or not well represented in clinical trials. Journal of the American College of Cardiology. 2014;64:1143-1177. DOI: 10.1016/j.jacc.2014.04.008

[167] Moss AJ, Greenberg H, Case RB, Zareba W, Hall WJ, Brown MW, Daubert JP, McNitt S, Andrews ML, Elkin AD, Multicenter Automatic Defibrillator Implantation Trial-II (MADIT-II) Research Group. Long-term clinical course of patients after termination of ven-tricular tachyarrhythmia by an implanted defibrillator. Circulation. 2004;110:3760-3765. DOI: 10.1161/01.CIR.0000150390.04704.B7

[168] Baerman JM, Kirsh MM, de Buitleir M, Hyatt L, Juni JE, Pitt B, Morady F. Natural his-tory and determinants of conduction defects following coronary artery bypass surgery. The Annals of Thoracic Surgery. 1987;44:150-153 PMID: 3497615

[169] Goldman BS, Hill TJ, Weisel RD, Scully HE, Mickleborough LL, Pym J, Baird RJ. Permanent pacing after open-heart sugery: Acquired heart disease. Pacing and Clinical Electrophysiology. 1984;7:367-371. DOI: 10.1111/j.1540-8159.1984.tb04919.x

[170] Emlein G, Huang SK, Pires LA, Rofino K, Okike ON, Vander Salm TJ. Prolonged bradyarrhythmias after isolated coronary artery bypass graft surgery. American Heart Journal. 1993;126:1084-1090. DOI: 10.1016/0002-8703(93)90658-V

[171] Al-Ghamdi B, Mallawi Y, Shafquat A, Ledesma A, AlRuwaili N, Shoukri M, Khan S, Al Saneia A. Predictors of permanent pacemaker implantation after coronary artery bypass grafting and valve surgery in adult patients in current surgical era. Cardiology Research. 2016;7:123-129. DOI: http://dx.doi.org/10.14740/cr480w

[172] Miriam S, Leonardo B, Solari Gabriel S. Pacemaker following adult cardiac surgery. In: Min M, editor. Cardiac Pacemakers–Biological Aspects, Clinical Applications and Possible Complications. Croatia: InTech; 2011. pp. 135-160. DOI: 10.5772/23402

[173] Raza SS, Li JM, John R, Chen LY, Tholakanahalli VN, Mbai M, Adabag AS. Long-term mortality and pacing outcomes of patients with permanent pacemaker implantation after cardiac surgery. Pacing and Clinical Electrophysiology. 2011;**34**:331-338. DOI: 10.1111/j.1540-8159.2010.02972.x

[174] Gordon RS, Ivanov J, Cohen G, Ralph-Edwards AL. Permanent cardiac pacing after a cardiac operation: Predictoing the use of permanent pacemakers. The Annals of Thoracic Surgery 1998;**66**:1698-1704. DOI: http://dx.doi.org/10.1016/S0003-4975(98)00889-3

[175] Limongelli G, Ducceschi V, D'Andrea A, Renzulli A, Sarubbi B, De Feo M, Cerasuolo F, Calabrò R, Cotrufo M. Risk factors for pacemaker implantation following aortic valve replacement: A single centre experience. Heart. 2003;**89**:901-904. DOI: http://dx.doi.org/10.1136/heart.89.8.901

[176] Erdogan O, Augostini R, Saliba W, Juratli N, Wilkoff BL. Transiliac permanent pacemaker implantation after extraction of infected pectoral pacemaker systems. The American Journal of Cardiology. 1999;**84**:474-475. DOI: http://dx.doi.org/10.1016/S0002-9149(99)00339-2

[177] Schurr UP, Berli J, Berdajs D, Häusler A, Dzemali O, Emmert M, Seifert B, Genoni M. Incidence and risk factors for pacemaker implantation following aortic valve replacement. Interactive Cardiovascular and Thoracic Surgery. 2010;**11**:556-560. DOI: 10.1510/icvts.2010.249904

[178] Nardi P, Pellegrino A, Scafuri A, Bellos K, De Propris S, Polisca P, Chiariello L. Permanent pacemaker implantation after isolated aortic valve replacement: Incidence, risk factors and surgical technical aspects. Journal of Cardiovascular Medicine (Hagerstown, Md.). 2010;**11**:14-19. DOI: 10.2459/JCM.0b013e32832f9fde

[179] Del Rizzo DF, Nishimura S, Lau C, Sever J, Goldman BS. Cardiac pacing following surgery for acquired heart disease. Journal of Cardiac Surgery. 1996;**11**:332-340. DOI: 10.1111/j.1540-8191.1996.tb00059.x

[180] Sachweh JS, Vazquez-Jimenez JF, Schondube FA, Daebritz SH, Dorge H, Muhler EG, Messmer BJ. Twenty years experience with pediatric pacing: Epicardial and transvenous stimulation. European Journal of Cardio-Thoracic Surgery. 2000;**17**:455-461. DOI: https://doi.org/10.1016/S1010-7940(00)00364-X

[181] Meimoun P, Zeghdi R, D'Attelis N, Berrebi A, Braunberger E, Deloche A, Fabiani JN, Carpentier A. Frequency, predictors, and consequences of atrioventricular block after mitral valve repair. The American Journal of Cardiology. 2002;**89**(9):1062-1066. DOI: http://dx.doi.org/10.1016/S0002-9149(02)02276-2

[182] Heinz G, Kratochwill C, Buxbaum P, Laufer G, Kreiner G, Siostrzonek P, Gasic S, Derfler K, Gössinger H. Immediate normalization of profound sinus node dysfunction by aminophylline after cardiac transplantation. The American Journal of Cardiology. 1993;**71**:346-349. DOI: https://doi.org/10.1016/0002-9149(93)90805-M

[183] Haught WH, Bertolet BD, Conti JB, Curtis AB, Mills RM. Theophylline reverses high-grade atrioventricular block resulting from cardiac transplant rejection. American Heart Journal. 1994;**128**:1255-1257. DOI: http://dx.doi.org/10.1016/0002-8703(94)90764-1

[184] European Society of Cardiology (ESC), European Heart Rhythm Association (EHRA), Brignole M, Auricchio A, Baron-Esquivias G, Bordachar P, Boriani G, Breithardt OA, Cleland J, Deharo JC, Delgado V, Elliott PM, Gorenek B, Israel CW, Leclercq C, Linde C, Mont L, Padeletti L, Sutton R, Vardas PE. 2013 ESC guidelines on cardiac pacing and cardiac resynchronization therapy: The task force on cardiac pacing and resynchronization therapy of the European Society of Cardiology (ESC). Developed in collaboration with the European heart rhythm association (EHRA). Europace. 2013;**15**:1070-1118. DOI: 10.1093/europace/eut206

9

Coronary CT Angiography and the Napkin-ring Sign Indicates High-Risk Atherosclerotic Lesions

Lucia Agoston-Coldea, Carmen Cionca and Silvia Lupu

Abstract

Coronary computed tomography angiography (CCTA) is used extensively nowadays as a non-invasive imaging method for the evaluation of patients suspected of coronary artery disease, providing data on calcium burden, the presence of coronary artery stenoses, but also, more recently, on coronary atherosclerotic plaque morphology and composition. Plaque morphology analysis by CCTA aims to accurately identify vulnerable plaques, in an attempt to reduce the number of ischemic events triggered by high-risk atherosclerotic lesions. Recent research provides CCTA descriptions of vulnerable plaques and a particular radiological sign shows promising perspectives. The napkin-ring sign refers to a rupture-prone plaque in a coronary artery, comprising a necrotic core covered by a thin cap fibro-atheroma. The napkin-ring sign is described on CCTA in cross-sectional images of coronary arteries as a central low-attenuation area surrounded by an open ring area of high attenuation, having a high specificity and positive predictive value for the presence of advanced lesions. These lesions have been designated as vulnerable plaques, indicating an increased probability of rupture, and were shown to correlate with a higher incidence of cardiovascular events. In acute coronary syndromes, the location of the napkin-ring sign was shown to correspond to the culprit lesions. The aim of the current paper is to provide an overview of the current literature on available methods for quantitative measurement of atherosclerotic plaque features from CCTA and to discuss the clinical implications of the napkin-ring sign as detected by CCTA.

Keywords: Coronary computed tomography angiography, Coronary artery plaque, Napkin-ring sign, Plaque quantification, Plaque characterization

1. Introduction

The development of atherosclerosis by lipoprotein storage, inflammation, muscle cell prolif-eration, necrosis, apoptosis, calcification, and fibrosis in the arterial wall triggers important changes in the coronary vessels, leading to coronary artery disease (CAD). In fact, atheroscle-rosis is the main etiology of CAD, and plaque rupture followed by intraluminal thrombosis is the most common cause of acute coronary events, including sudden coronary death [1, 2]. For that reason, the early and accurate characterization and quantification of atherosclerotic plaques is valuable for preventing and managing acute coronary syndrome (ACS) [3]. In everyday clinical practice, major acute ischemic cardiac events involve plaque rupture in thin-cap fibroatheromas, which are considered vulnerable plaques; these rupture-prone athero-sclerotic lesions usually contain a high level of lipids and have a large necrotic core, numerous inflammatory cells, and a thin, vulnerable fibrotic cap [4]. Vulnerable atherosclerotic plaques can be characterized by several invasive and non-invasive methods that are either fully validated, pending validation, or still under scrutiny for clinical practice. Among non-invasive methods, coronary computed tomography angiography (CCTA) by multi-detector computed tomography (MDCT) is currently the preferred modality for evaluating the extent of CAD, providing the advantage of accurate assessment of coronary atherosclerotic plaque morphol-ogy and composition. In two recent multicenter trials [5, 6], CCTA was shown to have excellent sensitivity (95–99%) and negative predictive value (97–99%), although rather low specificity (64–83%) for identifying patients with at least one coronary artery stenosis among individuals at low to intermediate risk for CAD. Moreover, CCTA imaging of atherosclerotic plaques was found to correlate well with invasive assessment by intravascular ultrasound (IVUS) [7, 8, 9].

2. Role of MDCT in the detection of plaque morphology and composition

2.1. Plaque characteristics

2.1.1. Plaque morphology and composition

Pathophysiologically, a subendothelial accumulation of lipoproteins generates inflammatory responses involving macrophages and T-cells, leading to the further development of athero-sclerotic lesions [10]. Initially, atherosclerotic lesions were classified as fatty streaks, fibroa-theromas [11], and advanced plaques, complicated with hemorrhage, calcification, ulceration, and thrombosis [12]. Over the years, this classification became more complex and six types of atherosclerotic lesions have been defined by the American Heart Association (AHA) Consen-sus Group: type I - characterized by adaptive intimal thickening; type II - fatty streak; type III - transitional or intermediate lesions; type IV - advanced plaques (atheromas); type V - fibroatheroma or atheroma with thick fibrous cap; and type VI - complicated plaques with denuded surface, and/or hematoma/hemorrhage, and/or thrombosis [13]. The earliest lesions are represented by adaptive intimal thickening (AHA type I) and fatty streaks or intimal xanthoma, which are basically foam cell collections (AHA type II) [13]. AHA type III transitional lesions, described as pathological intimal thickening, represent the earliest stage of the progressive plaques and are considered precursor lesions of more advanced fibroatheroma. This type of lesions consists of multiple layers of proliferating smooth muscle cells near the lumen, with an increased quantity of lipids on the intimal medial border. Intimal xanthomas are lesions containing a large amount of foamy macrophages but without lipid acumulation outside the cell [14]. Type IV AHA, also called fibrous cap atheromas, are the first of the advanced lesions of coronary atherosclerosis [15] and are characterized by the presence of a necrotic core with a high amount of lipids surrounded by a fibrous cap containing smooth muscle cells, collagen, and proteoglicans, as well as inflammatory cells such as macrophages and lymphocytes. This type of lesion can cause significant artery stenosis and may be submitted to complications, namely surface disruption, thrombosis, and calcification. Fibrous cap plaques may be more or less prone to complications depending on the thickness of the cap: fibroatheromas are more stable due to the rather thick fibrous cap, while thin-cap fibroatheromas characterize the typycal "vulnerable plaques" [15].

In fact, thin-cap fibroatheromas are very likely to lead to plaque rupture. Although they are not included as individual entities in the AHA consensus classification, plaque erosion and calcified nodules are also prone to coronary thrombosis. Erosions may occur on intimal thickening or fibroatheroma, whereas the notion of calcified nodules refers to eruptive fragments of calcium that protrude into the lumen, causing a thrombotic event [16]. Also, plaque ruptures may heal by wide accumulation of proteoglycans, having more reduced necrotic cores and more extensive areas of calcification. In their study on early coronary lesion progression near branch points, Nakashima et al. provided evidence endorsing the hypothesis that intimal thickening lesions with macrophages are more advanced [17].

Macrophage infiltration in lipid pools rich in cholesterol and the deterioration of the extracellular matrix believed to be induced by matrix metalloproteinase activity suggest early stages of the necrosis process and should be recognized. This particular feature, combined with macrophage destruction as a consequence of an anomalous phagocytic clearance of apoptotic cells, may contribute to the development of late plaque necrosis. In addition to that, an extended necrotic core is a strong predictor of complications [17, 18].

Thin-cap fibroatheromas are highly prone to plaque rupture due to their rather large necrotic core and thin, inflamed fibrous cap (<65 μm). The accumulation of an increased number of macrophages at the level of the cap is characteristic, although exceptions may occur. However, as a significant number of fatal coronary events are triggered by plaque rupture due to the impairment of the fibrous cap followed by thrombosis, early recognition of thin-cap fibroatheromas is crucial. The fibrous cap mainly contains type I collagen, variable numbers of macrophages and lymphocytes, and rather few alpha-actin positive smooth muscle cells. Fibrous cap disruption exposes the lipid-rich necrotic core, favoring the formation of local thrombi by platelet accumulation. Most plaque ruptures are reported in the proximal segments of the coronary arteries, near branch points, with the left anterior descending coronary artery being the most frequently affected, followed by the right and left circumflex coronary arteries [19]. Although the mechanisms behind plaque rupture are far from being fully understood, the increased activity of matrix metalloproteinases, excessive enzyme secretion by inflammatory cells, high shear stress, macrophage calcification, and iron build-up are recognized as implicated factors. Data are also beginning to pool on different gene expression in stable and unstable atherosclerotic plaques [20]. For instance, in one study, differential expression of 18 genes coding for metalloproteinase ADAMDEC1, retinoic acid receptor responser-1, cysteine protease legumain (a potential activator of matrix metalloproteinases), and cathepsins was shown to contribute to increased lesion vulnerability [20]. As previously mentioned, the extension of the necrotic core is also a main factor in plaque complication development, and intraplaque hemorrhage was shown to favor the accumulation of free cholesterol provided by red blood cells in these lesions [21]. As atherosclerotic lesions expand, more vasa vasorum infiltrate the plaque and become leaky, triggering intraplaque hemorrhage [22]. Morphologic studies have suggested that repeated ruptures are responsible for plaque progression beyond 40–50% cross-sectional luminal stenoses [23]. Three hystological types of lesions have been described in association with acute coronary events: rupture, erosion, and calcified nodule [13]. Ruptured coronary atherosclerotic plaques folowed by intraluminal thrombosis are the most common cause of acute myocardial infarction [24]. In fact, two-thirds of luminal thrombi in acute events result from ruptured atherosclerotic lesions characterized by a necrotic core covered by a thin layer of fibrous cap [4]. Ruptured plaques are characterized by a lipid-rich necrotic core (>40% of the total volume of the plaque), surrounded by a thin, fibrous cap with active inflammation (increased number of monocytes, macrophages, and sometimes even T-cells), endothelial denudation leading to superficial platelet aggregation, and the presence of hemodynamically significant coronary artery stenosis (>90%) [19]. Vulnerable plaques prone to rupture share most of the morphological characteristics with ruptured plaques, showing a large necrotic core, macrophage infiltration, and often an increased number of intraplaque vasa vasorum [4], but an intact, thin fibrous cap [13]. These lesions—called thin-cap fibroatheromas—are considered to be at high risk for rupture and subsequent ischemic events [4].

The destruction of the endothelium exposes the minimally inflammed intima containing smooth muscle cells and proteoglycans to circulating platelets, favoring thrombus formation. In a post-mortem study of 20 patients who died with acute myocardial infarction, plaque ruptures were found in 60% of lesions with thrombi, while the remainder of 40% only revealed superficial erosion [16]. Plaque erosion refers to the lack of endothelial cells on the luminal surface beneath the thrombus. Kramer et al. showed in their study that, when plaque erosion was the incriminated lesion, the thrombus was limited to the luminal portion of the plaque, and no ruptures were identified following serial sectioning of these lesions. In the same study, more than 85% of thrombi in erosions showed evidence of healing, such as acute inflammatory cell lysis, invasion by smooth muscle cells and/or endothelial cells, or organized layers of smooth muscle cells and proteoglycans with varying degrees of platelet/fibrin layering. By contrast, only half of the ruptured plaques showed signs of healing [25].

Beyond histopathological description, a clinically relevant definition of vulnerable plaques refers to the risk of developing future major cardiac events, which may also involve the presence of "vulnerable blood" (prone to hypercoagulability) or "vulnerable myocardium" (susceptible to arrhythmia), either due to acute or pre-existing ischemia and/or non-ischemic electrophysiological anomalies. The presence of one or more of these elements elevates the individual risk of the patients for cardiovascular events, turning them into "vulnerable patients".

Identifying vulnerable plaques is currently a major challenge, although recent progress in cardiovascular imaging raises new possibilities. As vulnerable plaques are prone to rupture and rapid evolution towards the development of ACS, [26, 27, 28] finding reliable imaging characteristics that could help detect unstable plaques are of the utmost importance. Early identification of such plaques could facilitate timely initiation of adequate primary prevention measures, thus diminishing the incidence of acute coronary events [29]. For this purpose, several imaging methods have been proposed, including IVUS, optical coherence tomography (OCT), magnetic resonance imaging (MRI), or MDCT (Table 1), with variable success [30, 31, 32]. However, the use of many of these methods is mainly confined to experimental studies and has not yet been validated for everyday clinical practice.

Non-invasive imaging methods	Advantages	Limitations
- MDCT	Measures local tissue attenuation to assess plaque morphology and composition	Patient exposure to ionizing radiation
		Implies contrast agent use
	Molecular imaging using new contrast agents is under study	May be hindered by artifacts (e.g., blooming)
	Identifies lumen narrowing accurately	The attenuation
	Can help characterize plaque morphology and composition (within limits)	spectrum of non-calcified plaque components (lipid and fibrous) can
	Has high spatial and temporal resolution	overlap
- Contrast-enhanced ultrasonography	Uses acoustically active microbubbles acting as pure intravascular tracers; when exposed to ultrasound, they produce a strong backscatter signal and specific nonlinear signal that differentiates them from surrounding tissues	Spatial resolution and penetration are limited
		Good application for coronary arteries
	Molecular imaging is available	
	There is no exposure to ionizing radiation	
	Has high temporal and spatial resolution	
	Allows neovasculature assessment	
- High-resolution magnetic resonace imaging	Uses different contrast weightings (T1, T2, proton-density, and time-of-flight) to evaluate plaque components	Contraindicated with many intracardiac devices
	Molecular imaging uses specific agents (paramagnetic nanoparticles targeting)	Cardiac motion
		Poor reproducibility
	Has high temporal and spatial resolution	Contrast agent
	Has high contrast resolution	Limited spatial resolution
		Time consuming reconstruction techniques
Invasive imaging methods		

Non-invasive imaging methods	Advantages	Limitations
- Coronary angiography	Identifies complex plaques, with irregular surface Quantifies stenoses accurately	Invasive Limited tissue penetration and spatial resolution
- IVUS		
Standard	Quantifies plaque volume, vascular remodeling, and neovascularization Characterizes plaque morphology and composition	Invasive Limited temporal resolution Limited spatial resolution prevents thin cap fibroatheroma quantification Low accuracy for detecting plaque composition by gray scale IVUS
IVUS elastography	Measures the local strain rate of vessel wall and plaque (fibrous plaques are stiffer than lipid-rich ones); high strain regions describe more vulnerable plaques	Invasive Limited spatial resolution Artefacted by cardiac motion
Virtual histology	Identifies the necrotic core, fibro-lipidic plaques, calcified, and non-calcified plaques	Invasive Limited spatial resolution
- Optical methods		
Angioscopy	Identifies lipid plaques, plaque rupture, erosion, and thrombosis	Invasive Limited tissue penetration and spatial resolution
OCT	Provides microscopic characterization of plaque morphology Identifies macrophages presence Allows accurate quantification of the fibrous plaque Highest spatial resolution of all imaging methods Can identify thin fibrous caps <65 μm The only technique for eroded plaques detection Accurate detection of plaque composition	Invasive Limited tissue penetration; however, the most relevant morphologic findings are primarily localized within the first 500 μm under lumen surface
Spectroscopy	Identifies the lipid core and evaluates the chemical structure, temperature and inflammation of the plaque	Invasive Limited tissue penetration Cardiac motion
- Termography	Quantifies plaque temperature Detects plaque inflammation and neoangiogenesis	Invasive Limited tissue penetration and spatial resolution The cooling effect of the blood leads to underestimated temperature differences
- Intravascular cardiac MRI	Quantifies the lipid content of the plaque	Invasive Prolonged duration

Non-invasive imaging methods	Advantages	Limitations
		Implies the use of contrast agents
Plasma markers of plaque vulnerability	Identifies blood hypercoagulability states (augmented platelet activation and aggregation, high levels of coagulation factors, low levels of anticoagulation factors, decreased endogenous fibrinolytic activity, thrombogenic factors)	

Table 1. Methods for the Identification and Characterization of Vulnerable Plaques

A possible imaging method for coronary artery plaque assessment is IVUS, which has been used to measure lumen area, plaque burden, and vascular remodeling [33, 34]; plaque burden and positive remodeling, in particular, can identify high-risk, thin-cap fibroatheromas during follow-up [34, 35, 36]. As suggested by IVUS-based studies, a vulnerable plaque is characterized by the presence of an extensive necrotic core surrounded by a thin-cap fibrous with macrophage infiltration, a large lipid pool, and several more specific traits such as positive remodeling or spotty calcifications [37, 38]. When such characteristics occur, there is an increased risk of fibrous rupture, exposing the thrombogenic lipid core, which leads to thrombus formation and the development of ACS. A more detailed analysis of coronary plaque composition has been provided by virtual histology (VH)-IVUS studies [39, 40, 41].

Another recently developed method for the assessment of coronary artery plaques quantification is intracoronary OCT that provides the advantage of very high resolution (approximately 10 to 20 μm), which is about 10-fold higher than that of IVUS [42, 43]. Unlike some other imaging methods, including CCTA [27, 44, 45], OCT can be used for measuring fibrous cap thickness and for detecting lipid content, which makes it useful for in vivo identification of thin-cap fibroatheromas and for evaluating plaque vulnerability [46]. For the time being, the correspondence between OCT- and IVUS-derived characteristics of thin-cap fibroatheromas, as well as the angiographic stenosis severity, is yet to be established.

As advanced coronary artery plaques have a high level of complexity, basic classifications that include non-calcified plaques, calcified plaques, and mixed plaques are rather crude and of limited use for establishing the potential risk for acute ischemic clinical events of individual lesions [4, 26, 47]. For that reason, some authors have attempted to provide more detailed descriptions of vulnerable plaques and to establish correlations between CCTA imaging characteristics (Figure 1) of the lesions and the risk for acute events. Motoyama et al. suggested that vulnerable plaques are characterized by positive remodeling, low attenuation plaque and spotty, limited calcification [44]. In later research, non-calcified plaques were more extensively characterized by modern MDCT and several authors described a ring-like attenuation of the non-calcified portion of the coronary atherosclerotic lesion, which is now called the napkin-ring sign [48, 49, 50]. The description of the napkin-ring sign has changed current classifications of non-calcified plaques, which are now classified in three categories: homogenous plaques, non-napkin-ring sign heterogeneous plaques, and napkin-ring sign heterogeneous plaques [49]. The napkin-ring sign corresponds to a morphological type of vulnerable plaque described on coronary CCTA (thin-cap fibroatheromas) comprising a necrotic, low attenuation core surrounded by a thin area of higher attenuation, which some believe may represent the thin peripheral fibrous cap (Figure 2) [26, 47]. However, in vulnerable plaques, the fibrous cap has extremely reduced thickness [48, 51], which makes it indistinguishable by non-invasive imaging methods; by contrast, the necrotic core may be visualized and quantified on thin sections (<0.6 mm) on modern CCTA [52, 53]. As the presence of the napkin-ring sign was shown to have a high predictive value for future cardiac events and is considered a valuable correlate of unstable plaques [49, 27, 20, 54, 55], its detection could add specificity to the CCTA assessment of vulnerable plaques.

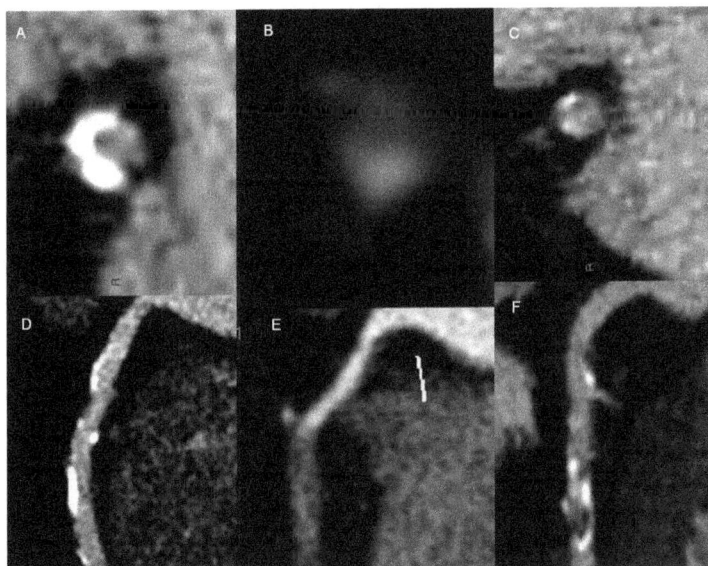

Figure 1. Different Types of Coronary Plaques by CCTA. The 3 main types of coronary plaques are shown: calcified plaques (A, D), non-calcified plaques (B, E) and partially calcified plaques (C, F), illustrated in curved planar reformatted and cross-sectional views.

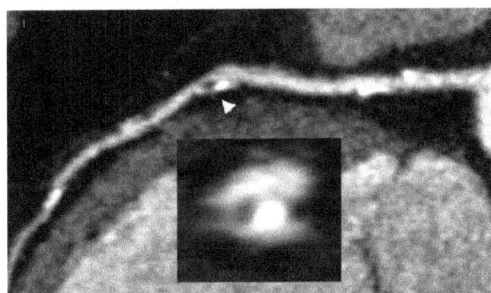

Figure 2. Representative CCTA Images with Napkin-ring Signs. An atherosclerotic plaque with positive remodeling, low attenuation plaque, and a napkin-ring sign in the proximal left anterior descending artery on computed tomography angiography. The boxed area indicates cross-sectional images of atherosclerotic plaque showing a napkin-ring sign.

However, in studies conducted over the last decade, CCTA was also shown to have excellent sensitivity for detecting, and particularly, for excluding coronary atherosclerosis in patients with symptoms suggesting either stable or acute CAD [56]. In addition to that, data from large prospective registries support the use of CAD absence/presence and extension evaluation by CCTA for prognostic purposes [53, 57, 58, 59, 60]. Recent studies conducted with more advanced scanners having 64 to 320 detector rows, and higher spatial (230 to 625 μm) and temporal (75 to 175 ms) resolution focused on identifying vulnerable coronary artery plaques and on establishing correlation between plaque characteristics and ischemic events [61]. Currently available spatial resolution of CCTA scanners approach the spatial resolution provided by invasive methods such as IVUS (100 μm) and invasive coronary angiography (200 μm). Moreover, spatial resolution reaching 0.3 mm in-plane in modern CCTA scanners allows a more accurate discrimination of the non-calcified portion of the plaques [62].

Some researchers [63, 64, 65] attempted to distinguish lipid-rich from fibrous plaque by CCTA based on attenuation criteria, as expressed by Hounsfield Units (HU), but conflicting results have been obtained. In addition to that, HU values cannot accurately discriminate between the types of plaques, mostly due to the small dimensions of the plaque, insufficient spatial resolution of CCTA, and reduced contrast difference between lipid-rich and fibrous plaques. In these studies, certified methods of coronary artery plaque quantification (such as IVUS and histology) were used for comparison to CCTA [63, 64, 65].

Despite current technical limitations, progress has been made in the non-invasive imaging assessment of coronary artery lesions by CCTA. Data from recent studies suggest that low attenuation (<30 HU) is more common to culprit lesions in acute coronary events, as well as to high-risk, vulnerable plaques [26, 27, 47, 66]. Currently, there is not enough data to support a valid assumption on the accuracy of CCTA for detecting non-calcified coronary plaques at high risk. Small studies comparing CCTA to IVUS reported sensitivities and specificities between 80 and 90% for the detection of coronary artery segments with plaque [8, 9, 67, 68]. Other studies demonstrated significant correlations between measurements of plaque cross-sectional area, volume of single plaques, and plaque volume per coronary segment on CCTA and IVUS [8, 69, 70, 71]. However, despite significant and quite high correlation coefficients, the limits of agreement were typically large in most studies, which betrays the limitations of CCTA, mainly imposed by the spatial resolution of the method. Plaque quantification is particularly challenging when plaques have low thickness. Reported interobserver variability is also unusually high (30% variability for plaque volume quantification) [9, 72, 73] and is very much influenced by image quality. In a research on 41 patients, the interobserver variability was 17±10% for the left anterior descending coronary artery, which was best, visualized with fewer artifacts, but escaladed to 29±13% for the left circumflex and 32±10% for the right coronary artery [73].

2.1.2. Low CT attenuation plaques

In CCTA studies investigating patients with ACS, several features of high-risk plaques have been described, such as low attenuation plaque, positive remodeling, and spotty calcification [74, 54]. Recent studies have also described a specific CCTA aspect of coronary artery lesions called the napkin-ring sign consisting of a low attenuation area surrounded by a rim-like area of higher CCTA attenuation [22, 47]. Speculations were made on the histological substrate of this aspect, as it was believed to be given by either a central lipid core within a fibrous cap, deep micro-calcifications, neo-vascularization, or the presence of intramural thrombus [22, 27]. Current criteria for the definition of the napkin-ring sign include the presence of a high attenuation ring around a certain coronary artery plaque and higher CCTA attenuation of the ring by comparison to the adjacent plaque, but no greater than 130 HU, in order to differentiate from calcium deposits [27, 47]. Plaques with rich necrotic core have been described as plaques of low attenuation; low attenuation areas were shown to correlate strongly with echolucent areas in IVUS [75]. In a large prospective study on more than 1000 patients, low attenuation plaques and positive remodeling were shown to correlate with the development of acute coronary events. In this group, 45 patients had both CCTA characteristics and 10 of them (22%) experienced an acute coronary event vs. only 4 (0.5%) of the patients who did not exhibit neither positive remodeling nor low attenuation plaques. Patients with normal CCTA did not have any coronary events at all (p<0.001). In this study, positive remodeling and/or low attenuation plaques were independent predictors of acute coronary events (hazard ratio: 23, 95% confidence interval: 7 to 75, p<0.001) [74].

A limitation of CCTA in quantifying atherosclerotic plaques may have its origin in the fact that intravascular attenuation significantly influences the attenuation of the plaques. Cademartiri et al. performed a phantom test that supports this hypothesis [76, 77] and Schroeder et al. also obtained similar results in their study [78]. Comparative studies between CCTA density and IVUS or histopathology suggest that lipid-rich plaques have lower CCTA density than fibrous plaques. However, low CCTA attenuation is not a constant finding in lipid-rich plaques, raising controversy over its ability to discriminate between lipid-rich and fibrous plaques. As mentioned above, some studies have reported that luminal density influences neighboring structures CCTA attenuation. Some authors reported that, when contrast medium is not used for examination, significant overlaps can occur between CCTA attenuation values of lipid-rich and fibrous plaques.

CCTA resolution is defined in terms of spatial, contrast and temporal resolution. Although significant technological progress has been made in CCTA, the spatial resolution of CCTA (0.5 mm) is still inferior to that of cardiac catheterization or IVUS. The 0.5 resolution is suboptimal, considering the fact that the average diameter of a coronary artery is 3–4 mm. CCTA density is influenced by the partial volume effect and contrast resolution has not improved despite other technological advances in MDCT [27]. CCTA attenuation values, measured in HU, are given by the amount of radiation absorbed by tissue in the voxel and density is directly proportional to the attenuation coefficient. A CCTA value of –1,000 HU corresponds to air, while 0 HU corresponds to water. Most soft tissues CCTA averages have values of 50 HU. Some tissues, such as bone, calcified tissues, or the iodine-rich tissue of the thyroid gland are >100 HU, whereas fat or fatty mixed tissue and lung tissue are <0 HU. If the value for a tissue type, with the exception of calcified or fatty tissues, deviates from the soft tissue attenuation, artifacts should be considered, particularly if contrast is used and the beam hardening effect is suspected; another element of confusion may be the presence of a near-by area of calcification or fat that may induce a partial volume effect. MIn addition to that, motion artifacts should be considered. CCTA values can also be influenced by tube voltage [27].

2.1.3. Spotty calcium in plaques

Besides plaque density (Figure 3), other CCTA features such as positive remodeling and spotty calcification can suggest plaque vulnerability. Positive remodeling is appreciated by referral to the remodeling index; obviously, expanded plaques have higher remodeling index, above the cut-off values, but borderline values can hamper interpretation, considering the narrow lumen of the coronary arteries, which barely averages 4 mm; a difference of 10% is less than 1 pixel on the CCTA image. Consequently, when the set cut-off value is near one, plaque expansion may be erroneously measured as positive. Also, the presence of spotty calcification can lead to overestimation of plaque expansion. As the presence of more calcium is considered to be an element of increased atherosclerotic plaque stability, low calcification plaques are regarded as more vulnerable [27].

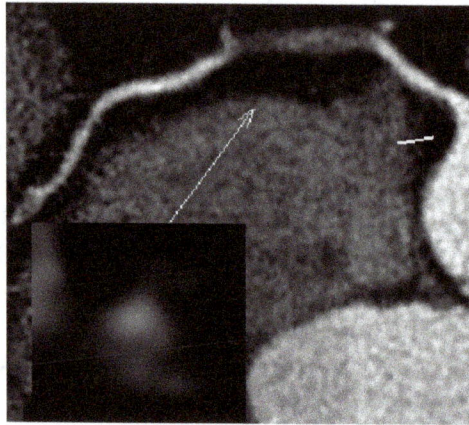

Figure 3. Curved Planar Reformation of the Coronary Artery in CCTA. The curved planar reformatted computed to-mography angiography image of the right coronary artery demonstrates two large, predominantly non-calcified athe-rosclerotic plaques with spotty calcification (arrowheads) in the proximal segment and mild of the right coronary artery.

However, pathological studies concluded that calcium is commonly encountered in ruptured plaques causing sudden cardiac death and that a few scattered small calcium deposits are often present in the fibrous cap of fibroatheromas [79]. The development of scattered small calcium around the necrotic core is believed to be triggered by osteogenic changes under the influence of inflammatory factors and oxidized lipids [80, 81]. The presence of spotty calcifications seems to induce mechanical instability at the interface with non-calcified plaque components [82]. Clinical studies have shown that: spotty calcification has been associated with an increased incidence of ischemic cardiovascular events [83] and, more accurately, that patients with ACSs have a different pattern of calcification when compared to those with stable angina [84]; spotty calcifications are more likely to be found in culprit lesions in patients with myocardial infarction than in patients with stable angina [38]; spotty calcification are more commonly encountered in patients with accelerated disease progression [85]; ruptured coronary plaques are associated with spotty calcification, particularly in deep locations and the number of deep calcium deposits is an independent predictor of culprit plaque ruptures in patients who had ACSs [84]; and superficial spotty calcifications in IVUS are associated with very late stent thrombosis after bare-metal stent implantation [86]. A possible caveat in CCTA imaging may be the fact that microcalcifications under the detection level of CCTA seem to induce very high plaque instability. However, the presence of calcification increases CCTA values, which seems to contradict the finding that low attenuation plaques are unstable.

2.2. Plaque quantification

Currently, MDCT with at least 64 detectors allows nearly motion-free visualization of the coronary arteries and accurate detection of significant stenosis, comparing well to coronary angiography at low heart rates [8, 87]. Contrast-enhanced scans are performed by injecting intravenously 80–100 ml of contrast agent at a flow rate of 6 ml/s followed by 70 ml of saline. The delay time is previously established using the bolus tracking technique with a region of interest positioned in the ascending aorta; a manually triggered threshold of 100 HU is specified for the main scanning. All scans are performed during a single breath-hold.

Non-contrast CCTA is also useful for atherosclerotic plaque description, allowing the calculation of the coronary artery calcium (CAC) score. The CAC is validated as a good marker of atherosclerotic burden and high values are associated with increased cardiovascular risk [88], However, despite relatively easy quantification, the CAC is hindered by several disadvantages, including the inability to identify small, scattered calcifications in non-calcified plaques, which may lead to the underestimation of disease severity and cardiovascular risk. Also, plaque morphology cannot be described on native calcium scans.

Quantitative measurements of coronary plaques aim to assess global atherosclerotic burden and provide detailed and specific descriptions of plaque morphology that could accurately evaluate the risk for cardiovascular events [70, 89, 90]. However, volumetric measurements of coronary artery plaques with manual tracing contours is strenuous and time-consuming; current software, such as AUTOPLAQ (APQ; Cedars-Sinai Medical Center, Los Angeles, CA), allow semi-automated quantification of both calcified and non-calcified plaques that has reduced the examination time and was shown to correlate very well to the IVUS assessment of the coronary plaque volume

[91]. Dey et al. [92] evaluated the accuracy of APQ and compared semi-automated quantification on CCTA using APQ to IVUS with manual tracing of the coronary artery plaque. Average examination time was significantly reduced by automated quantification. Manual IVUS required the longest processing time (15 to 35 minutes), followed by manual CCTA (5 to 15 minutes), while automated plaque segmentation and quantification took less than 20 seconds. There were no significant differences in plaque volumes calculation between IVUS compared with APQ, or between manual CCTA quantification and APQ. Interestingly, APQ quantification revealed smaller absolute differences from IVUS results than CT manual quantification. APQ has also been shown to have reliable interscan reproducibility of quantitative plaque measurements. Schuhbaeck et al. evaluated total plaque volume, volume of calcified and non-calcified plaque, and maximal remodeling index by performing CCTAs

twice in consecutive patients; using APQ there were no significant differences in any of the measurements between scans [93].

Another CCTA automated software for plaque quantification, QAngio (Medis, Netherland), has been developed and compared with IVUS. In their study, Boogers et al. [90] evaluated the accuracy of CCTA automated plaque quantification using a single algorithm to co-register CT and IVUS after having previously established anatomical markers; slice-by-slice comparisons of each location along the transverse axis of the coronary arteries have been made. The compared parameters included the percent lumen area stenosis, plaque burden, the degree of remodeling at the level of minimal lumen area, and the mean plaque burden for the whole coronary plaque. The study revealed significant correlations between the two methods regarding the quantification of lumen area stenosis, plaque burden at the level of the minimal lumen area, as well as mean plaque burden. However, CCTA failed to quantify all parameters as accurately as IVUS, underestimating minimal lesion area and overestimating lumen area stenosis. Moderate correlations were established between the two methods regarding coronary plaque remodeling. Automated plaque quantification methods are expected to reduce interobserver variability by comparison with manual quantification techniques. Several studies were conducted in order to assess the reproducibility of the results. Papadopoulou et al. [94] reported little inter- and intraobserver variability for lumen and vessel areas. Also, in an additional study inter- and intraobserver relative differences for lumen, vessel, plaque area, and plaque burden did not reach statistical significance. Automated plaque quantification proved, however, less reliable for compositional measurements of plaque attenuation values, demonstrating high inter-observer variability (12%), which is an important limiting factor. Despite this drawback, automated softwares can be used for evaluating coronary artery sclerosis progression, as demonstrated by Papadopoulou et al [95]. In another study, Blackmon et al. [96] tested the accuracy and interobserver variability for volumetric measurement of non-calcified lesions of another automated postprocessing software algorithm. Very strong correlations were found between manual measurements performed by highly experienced examiners and automated plaque volumetry, and interobserver variability was reduced when using the plaque analysis algorithm. As demonstrated by the aforementioned studies, automated softwares provide the major advantage of higher reproducibility, while also allowing faster quantifications, which make them elligible for more widespread use. CCTA is very accurate for stenosis detection [97] and for the measurement of calcified plaque burden [98, 99]. The amount of coronary calcification quantified by CCTA is a strong predictor of CAD [100, 101], but fails to accurately identify the site of stenosis. Moreover, even in modern CT scanners, spatial resolution is not sufficient to provide an accurate analysis of the fibrous cap by CCTA [102]. Also, histopathologically-based studies suggest that vulnerable plaques are enlarged in all three spatial dimensions [103] and that average measurements of the necrotic core, such as length and area [104] are beyond the plaque detection threshold for CCTA [105].

2.3. Functional plaque characteristics

Recently, some techniques have been developed for the purpose of analyzing functional parameters, as well as anatomical structures. CT-based fractional flow reserve (FFR-CT) and

CT perfusion allow the non-invasive hemodynamic assessment of coronary stenoses and increase the specificity of CCTA, which may greatly influence the management of CAD patients in the future [106].

2.3.1. Endothelial Shear Stress (ESS)

ESS refers to the tangential stress that is applied on the endothelial surface of the arterial wall by flowing blood friction and is expressed in units of force/unit area [107]. ESS is influenced by blood viscosity and the spatial gradient of blood velocity at the wall. When a fluid passes through a tube, its flow is influenced by the characteristics of the tube walls such as surface irregularities or obstructions. Fluid flow may be laminar or turbulent. Laminar flows are streamlined and may be either completely smooth ("undisturbed flows") or "disturbed", with areas of reversed flow. In turbulent flow, velocities vary continuously in a certain point in space [108]. The presence of low ESS favors the formation and development of coronary artery plaques, as well as their progression to high risk, vulnerable plaques. Local blood hemodynamics can influence atherosclerosis development for better or for worse. Therefore, an accurate in vivo quantification of plaque characteristics, local ESS, and vascular remodeling response would facilitate a better understanding of the mechanisms behind CAD progression, as well as clinical decision making regarding possible pre-emptive local interventions [109]. The evolution of each coronary artery plaque is individual and considerably influenced not only by the progression of atherosclerosis, but also by vascular remodeling. Extensive remodeling leads to the development of vulnerable plaques and is triggered by ESS. Persistent ESS favors local lipid build-up, inflammation, oxidative stress, and matrix breakdown, with subsequent plaque progression and further remodeling [109]. Advanced plaques in areas of severe stenosis are submitted to considerable shear stress that promotes plaque destabilization [110].

2.3.2. Fractional Flow Reserve (FFR)

FFR is calculated as the ratio between the maximum blood flow within a diseased coronay artery and the theoretical maximum flow in a normal coronary artery. An FFR of 1.0 is considered normal, while values of less than 0.75–0.80 are acknowledged by most as associated with myocardial ischemia [111]. FFR values >0.8 but <1 are considered indicative of a hemodinamically unsignificant stenosis, while values <0.75 reflect significant stenoses. In earlier works, values between 0.75–0.80 represented a grey area and were interpreted according to the clinical context. Investigators estimated that the cut-off value for FFR could be extended to 0.80, thus improving sensitivity without significantly compromising specificity. The cut-off value of 0.80 was already used in the FAME 1 and FAME 2 trials and proved to be clinically valid [112, 113]. This is now the recommended ischemic reference standard for the invasive assessment of myocardial ischemia [114]. Invasive coronary angiography is the established clinical standard for coronary artery disease assessment, with IVUS providing the advantage of intramural and transmural coronary artery imaging. OCT offers an even more accurate visualization of the coronary arteries [115]. The use of these additional invasive imaging methods can facilitate therapeutical decisions regarding revascularization and help guide percutaneous coronary interventions, leading to better postprocedural results. However, in current clinical practice, the reported rates of use for these techniques in assessing intermediate (40–70%) coronary stenoses are fairly low, 20.3% for IVUS and 6.1% for FFR [116].

In the Percutaneous Coronary Intervention of Functionally Non-significant Stenosis (DEFER) Study [117], investigators evaluated 181 patients with stable ischemic heart disease and FFR > 0.75 across an intermediate stenosis. These patients were randomized to either percutaneous coronary interventions or to deferral of percutaneous coronary interventions with medical treatment. At 5-year follow-up, patients in the deferred group had a significantly decreased (less than half) rate of death or myocardial infarction by comparison with the percutaneous coronary interventions group. In the Fractional Flow Reserve versus Angiography for Multivessel Evaluation (FAME) trial [113], 1,005 patients with multivessel disease were randomized to either FFR- or angiography-guided percutaneous coronary interventions. In patients with FFR-guided interventions, the composite rate of death, MI, or repeated revascularization at 1 year was significantly lower (13.2% vs. 18.3%, P<0.02). The Fractional Flow Reserve versus Angiography for Multivessel Evaluation 2 (FAME 2) trial [113] compared the outcomes of FFR-guided percutaneous coronary interventions with optimal medical therapy against optimal medical therapy alone in a group of 888 patients with stable ischemic heart disease. In this trial, unlike in others such as COURAGE, only patients having at least one lesion with FFR <0.80 were enrolled [118].

FFR assessment of lesions with 50% to 70% diameter narrowing revealed that only 35% of the lesions were hemodynamically significant. Interestingly, in severe lesions with 71% to 90% diameter stenoses, 20% were not hemodynamically significant based on FFR and did not require percutaneous coronary interventions. These results endorse the hypothesis that FFR can have essential clinical implications regarding revascularization decisions even in more severe angiographic stenoses and, particularly when noninvasive data is discordant with coronary angiography [119]. In patients with multivessel coronary artery disease, FFR can be performed, allowing an accurate determination of the Functional SYNTAX Score, and subsequently, a better selection of patients that could benefit from percutaneous coronary intervention rather than being submitted to coronary artery by-pass graft [120]. The use of CCTA for non-invasive anatomic assessment has increased considerably and the method is considered an accurate tool for detecting or excluding CAD [6, 5]. FFR-CT is a recently developed method based on computational fluid dynamics to calculate coronary blood flow, pressure, and FFR based on routinely acquired CCTA datasets [121, 122, 123, 124, 125, 126, 127, 128, 129].

3. Clinical implications of napkin-ring sign plaque for prognosis and management

Recent research has shown that the napkin-ring sign is associated with future cardiac events, frequently corresponding to the culprit lesion in ACS [53]. In the study by Otsuka et al., 895 patients were evaluated by CCTA and followed up for 2.3±0.8 years; in this population, the presence of the napkin-ring sign on CCTA was strongly associated with ACS events: 24 patients (2.6%) experienced ACS events, of which 41% developed plaques with napkin-ring sign during the follow-up period [53]. Kashiwagi et al. conducted a CCTA-based study on 273 patients with either ACS or stable angina. In their research, the authors described the napkin-ring sign as the presence of a ring of high attenuation and the CT attenuation of a ring presenting higher than those of the adjacent plaque and no greater than 130 HU. The napkin-ring sign was more frequently encountered in culprit lesions (12.7% vs. 2.8%, p<0.01). Moreover, napkin-ring sign plaques were associated with a higher remodeling index and lower CT attenuation (1.15 ± 0.12 vs. 1.02 ± 0.12, p<0.01 and 39.9 ± 22.8 HU vs.72.7 ± 26.6 HU, p<0.01) [50]. Similar results were obtained in another study in which the napkin-ring sign was more common in patients developing ACS than in those with stable angina [28].

Besides the napkin-ring sign, other imaging characteristics such as large plaque volume, low CT attenuation, positive remodeling, and spotty calcification were proved to be correlated with a higher risk of acute events [130]. Motoyama et al. found that positive remodeling and low attenuation correlated best with the development of ACS, [74] which is consistent with results from other studies [131, 132]. Considering the results of the previously mentioned studies, one can conclude that the identification of CCTA aspects suggesting vulnerable lesions may be useful for several reasons. Firstly, although statins are known to reduce the incidence of acute cardiovascular events [133], proving their effect on a certain individual is challenging. CCTA may help identify coronary artery lesions regression, but, as it is not routinely performed, there is not enough data to support this hypothesis. Risk stratification in asymptomatic individuals has also been taken into account as a possible use for CCTA, but the actual ability of MDCT for detecting small non-stenotic plaques is yet to be established [134].

In conclusion CCTA is used extensively nowadays as a non-invasive imaging method for the evaluation of patients suspected of CAD and the napkin-ring sign described on CCTA has been designated as a valid element for identifying vulnerable plaques, indicating an increased probability of rupture, and was shown to correlate with a higher incidence of cardiovascular events.

Author details

Lucia Agoston-Coldea[1,2], Carmen Cionca[2] and Silvia Lupu[3]

1 Iuliu Hatieganu University of Medicine and Pharmacy, Cluj-Napoca, Romania

2 Hiperdia Diagnostic Imaging Center, Cluj-Napoca, Romania

3 University of Medicine and Pharmacy of Targu Mures, Romania

References

[1] Naghavi M, Libby P, Falk E, Casscells SW, Litovsky S, Rumberger J, Badimon JJ, Stefanadis C, Moreno P, Pasterkamp G, Fayad Z, Stone PH, Waxman S, Raggi P, Madjid M, Zarrabi A, Burke A, Yuan C, Fitzgerald PJ, Siscovick DS, de Korte CL, Aikawa M, Juhani Airaksinen KE, Assmann G, Becker CR, Chesebro JH, Farb A, Galis ZS, Jackson C, Jang IK, Koenig W, Lodder RA, March K, Demirovic J, Navab M, Priori SG, Rekhter MD, Bahr R, Grundy SM, Mehran R, Colombo A, Boerwinkle E, Ballantyne C, Insull W Jr, Schwartz RS, Vogel R, Serruys PW, Hansson GK, Faxon DP, Kaul S, Drexler H, Greenland P, Muller JE, Virmani R, Ridker PM, Zipes DP, Shah PK, Willerson JT. From vulnerable plaque to vulnerable patient: A call for new definitions and risk assessment strategies: Part I. Circulation. 2003;108:1664-1672. DOI: 10.1161/01.CIR.0000087480.94275.97.

[2] Naghavi M, Libby P, Falk E, Casscells SW, Litovsky S, Rumberger J, Badimon JJ, Stefanadis C, Moreno P, Pasterkamp G, Fayad Z, Stone PH, Waxman S, Raggi P, Madjid M, Zarrabi A, Burke A, Yuan C, Fitzgerald PJ, Siscovick DS, de Korte CL, Aikawa M, Airaksinen KE, Assmann G, Becker CR, Chesebro JH, Farb A, Galis ZS, Jackson C, Jang IK, Koenig W, Lodder RA, March K, Demirovic J, Navab M, Priori SG, Rekhter MD, Bahr R, Grundy SM, Mehran R, Colombo A, Boerwinkle E, Ballantyne C, Insull W Jr, Schwartz RS, Vogel R, Serruys PW, Hansson GK, Faxon DP, Kaul S, Drexler H, Greenland P, Muller JE, Virmani R, Ridker PM, Zipes DP, Shah PK, Willerson JT. From vulnerable plaque to vulnerable patient: A call for new definitions and risk assessment strategies: Part II. Circulation. 2003;108:1772-1778. DOI: 10.1161/01.CIR.0000087481.55887.C9.

[3] Taylor AJ, Merz CN, Udelson JE. 34th Bethesda Conference: Executive summary — can atherosclerosis imaging techniques improve the detection of patients at risk for ischemic heart disease? J Am Coll Cardiol. 2003;41:1860-1862. DOI:10.1016/ S0735-1097(03)00363-2.

[4] Virmani R, Burke AP, Farb A, Kolodgie FD. Pathology of the vulnerable plaque. J Am Coll Cardiol. 2006;47:C13-18. DOI:10.1016/ j.jacc.2005.10.065.

[5] Budoff MJ, Dowe D, Jollis JG, Gitter M, Sutherland J, Halamert E, Scherer M, Bellinger R, Martin A, Benton R, Delago A, Min JK. Diagnostic performance of 64-multidetector-row coronary computed tomographic angiography for evaluation of coronary artery stenosis in individuals without known coronary artery disease. J Am Coll Cardiol. 2008;52:1724-1732. DOI: 10.1016/j.jacc.2008.07.031.

[6] Meijboom WB, Meijs MF, Schuijf JD, Cramer MJ, Mollet NR, van Mieghem CA, Nieman K, van Werkhoven JM, Pundziute G, Weustink AC, de Vos AM, Pugliese F, Rensing B, Jukema JW, Bax JJ, Prokop M, Doevendans PA, Hunink MG, Krestin GP, de Feyter PJ. Diagnostic accuracy of 64-slice computed tomography coronary angiogra-

phy: A prospective, multicenter, multivendor study. J Am Coll Cardiol. 2008;52:2135-2144. DOI: 10.1016/ j.jacc. 2008.08.058.

[7] Pundziute G, Schuijf JD, Jukema JW, Decramer I, Sarno G, Vanhoenacker PK, Boersma E, Reiber JH, Schalij MJ, Wijns W, Bax JJ. Evaluation of plaque characteristics in acute coronary syndromes: Non-invasive assessment with multi-slice computed tomography and invasive evaluation with intravascular ultrasound radiofrequency data analysis. Eur Heart J. 2008;29:2373-2381. DOI: 10.1093/eurheartj/ehn356.

[8] Achenbach S, Moselewski F, Ropers D, Ferencik M, Hoffmann U, MacNeill B, Pohle K, Baum U, Anders K, Jang IK, Daniel WG, Brady TJ. Detection of calcified and non-calcified coronary atherosclerotic plaque by contrast-enhanced, submillimeter multidetector spiral computed tomography: A segment-based comparison with intravascular ultrasound. Circulation. 2004;109:14-17. DOI: 10.1161/01.CIR. 0000111517.69230.0F.

[9] Petranovic M, Soni A, Bezzera H, Loureiro R, Sarwar A, Raffel C, Pomerantsev E, Jang IK, Brady TJ, Achenbach S, Cury RC. Assessment of nonstenotic coronary lesions by 64-slice multidetector computed tomography in comparison to intravascular ultrasound: Evaluation of nonculprit coronary lesions. J Cardiovasc Comput Tomogr. 2009;3:24-31. DOI: 10.1016/j.jcct.2008.12.005.

[10] Duewell P, Kono H, Rayner KJ, Sirois CM, Vladimer G, Bauernfeind FG, Abela GS, Franchi L, Nuñez G, Schnurr M, Espevik T, Lien E, Fitzgerald KA, Rock KL, Moore KJ, Wright SD, Hornung V, Latz E. NLRP3 inflammasomes are required for atherogenesis and activated by cholesterol crystals. Nature. 2010;464:1357-1361. DOI: 10.1038/nature08938.

[11] Stary HC, Chandler AB, Glagov S, Guyton JR, Insull W Jr, Rosenfeld ME, Schaffer SA, Schwartz CJ, Wagner WD, Wissler RW. A definition of initial, fatty streak, and intermediate lesions of atherosclerosis. A report from the Committee on Vascular Lesions of the Council on Arteriosclerosis, American Heart Association. Circulation. 1994;89:2462-2478. DOI: 10.1161/01.CIR.89.5.2462.

[12] Stary HC, Chandler AB, Dinsmore RE, Fuster V, Glagov S, Insull W Jr, Rosenfeld ME, Schwartz CJ, Wagner WD, Wissler RW. A definition of advanced types of atherosclerotic lesions and a histological classification of atherosclerosis. A report from the Committee on Vascular Lesions of the Council on Arteriosclerosis, American Heart Association. Arterioscler Thromb Vasc Biol. 1995;15:1512-1531. DOI: 10.1161/01.ATV.15.9.1512.

[13] Virmani R, Kolodgie FD, Burke AP, Farb A, Schwartz SM. Lessons from sudden coronary death: A comprehensive morphological classification scheme for atherosclerotic lesions. Arterioscler Thromb Vasc Biol. 2000;20:1262-1275. DOI: 10.1161/01.ATV. 20.5.1262.

[14] Nakashima Y, Wight TN, Sueishi K. Early atherosclerosis in humans: Role of diffuse intimal thickening and extracellular matrix proteoglycans. Cardiovasc Res. 2008;79:14-23. DOI: 10.1093/cvr/cvn099.

[15] Liao X, Sluimer JC, Wang Y, Subramanian M, Brown K, Pattison JS, Robbins J, Martinez J, Tabas I. Macrophage autophagy plays a protective role in advanced atherosclerosis. Cell Metab. 2012;15:545-553. DOI: 10.1016/j.cmet.2012.01.022.

[16] van der Wal AC, Becker AE, van der Loos CM, Das PK. Site of intimal rupture or erosion of thrombosed coronary atherosclerotic plaques is characterized by an inflammatory process irrespective of the dominant plaque morphology. Circulation. 1994;89:36-44. DOI: 10.1161/01.CIR.89.1.36.

[17] Nakashima Y, Fujii H, Sumiyoshi S, Wight TN, Sueishi K. Early human atherosclerosis: Accumulation of lipid and proteoglycans in intimal thickenings followed by macrophage infiltration. Arterioscler Thromb Vasc Biol. 2007;27:1159-1165. DOI: 10.1161/ATVBAHA.106.134080.

[18] Ohayon J, Finet G, Gharib AM, Herzka DA, Tracqui P, Heroux J, Rioufol G, Kotys MS, Elagha A, Pettigrew RI. Necrotic core thickness and positive arterial remodeling index: emergent biomechanical factors for evaluating the risk of plaque rupture. Am J Physiol Heart Circ Physiol. 2008;295:H717-727. DOI: 10.1152/ajpheart.00005.2008.

[19] Dhawan SS, Avati Nanjundappa RP, Branch JR, Taylor WR, Quyyumi AA, Jo H, McDaniel MC, Suo J, Giddens D, Samady H. Shear stress and plaque development. Expert Rev Cardiovasc Ther. 2010;8:545-556. DOI: 10.1586/erc.10.28.

[20] Papaspyridonos M, Smith A, Burnand KG, Taylor P, Padayachee S, Suckling KE, James CH, Greaves DR, Patel L. Novel candidate genes in unstable areas of human atherosclerotic plaques. Arterioscler Thromb Vasc Biol. 2006;26:1837-1844. DOI: 10.1161/01.ATV.0000229695.68416.76.

[21] Kolodgie FD, Gold HK, Burke AP, Fowler DR, Kruth HS, Weber DK, Farb A, Guerrero LJ, Hayase M, Kutys R, Narula J, Finn AV, Virmani R. Intraplaque hemorrhage and progression of coronary atheroma. N Engl J Med. 2003;349:2316-2325. DOI: 10.1056/NEJMoa035655.

[22] Sluimer JC, Kolodgie FD, Bijnens AP, Maxfield K, Pacheco E, Kutys B, Duimel H, Frederik PM, van Hinsbergh VW, Virmani R, Daemen MJ. Thin-walled microvessels in human coronary atherosclerotic plaques show incomplete endothelial junctions relevance of compromised structural integrity for intraplaque microvascular leakage. J Am Coll Cardiol. 2009;53:1517-1527. DOI: 10.1016/j.jacc.2008.12.056.

[23] Mann J, Davies MJ. Mechanisms of progression in native coronary artery disease: Role of healed plaque disruption. Heart. 1999;82:265-268. DOI:10.1136/hrt.82.3.265.

[24] Arbustini E, Dal Bello B, Morbini P, Burke AP, Bocciarelli M, Specchia G, Virmani R. Plaque erosion is a major substrate for coronary thrombosis in acute myocardial infarction. Heart. 1999;82:269-272. DOI:10.1136/ hrt.82.3.269.

[25] Kramer MC, Rittersma SZ, de Winter RJ, Ladich ER, Fowler DR, Liang YH, Kutys R, Carter-Monroe N, Kolodgie FD, van der Wal AC, Virmani R. Relationship of thrombus healing to underlying plaque morphology in sudden coronary death. J Am Coll Cardiol. 2010;55:122-132. DOI: 10.1016/j.jacc.2009.09.007.

[26] Maurovich-Horvat P, Hoffmann U, Vorpahl M, Nakano M, Virmani R, Alkadhi H. The napkin-ring sign: CT signature of high risk coronary plaques? J Am Coll Cardiol Img. 2010;3:440-444. DOI: 10.1016/j.jcmg.2010.02.003.

[27] Tanaka A, Shimada K, Yoshida K, Jissyo S, Tanaka H, Sakamoto M, Matsuba K, Imanishi T, Akasaka T, Yoshikawa J. Non-invasive assessment of plaque rupture by 64-slice multidetector computed tomography—comparison with intravascular ultrasound. Circ J. 2008;72:1276-1281. DOI: 10.1253/circj.72.1276.

[28] Pflederer T, Marwan M, Schepis T, Ropers D, Seltmann M, Muschiol G, Daniel WG, Achenbach S. Characterization of culprit lesions in acute coronary syndromes using coronary dual-source CT angiography. Atherosclerosis. 2010;211:437-444. DOI: 10.1016/j.atherosclerosis.2010.02.001.

[29] Aziz K, Berger K, Claycombe K, Huang R, Patel R, Abela GS. Noninvasive detection and localization of vulnerable plaque and arterial thrombosis with computed tomography angiography/positron emission tomography. Circulation. 2008;117:2061-2070. DOI: 10.1161/CirculationAHA.106.652313.

[30] Youssef G, Budoff M. Role of Computed Tomography Coronary Angiography in the Detection of Vulnerable Plaque, Where Does it Stand Among Others? Angiol. 2013:1:2. DOI: 10.4172/2329-9495.1000111.

[31] Vancraeynest D, Pasquet A, Roelants V, Gerber BL, Vanoverschelde JL. Imaging the vulnerable plaque. J Am Coll Cardiol. 2011;57:1961-1979. DOI: 10.1016/j.jacc.2011.02.018.

[32] Toutouzas K, Stathogiannis K, Synetos A, Karanasos A, Stefanadis C. Vulnerable atherosclerotic plaque: From the basic research laboratory to the clinic. Cardiology. 2012;123:248-253. DOI: 10.1159/000345291.

[33] Hong MK, Mintz GS, Lee CW, Kim YH, Lee SW, Song JM, Han KH, Kang DH, Song JK, Kim JJ, Park SW, Park SJ. Comparison of coronary plaque rupture between stable angina and acute myocardial infarction: A three-vessel intravascular ultrasound study in 235 patients. Circulation. 2004;110:928-933. DOI: 10.1161/ 01.CIR.0000139858.69915.2E.

[34] Stone GW, Maehara A, Lansky AJ, de Bruyne B, Cristea E, Mintz GS, Mehran R, McPherson J, Farhat N, Marso SP, Parise H, Templin B, White R, Zhang Z, Serruys

PW; PROSPECT Investigators. A prospective natural-history study of coronary atherosclerosis. N Engl J Med. 2011;364:226-235. DOI: 10.1056/NEJMoa1002358.

[35] Cheng JM, Garcia-Garcia HM, de Boer SP, Kardys I, Heo JH, Akkerhuis KM, Oemrawsingh RM, van Domburg RT, Ligthart J, Witberg KT, Regar E, Serruys PW, van Geuns RJ, Boersma E. In vivo detection of high-risk coronary plaques by radiofrequency intravascular ultrasound and cardiovascular outcome: Results of the ATHEROREMO-IVUS study. Eur Heart J. 2014;35:639-647. DOI:10.1093/eurheartj/eht484.

[36] Tian J, Dauerman H, Toma C, Samady H, Itoh T, Kuramitsu S, Domei T, Jia H, Vergallo R, Soeda T, Hu S, Minami Y, Lee H, Yu B, Jang IK. Prevalence and characteristics of TCFA and degree of coronary artery stenosis: An OCT, IVUS, and angiographic study. J Am Coll Cardiol. 2014;64:672-680. DOI:10.1016/j.jacc.2014.05.052.

[37] Schoenhagen P, Ziada KM, Kapadia SR, Crowe TD, Nissen SE, Tuzcu EM. Extent and direction of arterial remodeling in stable versus unstable coronary syndromes: an intravascular ultrasound study. Circulation. 2000;101:598-603. DOI: 10.1161/01.CIR. 101.6.598.

[38] Ehara S, Kobayashi Y, Yoshiyama M, Shimada K, Shimada Y, Fukuda D, Nakamura Y, Yamashita H, Yamagishi H, Takeuchi K, Naruko T, Haze K, Becker AE, Yoshikawa J, Ueda M. Spotty calcification typifies the culprit plaque in patients with acute myocardial infarction: An intravascular ultrasound study. Circulation. 2004;110:3424-3429. DOI: 10.1161/01.CIR.0000148131.41425.E9.

[39] Rodriguez-Granillo GA, García-García HM, Mc Fadden EP, Valgimigli M, Aoki J, de Feyter P, Serruys PW. In vivo intravascular ultrasound-derived thin-cap fibroatheroma detection using ultrasound radiofrequency data analysis. J Am Coll Cardiol. 2005;46:2038-2042. DOI:10.1016/j.jacc.2005.07.064.

[40] Hong MK, Mintz GS, Lee CW, Suh J, Kim JH, Park DW, Lee SW, Kim YH, Cheong SS, Kim JJ, Park SW, Park SJ. Comparison of virtual histology to intravascular ultrasound of culprit coronary lesions in acute coronary syndrome and target coronary lesions instable angina pectoris. Am J Cardiol. 2007;100:953-999. DOI: 10.1016/j.amjcard.2007.04.034.

[41] Hong YJ, Jeong MH, Choi YH, Park SY, Rhew SH, Jeong HC, Cho JY, Jang SY, Lee KH, Park KH, Sim DS, Yoon NS, Yoon HJ, Kim KH, Park HW, Kim JH, Ahn Y, Cho JG, Park JC, Kang JC. Comparison of Coronary Plaque Components between Non-Culprit Lesions in Patients with Acute Coronary Syndrome and Target Lesions in Patients with Stable Angina: Virtual Histology-Intravascular Ultrasound Analysis. Korean Circ J. 2013;43:607-614. DOI: 10.4070/kcj.2013.43.9.607.

[42] Patwari P, Weissman NJ, Boppart SA, Jesser C, Stamper D, Fujimoto JG, Brezinski ME. Assessment of coronary plaque with optical coherence tomography and high-

frequency ultrasound. Am J Cardiol. 2000;85:641-644. DOI: 10.1016/ S0002-9149(99)00825-5.

[43] Kume T, Akasaka T, Kawamoto T, Watanabe N, Toyota E, Neishi Y, Sukmawan R, Sadahira Y, Yoshida K. Assessment of coronary intima media thickness by optical co-herence tomography: comparison with intravascular ultrasound. Circ J. 2005;69:903-907. DOI:10.1253/circj.69.903.

[44] Motoyama S, Kondo T, Sarai M, Sugiura A, Harigaya H, Sato T, Inoue K, Okumura M, Ishii J, Anno H, Virmani R, Ozaki Y, Hishida H, Narula J. Multislice computed tomographic characteristics of coronary lesions in acute coronary syndromes. J Am Coll Cardiol. 2007;50:319-326. DOI:10.1016/j.jacc.2007.03.044.

[45] Hoffmann U, Moselewski F, Nieman K, Jang IK, Ferencik M, Rahman AM, Cury RC, Abbara S, Joneidi-Jafari H, Achenbach S, Brady TJ. Noninvasive assessment of pla-que morphology and composition in culprit and stable lesions in acute coronary syn drome and stable lesions in stable angina by multidetector computed tomography. J Am Coll Cardiol. 2006;47:1655-1662. DOI:10.1016/j.jacc.2006.01.041.

[46] Tearney GJ, Regar E, Akasaka T, Adriaenssens T, Barlis P, Bezerra HG, Bouma B, Bruining N, Cho JM, Chowdhary S, Costa MA, de Silva R, Dijkstra J, Di Mario C, Du-dek D, Falk E, Feldman MD, Fitzgerald P, Garcia-Garcia HM, Gonzalo N, Granada JF, Guagliumi G, Holm NR, Honda Y, Ikeno F, Kawasaki M, Kochman J, Koltowski L, Kubo T, Kume T, Kyono H, Lam CC, Lamouche G, Lee DP, Leon MB, Maehara A, Manfrini O, Mintz GS, Mizuno K, Morel MA, Nadkarni S, Okura H, Otake H, Pietra-sik A, Prati F, Räber L, Radu MD, Rieber J, Riga M, Rollins A, Rosenberg M, Sirbu V, Serruys PW, Shimada K, Shinke T, Shite J, Siegel E, Sonoda S, Suter M, Takarada S, Tanaka A, Terashima M, Thim T, Uemura S, Ughi GJ, van Beusekom HM, van der Steen AF, van Es GA, van Soest G, Virmani R, Waxman S, Weissman NJ, Weisz G. International Working Group for Intravascular Optical Coherence Tomography (IWG-IVOCT). Consensus standards for acquisition, measurement, and reporting of intravascular optical coherence tomography studies: A report from the International Working Group for Intravascular Optical Coherence Tomography Standardization and Validation. J Am Coll Cardiol. 2012;59:1058-1072. DOI: 10.1016/j.jacc.2011.09.079.

[47] Kashiwagi M, Tanaka A, Kitabata H, Tsujioka H, Kataiwa H, Komukai K, Tanimoto T, Takemoto K, Takarada S, Kubo T, Hirata K, Nakamura N, Mizukoshi M, Imanishi T, Akasaka T. Feasibility of noninvasive assessment of thin-cap fibroatheroma by multidetector computed tomography. J Am Coll Cardiol Img. 2009;2:1412-1419. DOI: 10.1016/j.jcmg.2009.09.012.

[48] Narula J, Garg P, Achenbach S, Motoyama S, Virmani R, Strauss HW. Arithmetic of vulnerable plaques for noninvasive imaging. Nat Clin Pract Cardiovasc Med. 2008;5 Suppl 2:S2-10. DOI: 10.1038/ncpcardio1247.

[49] Maurovich-Horvat P, Schlett CL, Alkadhi H, Nakano M, Otsuka F, Stolzmann P, Scheffel H, Ferencik M, Kriegel MF, Seifarth H, Virmani R, Hoffmann U. The napkin

ring sign indicates advanced atherosclerotic lesions in coronary CT angiography. JACC Cardiovasc Imaging. 2012;5:1243-1252. DOI:10.1016/j.jcmg.2012.03.019.

[50] Kashiwagi M, Tanaka A, Shimada K, Kitabata H, Komukai K, Nishiguchi T, Ozaki Y,Tanimoto T, Kubo T, Hirata K, Mizukoshi M, Akasaka T. Distribution, frequency and clinical implications of napkin-ring sign assessed by multidetector computed tomography. J Cardiol. 2013;61:399-403. DOI: 10.1016/j.jjcc.2013.01.004.

[51] Seifarth H, Schlett CL, Nakano M, Otsuka F, Károlyi M, Liew G, Maurovich-Horvat P, Alkadhi H, Virmani R, Hoffmann U. Histopathological correlates of the napkin-ring sign plaque in coronary CT angiography. Atherosclerosis. 2012;224:90-96. DOI: 10.1016/j.atherosclerosis.2012.06.021.

[52] Hamon M, Morello R, Riddell JW, Hamon M: Coronary arteries. diagnostic performance of 16- versus 64-section spiral CT compared with invasive coronary angiography—meta-analysis. Radiology. 2007;245:720-731. DOI:10.1148/radiol. 2453061899.

[53] Otsuka K, Fukuda S, Tanaka A, Nakanishi K, Taguchi H, Yoshikawa J, Shimada K, Yoshiyama M. Napkin-ring sign on coronary CT angiography for the prediction of acute coronary syndrome. JACC Cardiovasc Imaging. 2013;6:448-457. DOI: 10.1016/j.jcmg. 2012.09.016.

[54] Fujimoto S, Kondo T, Narula J. Evaluation of plaque morphology by coronary CT angiography. Cardiol Clin. 2012;30:69-75. DOI: 10.1016/j.ccl.2011.10.002.

[55] Narula J, Achenbach S. Napkin-ring necrotic cores: Defining circumferential extent of necrotic cores in unstable plaques. JACC Cardiovasc Imaging. 2009;2:1436-1438. DOI: 10.1016/j.jcmg.2009.10.004.

[56] Raff GL, Gallagher MJ, O'Neill WW, Goldstein JA. Diagnostic accuracy of noninvasive coronary angiography using 64-slice spiral computed tomography. J Am Coll Cardiol. 2005;46:552-557. DOI:10.1016/j.jacc.2005.05.056.

[57] Hadamitzky M, Freissmuth B, Meyer T, Hein F, Kastrati A, Martinoff S, Schömig A, Hausleiter J. Prognostic value of coronary computed tomographic angiography for prediction of cardiac events in patients with suspected coronary artery disease. JACC Cardiovasc Imaging. 2009;2:404-411. DOI: 10.1016/j.jcmg.2008.11.015.

[58] Chow BJ, Wells GA, Chen L, Yam Y, Galiwango P, Abraham A, Sheth T, Dennie C, Beanlands RS, Ruddy TD. Prognostic value of 64- slice cardiac computed tomography severity of coronary artery disease, coronary atherosclerosis, and left ventricular ejection fraction. J Am Coll Cardiol. 2010;55:1017-1028. DOI: 10.1016/j.jacc. 2009.10.039.

[59] Kristensen TS, Kofoed KF, Kühl JT, Nielsen WB, Nielsen MB, Kelbæk H. Prognostic implications of nonobstructive coronary plaques in patients with non-ST-segment elevation myocardial infarction: A multidetector computed tomography study. J Am Coll Cardiol. 2011;58:502-509. DOI: 10.1016/ j.jacc.2011.01.058.

[60]   Abdulla J, Asferg C, Kofoed KF. Prognostic value of absence or presence of coronary artery disease determined by 64-slice computed tomography coronary angiography a systematic review and meta-analysis. Int J Cardiovasc Imaging. 2011;27:413-420. DOI: 10.1007/s10554-010-9652-x.

[61]   Voros S. What are the potential advantagesand disadvantages of volumetric CT scanning? J Cardiovasc Comput Tomogr. 2009;3:67-70. DOI: 10.1016/j.jcct.2008.12.010.

[62]   Kristanto W, van Ooijen PM, Greuter MJ, Groen JM, Vliegenthart R, Oudkerk M. Non-calcified coronary atherosclerotic plaque visualization on CT: Effects of contrast-enhancement and lipid-content fractions. Int J Cardiovasc Imaging. 2013;29:1137-1148. DOI 10.1007/s10554-012-0176-4.

[63]   Becker CR, Nikolaou K, Muders M, Babaryka G, Crispin A, Schoepf UJ, Loehrs U, Reiser MF. Ex vivo coronary atherosclerotic plaque characterization with multi-detector-row CT. Eur Radiol. 2003;13:2094-2098. DOI: 10.1007/ s00330-003-1889-5.

[64]   Pohle K, Achenbach S, Macneill B, Ropers D, Ferencik M, Moselewski F, Hoffmann U, Brady TJ, Jang IK, Daniel WG. Characterization of non-calcified coronary atherosclerotic plaque by multi-detector row CT: Comparison to IVUS. Atherosclerosis. 2007;190:174-180. DOI: 10.1016/j.atherosclerosis.2006.01.013.

[65]   Schroeder S, Kuettner A, Wojak T, Janzen J, Heuschmid M, Athanasiou T, Beck T, Burgstahler C, Herdeg C, Claussen CD, Kopp AF. Non-invasive evaluation of atherosclerosis with contrast enhanced 16 slice spiral computed tomography: Results of ex vivo investigations. Heart. 2004;90:1471-1475. DOI:10.1136/hrt.2004.037861.

[66]   Nakazawa G, Tanabe K, Onuma Y, Yachi S, Aoki J, Yamamoto H, Higashikuni Y, Yagishita A, Nakajima H, Hara K. Efficacy of culprit plaque assessment by 64-slice multidetector computed tomography to predict transient no-reflow phenomenon during percutaneous coronary intervention. Am Heart J. 2008;155:1150-1157. DOI: 10.1016/ j.ahj.2008.01.006.

[67]   Leber AW, Becker A, Knez A, von Ziegler F, Sirol M, Nikolaou K, Ohnesorge B, Fayad ZA, Becker CR, Reiser M, Steinbeck G, Boekstegers P. Accuracy of 64-slice computed tomography to classify and quantify plaque volumes in the proximal coronary system: A comparative study using intravascular ultrasound. J Am Coll Cardiol. 2006;47:672-677. DOI:10.1016/j.jacc.2005.10.058.

[68]   Sun J, Zhang Z, Lu B, Yu W, Yang Y, Zhou Y, Wang Y, Fan Z. Identification and quantification of coronary atherosclerotic plaques: A comparison of 64-MDCT and intravascular ultrasound. Am J Roentgenol. 2008;190:748-754. DOI: 10.2214/AJR. 07.2763.

[69]   Schepis T, Marwan M, Pflederer T, Seltmann M, Ropers D, Daniel WG, Achenbach S. Quantification of noncalcified coronary atherosclerotic plaques with Dual Source Computed Tomography: Comparison to intravascular ultrasound. Heart. 2010;96:610-615. DOI: 10.1136/hrt.2009.184226.

[70] Otsuka M, Bruining N, Van Pelt NC, Mollet NR, Ligthart JM, Vourvouri E, Hamers R, De Jaegere P, Wijns W, Van Domburg RT, Stone GW, Veldhof S, Verheye S, Dudek D, Serruys PW, Krestin GP, De Feyter PJ. Quantification of coronary plaque by 64-slice computed tomography: A comparison with quantitative intracoronary ultrasound. Invest Radiol. 2008;43:314-321. DOI: 10.1097/RLI.0b013e31816a88a9.

[71] Springer I, Dewey M. Comparison of multislice computed tomography with intravascular ultrasound for detection and characterization of coronary artery plaques: a systematic review. Eur J Radiol. 2009;71:275-282. DOI: 10.1016/j.ejrad.2008.04.035.

[72] Hoffmann H, Frieler K, Hamm B, Dewey M. Intra- and interobserver variability in detection and assessment of calcified and noncalcified coronary artery plaques using 64-slice computed tomography: Variability in coronary plaque measurement using MSCT. Int J Cardiovasc Imaging. 2008;24:735-742. DOI: 10.1007/s10554-008-9299-z.

[73] Pflederer T, Schmid M, Ropers D, Ropers U, Komatsu S, Daniel WG, Achenbach S. Interobserver variability of 64-slice computed tomography for the quantification of non-calcified coronary atherosclerotic plaque. Rofo. 2007;179:953-957. DOI: 10.1055/s-2007-963113.

[74] Motoyama S, Sarai M, Harigaya H, Anno H, Inoue K, Hara T, Naruse H, Ishii J, Hishida H, Wong ND, Virmani R, Kondo T, Ozaki Y, Narula J. Computed tomographic angiography characteristics of atherosclerotic plaques subsequently resulting in acute coronary syndrome. J Am Coll Cardiol. 2009;54:49-57. DOI: 10.1016/j.jacc.2009.02.068.

[75] Motoyama S, Kondo T, Anno H, Sugiura A, Ito Y, Mori K, Ishii J, Sato T, Inoue K, Sarai M, Hishida H, Narula J. Atherosclerotic plaque characterization by 0.5-mm-slice multislice computed tomographic imaging. Circ J. 2007;71:363-366. DOI: 10.1253/circj.71.363.

[76] Cademartiri F, Mollet NR, Runza G, Bruining N, Hamers R, Somers P, Knaapen M, Verheye S, Midiri M, Krestin GP, de Feyter PJ: Influence of intracoronary attenuation on coronary plaque measurements using multislice computed tomography: observations in an ex vivo model of coronary computed tomography angiography. Eur Radiol. 2005;15:1426-1431. DOI: 10.1007/s00330-005-2697-x.

[77] Cademartiri F, La Grutta L, Runza G, Palumbo A, Maffei E, Mollet NR, Bartolotta TV, Somers P, Knaapen M, Verheye S, Midiri M, Hamers R, Bruining N: Influence of convolution filtering on coronary plaque attenuation values: observations in an ex vivo model of multislice computed tomography coronary angiography. Eur Radiol. 2007;17:1842-1849. DOI: 10.1007/s00330-006-0548-z.

[78] Schroeder S, Flohr T, Kopp AF, Meisner C, Kuettner A, Herdeg C, Baumbach A, Ohnesorge B. Accuracy of density measurements within plaque located in artificial coronary arteries by X-ray multislice CT: Results of a phantom study. J Comput Assist Tomogr. 2001;25:900-906.

[79] Falk E, Nakano M, Bentzon JF, Finn AV, Virmani R. Update on acute coronary syndromes: The pathologists' view. Eur Heart J. 2013;34:719-728. DOI: 10.1093/eurheartj/ehs411.

[80] Aikawa E, Nahrendorf M, Figueiredo JL, Swirski FK, Shtatland T, Kohler RH, Jaffer FA, Aikawa M, Weissleder R. Osteogenesis associates with inflammation in early-stage atherosclerosis evaluated by molecular imaging in vivo. Circulation. 2007;116:2841-2850. DOI: 10.1161/CIRCULATIONAHA.107.732867.

[81] Flammer AJ, Gössl M, Widmer RJ, Reriani M, Lennon R, Loeffler D, Shonyo S, Simari RD, Lerman LO, Khosla S, Lerman A. Osteocalcin positive CD133þ/CD34-/KDRþ progenitor cells as an independent marker for unstable atherosclerosis. Eur Heart J. 2012;33:2963-2969. DOI: 10.1093/eurheartj/ehs234.

[82] Johnson RC, Leopold JA, Loscalzo J. Vascular calcification: Pathobiological mechanisms and clinical implications. Circ Res. 2006;99:1044-1059. DOI: 10.1161/01.RES. 0000249379.55535.21.

[83] Watabe H, Sato A, Akiyama D, Kakefuda Y, Adachi T, Ojima E, Hoshi T, Murakoshi N, Ishizu T, Seo Y, Aonuma K. Impact of coronary plaquecomposition on cardiac troponin elevation after percutaneous coronary intervention in stable angina pectoris: a computed tomography analysis. J Am Coll Cardiol. 2012;59:1881-1888. DOI: 10.1016/j.jacc.2012.01.051.

[84] Fujii K, Carlier SG, Mintz GS, Takebayashi H, Yasuda T, Costa RA, Moussa I, Dangas G, Mehran R, Lansky AJ, Kreps EM, Collins M, Stone GW, Moses JW, Leon MB. Intravascular ultrasound study of patterns of calcium in ruptured coronary plaques. Am J Cardiol. 2005;96:352-357. DOI: 10.1016/j.amjcard.2005.03.074.

[85] Kataoka Y, Wolski K, Uno K, Puri R, Tuzcu EM, Nissen SE, Nicholls SJ. Spotty calcification as a marker of accelerated progression of coronary atherosclerosis: Insights from serial intravascular ultrasound. J Am Coll Cardiol. 2012;59:1592-1597. DOI: 10.1016/j.jacc.2012.03.012.

[86] Yumoto K, Anzai T, Aoki H, Inoue A, Funada S, Nishiyama H, Tanaka S, Kowase S, Shirai Y, Kurosaki K, Nogami A, Daida H, Kato K. Calcified plaque rupture and very late stent thrombosis after bare-metal stent implantation. Cardiovasc Interv Ther. 2011;26:252-259. DOI: 10.1007/s12928-011-0070-3.

[87] Nieman K, Cademartiri F, Lemos PA, Raaijmakers R, Pattynama PM, de Feyter PJ. Reliable noninvasive coronary angiography with fast submillimeter multislice spiral computed tomography. Circulation. 2002;106:2051-2054. DOI: 10.1161/01.CIR. 0000037222.58317.3D.

[88] Sangiorgi G, Rumberger JA, Severson A, Edwards WD, Gregoire J, Fitzpatrick LA, Schwartz RS. Arterial calcification and not lumen stenosis is highly correlated with atherosclerotic plaque burden in humans: a histologic study of 723 coronary artery

segments using nondecalcifying methodology. J Am Coll Cardiol. 1998;31:126-133. DOI: 10.1016/S0735-1097(97)00443-9.

[89] Brodoefel H, Burgstahler C, Sabir A, Yam CS, Khosa F, Claussen CD, Clouse ME. Coronary plaque quantification by voxel analysis: Dual-source MDCT angiography versus intravascular sonography. AJR Am J Roentgenol. 2009;192:W84-89. DOI: 10.2214/AJR.08.1381.

[90] Boogers MJ, Broersen A, van Velzen JE, de Graaf FR, El-Naggar HM, Kitslaar PH, Dijkstra J, Delgado V, Boersma E, de Roos A, Schuijf JD, Schalij MJ, Reiber JH, Bax JJ, Jukema JW. Automated quantification of coronary plaque with computed tomography: Comparison with intravascular ultrasound using a dedicated registration algorithm for fusion-based quantification. Eur Heart J. 2012;33:1007-1016. DOI: 10.1093/eurheartj/ehr465.

[91] Dey D, Cheng VY, Slomka PJ, Nakazato R, Ramesh A, Gurudevan S, Germano G, Berman DS. Automated 3-dimensional quantification of noncalcified and calcified coronary plaque from coronary CT angiography. J Cardiovasc Comput Tomogr. 2009;3:372-382. DOI: 10.1016/j.jcct.2009.09.004.

[92] Dey D, Schepis T, Marwan M, Slomka PJ, Berman DS, Achenbach S. Automated three dimensional quantification of noncalcified coronary plaque from coronary CT angiography: Comparison with intravascular US. Radiology. 2010;257:516-522. DOI: 10.1148/radiol.10100681.

[93] Schuhbaeck A, Dey D, Otaki Y, Slomka P, Kral BG, Achenbach S, Berman DS, Fishman EK, Lai S, Lai H. Interscan reproducibility of quantitative coronary plaque volume and composition from CT coronary angiography using an automated method. Eur Radiol. 2014;24:2300-8. DOI: 10.1007/s00330-014-3253-3.

[94] Papadopoulou SL, Neefjes LA, Garcia-Garcia HM, Flu WJ, Rossi A, Dharampal AS, Kitslaar PH, Mollet NR, Veldhof S, Nieman K, Stone GW, Serruys PW, Krestin GP, de Feyter PJ. Natural history of coronary atherosclerosis by multislice computed tomography. JACC Cardiovasc Imaging. 2012;5(3 Suppl):S28-37. DOI: 10.1016/j.jcmg.2012.01.009.

[95] Papadopoulou SL, Garcia-Garcia HM, Rossi A, Girasis C, Dharampal AS, Kitslaar PH, Krestin GP, de Feyter PJ. Reproducibility of computed tomography angiography data analysis using semiautomated plaque quantification software: implications for the design of longitudinal studies. Int J Cardiovasc Imaging. 2013;29:1095-104. DOI: 10.1007/s10554-012-0167-5.

[96] Blackmon KN, Streck J, Thilo C, Bastarrika G, Costello P, Schoepf UJ. Reproducibility of automated noncalcified coronary artery plaque burden assessment at coronary CT angiography. J Thorac Imaging. 2009;24:96-102. DOI: 10.1097/RTI.0b013e31819b674b.

[97] Leber AW, Johnson T, Becker A, von Ziegler F, Tittus J, Nikolaou K, Reiser M, Steinbeck G, Becker CR, Knez A. Diagnostic accuracy of dual-source multi-slice CT-coro-

nary angiography in patients with an intermediate pretest likelihood for coronary artery disease. Eur Heart J. 2007;28:2354-2360. DOI: 10.1093/eurheartj/ehm294.

[98]   Agatston AS, Janowitz WR, Hildner FJ, Zusmer NR, Viamonte M Jr, Detrano R. Quantification of coronary artery calcium using ultrafast computed tomography. J Am Coll Cardiol. 1990;15:827-832. DOI:10.1016/0735-1097(90)90282-T.

[99]   Oudkerk M, Stillman AE, Halliburton SS, Kalender WA, Möhlenkamp S, McCol-lough CH, Vliegenthart R, Shaw LJ, Stanford W, Taylor AJ, van Ooijen PM, Wexler L, Raggi P. Coronary artery calcium screening: Current status and recommendations from the European Society of Cardiac Radiology and North American Society for Cardiovascular Imaging. Eur Radiol. 2008;18:2785-807. DOI: 10.1007/s00330-008-1095-6.

[100] Greenland P, LaBree L, Azen SP, Doherty TM, Detrano RC. Coronary artery calcium score combined with Framingham score for risk prediction in asymptomatic individ-uals. JAMA. 2004;291:210-215. DOI: 10.1001/jama.291.2.210.

[101] Vliegenthart R, Oudkerk M, Hofman A Oei HH, van Dijck W, van Rooij FJ, Witteman JC. Coronary calcification improves cardiovascular risk prediction in the elderly. Cir-culation. 2005;112:572-527. DOI: 10.1161/CIRCULATIONAHA.104.488916.

[102] Achenbach S. Can CT detect the vulnerable coronary plaque? Int J Cardiovasc Imag-ing. 2008;24:311-312. DOI: 10.1007/s10554-007-9281-1.

[103] Kolodgie FD, Burke AP, Farb A, Gold HK, Yuan J, Narula J, Finn AV, Virmani R. The thin-cap fibroatheroma: A type of vulnerable plaque: The major precursor lesion to acute coronary syndromes. Curr Opin Cardiol. 2011;16:285-292.

[104] Heidenreich PA, Trogdon JG, Khavjou OA, Butler J, Dracup K, Ezekowitz MD, Fin-kelstein EA, Hong Y, Johnston SC, Khera A, Lloyd-Jones DM, Nelson SA, Nichol G, Orenstein D, Wilson PW, Woo YJ. Forecasting the future of cardiovascular disease in the United States: a policy statement from the American Heart Association. Circula-tion. 2011;123:933-944. DOI: 10.1161/ CIR.0b013e31820a55f5.

[105] van der Giessen AG, Toepker MH, Donelly PM, Bamberg F, Schlett CL, Raffle C, Irl-beck T, Lee H, van Walsum T, Maurovich-Horvat P, Gijsen FJ, Wentzel JJ, Hoffmann U. Reproducibility, accuracy, and predictors of accuracy for the detection of coronary atherosclerotic plaque composition by computed tomography: An ex vivo compari-son to intravascular ultrasound. Invest Radiol. 2010;45:693-701. DOI: 10.1097/RLI. 0b013e3181e0a541.

[106] Schulman-Marcus J, Danad I, Truong QA: State-of-the-Art Updates on Cardiac Com-puted Tomographic Angiography for Assessing Coronary Artery Disease. Curr Treat Options Cardiovasc Med. 2015;17:398. DOI: 10.1007/s11936-015-0398-6.

[107] Wentzel JJ, Janssen E, Vos J, Schuurbiers JC, Krams R, Serruys PW, de Feyter PJ, Slag-er CJ. Extension of increased atherosclerotic wall thickness into high shear stress re-

gions is associated with loss of compensatory remodeling. Circulation. 2003;108:17-23. DOI: 10.1161/01.CIR.0000078637.21322.D3.

[108] Feldman CL, Ilegbusi OJ, Hu Z, Nesto R, Waxman S, Stone PH. Determination of in vivo velocity and endothelial shear stress patterns with phasic flow in human coronary arteries: A methodology to predict progression of coronary atherosclerosis. Am Heart J 2002; 143:931-939. DOI: 10.1067/mhj.2002.123118.

[109] Chatzizisis YS, Coskun AU, Jonas M, Edelman ER, Feldman CL, Stone PH. Role of endothelial shear stress in the natural history of coronary atherosclerosis and vascular remodeling: Molecular, cellular, and vascular behavior J Am Coll Cardiol. 2007;49:2379-2393. DOI:10.1016/j.jacc.2007.02.059.

[110] Wentzel JJ, Chatzizisis YS, Gijsen FJ, Giannoglou GD, Feldman CL, Stone PH. Endothelial shear stress in the evolution of coronary atherosclerotic plaque and vascular remodelling: Current understanding and remaining questions. Cardiovasc Res. 2012;96:234-243. DOI: 10.1093/cvr/cvs217.

[111] Pijls NH, De Bruyne B, Peels K, Van Der Voort PH, Bonnier HJ, Bartunek J Koolen JJ, Koolen JJ. Measurement of fractional flow reserve to assess the functional severity of coronary-artery stenoses. N Engl J Med. 1996;334:1703-1708. DOI: 10.1056/NEJM199606273342604.

[112] Tonino PA, De Bruyne B, Pijls NH, Siebert U, Ikeno F, van' t Veer M, Klauss V, Manoharan G, Engstrøm T, Oldroyd KG, Ver Lee PN, MacCarthy PA, Fearon WF. Fractional flow reserve versus angiography for guiding percutaneous coronary intervention. N Engl J Med. 2009;360:213-224. DOI: 10.1056/NEJMoa0807611.

[113] De Bruyne B, Pijls NH, Kalesan B, Barbato E, Tonino PA, Piroth Z, Jagic N, Möbius-Winkler S, Rioufol G, Witt N, Kala P, MacCarthy P, Engström T, Oldroyd KG, Mavromatis K, Manoharan G, Verlee P, Frobert O, Curzen N, Johnson JB, Jüni P, Fearon WF. Fractional flow reserve-guided PCI versus medical therapy in stable coronary disease. N Engl J Med. 2012;367:991-1001. DOI: 10.1056/NEJMoa1205361.

[114] Melikian N, De Bondt P, Tonino P, De Winter O, Wyffels Bartunek J, Heyndrickx GR, Fearon WF, Pijils NHJ, Wijns W, De Bruyne B. Fractional flow research and myocardial perfusion imaging in patients with angiographic multivessel coronary artery disease. JACC Cardiovasc Interv. 2010;3:307-314. DOI: 10.1016/j.jcin.2009.12.010.

[115] Christou MA, Siontis GC, Katritsis DG, Ioannidis JP. Metaanalysis of fractional flow reserve versus quantitative coronary angiography and noninvasive imaging for evaluation of myocardial ischemia. Am J Cardiol. 2007;99:450-456. DOI: 10.1016/j.amjcard.2006.09.092.

[116] Dattilo PB, Prasad A, Honeycutt E, Wang TY, Messenger JC. Contemporary patterns of fractional flow reserve and intravascular ultrasound use among patients undergoing percutaneous coronary intervention in the United States: Insights from the Na-

tional Cardiovascular Data Registry. J Am Coll Cardiol. 2012;60:2337-2339. DOI: 10.1016/j.jacc.2012.08.990.

[117] Pijls NH, van Schaardenburgh P, Manoharan G, Boersma E, Bech JW, et al. Percutaneous coronary intervention of functionally nonsignificant stenosis: 5-year follow-up of the DEFER Study. J Am Coll Cardiol. 2007;49:2105-2111. DOI:10.1016/j.jacc.2007.01.087.

[118] Boden WE, O'Rourke RA, Teo KK, Hartigan PM, Maron DJ, Kostuk WJ, Knudtson M, Dada M, Casperson P, Harris CL, Chaitman BR, Shaw L, Gosselin G, Nawaz S, Title LM, Gau G, Blaustein AS, Booth DC, Bates ER, Spertus JA, Berman DS, Mancini GB, Weintraub WS. Optimal medical therapy with or without PCI for stable coronary disease. N Engl J Med. 2007;356:1503-1516. DOI: 10.1056/NEJMoa070829.

[119] Lotfi A, Jeremias A, Fearon WF, Feldman MD, Mehran R, Messenger JC, Grines CL, Dean LS, Kern MJ, Klein LW. Expert Consensus Statement on the Use of Fractional Flow Reserve, Intravascular Ultrasound, and Optical Coherence Tomography: A Consensus Statement of the Society of Cardiovascular Angiography and Interventions. Catheter Cardiovasc Interv. 2014;83:509-518. DOI: 10.1002/ccd.25222.

[120] Nam CW, Mangiacapra F, Entjes R, Chung IS, Sels JW, Tonino PA, De Bruyne B, Pijls NH, Fearon WF; FAME Study Investigators. Functional SYNTAX Score for risk assessment in multivessel coronary artery disease. J Am Coll Cardiol. 2011;58:1211-1218. DOI: 10.1016/j.jacc.2011.06.020.

[121] Koo BK, Erglis A, Doh JH, Daniels DV, Jegere S, Kim HS, Dunning A, DeFrance T, Lansky A, Leipsic J, Min JK. Diagnosis of ischemia-causing coronary stenoses by noninvasive fractional flow reserve computed from coronary computed tomographic angiograms. Results from the prospective multicenter DISCOVER-FLOW (Diagnosis of Ischemia-Causing Stenoses Obtained Via Noninvasive Fractional Flow Reserve) study. J Am Coll Cardiol. 2011;58:1989-1997. DOI: 10.1016/j.jacc. 2011.06.066.

[122] Taylor CA, Fonte TA, Min JK. Computational fluid dynamics applied to cardiac computed tomography for noninvasive quantification of fractional flow reserve: Scientific basis. J Am Coll Cardiol. 2013;61:2233-2241. DOI: 10.1016/j.jacc.2012.11.083.

[123] Min JK, Leipsic J, Pencina MJ, Berman DS, Koo BK, van Mieghem C, Erglis A, Lin FY, Dunning AM, Apruzzese P, Budoff MJ, Cole JH, Jaffer FA, Leon MB, Malpeso J, Mancini GB, Park SJ, Schwartz RS, Shaw LJ, Mauri L. Diagnostic accuracy of fractional flow reserve from anatomic CT angiography. JAMA. 2012;308:1237-1245. DOI: 10.1001/2012.jama.11274.

[124] Nørgaard BL, Leipsic J, Gaur S, Seneviratne S, Ko BS, Ito H, Jensen JM, Mauri L, De Bruyne B, Bezerra H, Osawa K, Marwan M, Naber C, Erglis A, Park SJ, Christiansen EH, Kaltoft A, Lassen JF, Bøtker HE, Achenbach S; NXT Trial Study Group. Diagnostic performance of noninvasive fractional flow reserve derived from coronary computed tomography angiography in suspected coronary artery disease: the NXT trial

(Analysis of Coronary Blood Flow Using CT Angiography: Next Steps). J Am Coll Cardiol. 2014;63:1145-1155. DOI:10.1016/j.jacc.2013.11.043.

[125]   Abbara S, Arbab-Zadeh A, Callister TQ, Desai MY, Mamuya W, Thomson L, Weigold WG. SCCT guidelines for performance of coronary computed tomographic angiography: A report of the Society of Cardiovascular Computed Tomography Guidelines Committee. J Cardiovasc Comput Tomogr. 2009;3:190-204. DOI:10.1016/ j.jcct.2009.03. 004.

[126]   Leipsic J, Yang TH, Thompson A, Koo BK, Mancini GB, Taylor C, Budoff MJ, Park HB, Berman DS, Min JK. Technical factors and patient preparation prior to coronary CT angiography and diagnostic performance of non-invasive fractional flow reserve: Results from the determination of fractional flow reserve by anatomic computed angiography (DeFACTO) study. AJR Am J Roentgenol. 2014;202:989-994. DOI:10.2214/ AJR.13.11441.

[127]   Patel MR. Detecting obstructive coronary disease with CT angiography and noninvasive fractional flow reserve. JAMA. 2012;308:1269-1270. DOI: 10.1001/2012.jama. 11383.

[128]   Montalescot G, Sechtem U, Achenbach S, Andreotti F, Arden C, Budaj A, Bugiardini R, Crea F, Cuisset T, Di Mario C, Ferreira JR, Gersh BJ, Gitt AK, Hulot JS, Marx N, Opie LH, Pfisterer M, Prescott E, Ruschitzka F, Sabaté M, Senior R, Taggart DP, van der Wall EE, Vrints CJ; ESC Committee for Practice Guidelines, Zamorano JL, Achenbach S, Baumgartner H, Bax JJ, Bueno H, Dean V, Deaton C, Erol C, Fagard R, Ferrari R, Hasdai D, Hoes AW, Kirchhof P, Knuuti J, Kolh P, Lancellotti P, Linhart A, Nihoyannopoulos P, Piepoli MF, Ponikowski P, Sirnes PA, Tamargo JL, Tendera M, Torbicki A, Wijns W, Windecker S; Document Reviewers, Knuuti J, Valgimigli M, Bueno H, Claeys MJ, Donner-Banzhoff N, Erol C, Frank H, Funck-Brentano C, Gaemperli O, Gonzalez-Juanatey JR, Hamilos M, Hasdai D, Husted S, James SK, Kervinen K, Kolh P, Kristensen SD, Lancellotti P, Maggioni AP, Piepoli MF, Pries AR, Romeo F, Rydén L, Simoons ML, Sirnes PA, Steg PG, Timmis A, Wijns W, Windecker S, Yildirir A, Zamorano JL. 2013 ESC guidelines on the management of stable coronary artery disease: The task force on the management of stable coronary artery disease of the European Society of Cardiology. Eur Heart J. 2013;34:2949-3003. DOI: 10.1093/ eurheartj/eht296.

[129]   Tonino PA, Fearon WF, De Bruyne B, Oldroyd KG, Leesar MA, Ver Lee PN, Maccarthy PA, Van't Veer M, Pijls NH. Angiographic versus functional severity of coronary artery stenoses in the FAME study fractional flow reserve versus angiography in multivessel evaluation. J Am Coll Cardiol. 2010;55:2816-2821. DOI: 10.1016/ j.jacc. 2009.11.096.

[130]   Maurovich-Horvat P, Ferencik M, Voros S, Merkely B, Hoffmann U. Comprehensive plaque assessment by coronary CT angiography. Nat Rev Cardiol. 2014;11:390-402. DOI: 10.1038/nrcardio.2014.60.

[131] Nakanishi K, Fukuda S, Shimada K, Ehara S, Inanami H, Matsumoto K, Taguchi H, Muro T, Yoshikawa J, Yoshiyama M. Non-obstructive low attenuation coronary plaque predicts three-year acute coronary syndrome events in patients with hypertension: multidetector computed tomographic study. J Cardiol. 2012;59:167-175. DOI: 10.1016/j.jjcc. 2011.11.010.

[132] Utsunomiya M, Hara H, Moroi M, Sugi K, Nakamura M. Relationship between tissue characterization with 40 MHz intravascular ultrasound imaging and 64-slice computed tomography. J Cardiol 2011;57:297-302. DOI: 10.1016/j.jjcc.2011.01.016.

[133] Ridker PM, Danielson E, Fonseca FA, Genest J, Gotto Jr AM, Kastelein JJ, Koenig W, Libby P, Lorenzatti AJ, MacFadyen JG, Nordestgaard BG, Shepherd J, Willerson JT, Glynn RJ, JUPITER Study Group. Rosuvastatin to prevent vascular events in men and women with elevated C-reactive protein. N Engl J Med. 2008;359:2195-2207. DOI: 10.1056/NEJMoa0807646.

[134] Fayad ZA, Fuster V, Nikolaou K, Becker C. Computed tomography and magnetic resonance imaging for noninvasive coronary angiography and plaque imaging: Current and potential future concepts. Circulation. 2002;106:2026-2034. DOI: 10.1161/01.CIR.0000034392.34211.FC.

Permissions

All chapters in this book were first published in CABGS&CAD, by InTech Open; hereby published with permission under the Creative Commons Attribution License or equivalent. Every chapter published in this book has been scrutinized by our experts. Their significance has been extensively debated. The topics covered herein carry significant findings which will fuel the growth of the discipline. They may even be implemented as practical applications or may be referred to as a beginning point for another development.

The contributors of this book come from diverse backgrounds, making this book a truly international effort. This book will bring forth new frontiers with its revolutionizing research information and detailed analysis of the nascent developments around the world.

We would like to thank all the contributing authors for lending their expertise to make the book truly unique. They have played a crucial role in the development of this book. Without their invaluable contributions this book wouldn't have been possible. They have made vital efforts to compile up to date information on the varied aspects of this subject to make this book a valuable addition to the collection of many professionals and students.

This book was conceptualized with the vision of imparting up-to-date information and advanced data in this field. To ensure the same, a matchless editorial board was set up. Every individual on the board went through rigorous rounds of assessment to prove their worth. After which they invested a large part of their time researching and compiling the most relevant data for our readers.

The editorial board has been involved in producing this book since its inception. They have spent rigorous hours researching and exploring the diverse topics which have resulted in the successful publishing of this book. They have passed on their knowledge of decades through this book. To expedite this challenging task, the publisher supported the team at every step. A small team of assistant editors was also appointed to further simplify the editing procedure and attain best results for the readers.

Apart from the editorial board, the designing team has also invested a significant amount of their time in understanding the subject and creating the most relevant covers. They scrutinized every image to scout for the most suitable representation of the subject and create an appropriate cover for the book.

The publishing team has been an ardent support to the editorial, designing and production team. Their endless efforts to recruit the best for this project, has resulted in the accomplishment of this book. They are a veteran in the field of academics and their pool of knowledge is as vast as their experience in printing. Their expertise and guidance has proved useful at every step. Their uncompromising quality standards have made this book an exceptional effort. Their encouragement from time to time has been an inspiration for everyone.

The publisher and the editorial board hope that this book will prove to be a valuable piece of knowledge for researchers, students, practitioners and scholars across the globe.

List of Contributors

David Fridman and John N. Makaryus
North Shore-LIJ Health System, Hofstra NSLIJ School of Medicine, Manhasset, NY, USA

Amgad N. Makaryus
North Shore-LIJ Health System, Hofstra NSLIJ School of Medicine, Manhasset, NY, USA
Department of Cardiology, NuHealth, Nassau University Medical Center, East Meadow, NY, USA

Amit Bhanvadia, Alina Masters and Samy I. McFarlane
Division of Endocrinology, Department of Medicine, SUNY Downstate Medical Center, Brooklyn, NY, USA

Erion Qaja
Wyckoff Heights Medical Center, Brooklyn, NY, USA

Allan Mattia and Frank Manetta
Department of Cardiovascular and Thoracic Surgery, Hofstra Northwell School of Medicine, Manhasset, NY, USA

Bezdenezhnykh Natalia Alexandrovna, Sumin Alexei Nikolaevich and Bezdenezhnykh Andrey Viktorovich
Federal State Budgetary Institution, Research Institute for Complex Issues of Cardiovascular Diseases, Kemerovo, Russian Federation

Barbarash Olga Leonidovna
Federal State Budgetary Institution, Research Institute for Complex Issues of Cardiovascular Diseases, Kemerovo, Russian Federation
Federal State Budgetary Institution of Higher Professional Education, Kemerovo State Medical Institution, Kemerovo, Russian Federation

Kaan Kırali and Yücel Özen
Department of Cardiovascular Surgery, Koşuyolu Herat and Research Hospital, Istanbul, Turkey

Terrence D. Ruddy
University of Ottawa Heart Institute, Ottawa, Canada

Punitha Arasaratnam
University of Ottawa Heart Institute, Ottawa, Canada
Ng Teng Fong General Hospital, Singapore

Marco Gennari, Sabrina Manganiello and Gabriella Ricciardi
Centro Cardiologico Monzino, IRCCS, Milan, Italy

Gianluca Polvani and Marco Agrifoglio
Centro Cardiologico Monzino, IRCCS, Milan, Italy
Department of Cardiovascular Sciences and Community Health, University of Milan, Italy

Tommaso Generali
San Donato Hospital, IRCCS, Italy

Kendal M. Endicott
Division of Cardiothoracic Surgery, The George Washington University, Washington, DC, USA

Gregory D. Trachiotis
Division of Cardiothoracic Surgery, Veterans Affairs Medical Center, Washington, DC, USA
Division of Cardiothoracic Surgery, The George Washington University, Washington, DC, USA

Bandar Al-Ghamdi
Heart Centre, King Faisal Specialist Hospital
and Research Centre, Riyadh, Saudi Arabia
College of Medicine, Alfaisal University,
Riyadh, Saudi Arabia

Lucia Agoston-Coldea
Iuliu Hatieganu University of Medicine and
Pharmacy, Cluj-Napoca, Romania
Hiperdia Diagnostic Imaging Center, Cluj-
Napoca, Romania

Carmen Cionca
Hiperdia Diagnostic Imaging Center, Cluj-
Napoca, Romania

Silvia Lupu
University of Medicine and Pharmacy of
Targu Mures, Romania

Index

www.ingramcontent.com/pod-product-compliance
Lightning Source LLC
Chambersburg PA
CBHW061956190326
41458CB00009B/2886

* 9 7 8 1 6 3 2 4 1 5 5 9 2 *